Study Guide to Accompany

Rosdahl & Kowalski's Textbook of Basic Nursing

EIGHTH EDITION

Lazette Nowicki, MSN, RN

Nursing Assistant Professor
Allied Health Department
Sacramento City College
Sacramento, California

STUDENT SELF STUDY CD-ROM AUTHOR

Eileen Klein, EdD, MSN, RN

Task Force Chair Health Sciences
Austin Community College
Austin, Texas

Visit the Lippincott Williams & Wilkins Website
http://www.lww.com

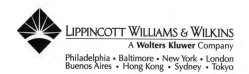

LIPPINCOTT WILLIAMS & WILKINS
A **Wolters Kluwer** Company

Philadelphia • Baltimore • New York • London
Buenos Aires • Hong Kong • Sydney • Tokyo

Ancillary Editor: Doris S. Wray
Compositor: LWW
Printer/Binder: Victor Graphics

ISBN: 0-7817-3430-4

9 8

Any procedure or practice described in this book should be applied by the health care practitioner under appropriate supervision in accordance with professional standards of care used with regard to the unique circumstances that apply in each practice situation. Care has been taken to confirm the accuracy of information presented and to describe generally accepted practices. However, the authors, editors, and publisher cannot accept any responsibility for errors or omissions or for any consequences from application of the information in this book and make no warranty, express or implied, with respect to the contents of the book.

Acknowledgments

To all the staff at Lippincott Williams & Wilkins, who have provided direction and support throughout this project.
To Karin McAndrews, who encouraged me to get involved with this project, and Doris Wray, for seeing me through the project.

To my husband, Craig, who provided his love, encouragement, and patience.
To my mother, Viola, and in memory of my father, Lester, who taught me the value of education and to believe in myself.
To my sister, Yvette, my mother-in-law, Mary, and my family and friends who have been a constant source of support and encouragement.

And finally, to the students for being the inspiration to write this book. I hope this book will enhance your educational experience as you begin your nursing career.

Contents

PART A
Foundations of Nursing

UNIT I
THE NATURE OF NURSING

1 The Origins of Nursing   1
2 Beginning Your Nursing Career   5
3 The Healthcare Delivery System   8
4 Legal and Ethical Aspects of Nursing   11

UNIT II
PERSONAL AND ENVIRONMENTAL HEALTH

5 Basic Human Needs   15
6 Health and Wellness   18
7 Community Health   22
8 Transcultural Healthcare   25

UNIT III
DEVELOPMENT THROUGHOUT THE LIFE CYCLE

9 The Family   28
10 Infancy and Childhood   31
11 Adolescence   35
12 Early and Middle Adulthood   38
13 Older Adulthood and Aging   40
14 Death and Dying   42

UNIT IV
STRUCTURE AND FUNCTION

15 Organization of the Human Body   44
16 The Integumentary System   48
17 Fluid and Electrolyte Balance   52
18 The Musculoskeletal System   56
19 The Nervous System   60
20 The Endocrine System   64
21 The Sensory System   68
22 The Cardiovascular System   72
23 The Hematologic and Lymphatic Systems   76
24 The Immune System   79
25 The Respiratory System   82
26 The Digestive System   85

27 The Urinary System   89
28 The Male Reproductive System   92
29 The Female Reproductive System   95

UNIT V
NUTRITION AND DIET THERAPY

30 Basic Nutrition   98
31 Transcultural and Social Aspects of Nutrition   103
32 Diet Therapy and Special Diets   105

PART B
Nursing Care Skills

UNIT VI
THE NURSING PROCESS

33 Introduction to the Nursing Process   109
34 Nursing Assessment   111
35 Diagnosis and Planning   113
36 Implementing and Evaluating Care   115
37 Documenting and Reporting   118

UNIT VII
SAFETY IN THE HEALTHCARE FACILITY

38 The Healthcare Facility Environment   121
39 Emergency Preparedness   124
40 Microbiology and Defense Against Disease   127
41 Medical Asepsis   130
42 Infection Control   133
43 Emergency Care and First Aid   136

UNIT VIII
CLIENT CARE

44 Therapeutic Communication Skills   142
45 Admission, Transfer, and Discharge   145
46 Vital Signs   148
47 Data Collection in Client Care   152
48 Body Mechanics and Positioning   156
49 Beds and Bed Making   160

50 Personal Hygiene and Skin Care   163
51 Elimination   166
52 Specimen Collection   170
53 Bandages and Binders   173
54 Heat and Cold Application   176
55 Client Comfort and Pain Management   178
56 Preoperative and Postoperative Care   181
57 Surgical Asepsis   185
58 Wound Care   187
59 Care of the Dying Person   190

UNIT IX
PHARMACOLOGY AND ADMINISTRATION OF MEDICATIONS

60 Review of Mathematics   193
61 Introduction to Pharmacology   196
62 Classification of Medications   199
63 Administration of Medications   203

PART C
Nursing Throughout the Life Cycle

UNIT X
MATERNAL AND NEWBORN NURSING

64 Normal Pregnancy   208
65 Normal Labor, Delivery, and Postpartum Care   213
66 Care of the Normal Newborn   217
67 High-Risk Pregnancy and Childbirth   222
68 The High-Risk Newborn   226
69 Sexuality, Fertility, and Sexually Transmitted Diseases   230

UNIT XI
PEDIATRIC NURSING

70 Fundamentals of Pediatric Nursing   234
71 Care of the Infant, Toddler, or Preschooler   237
72 Care of the School-Age Child or Adolescent   241
73 The Child or Adolescent With Special Needs   244

UNIT XII
ADULT CARE NURSING

74 Skin Disorders   247
75 Disorders in Fluid and Electrolyte Balance   253

76 Musculoskeletal Disorders   256
77 Nervous System Disorders   262
78 Endocrine Disorders   267
79 Sensory System Disorders   272
80 Cardiovascular Disorders   277
81 Blood and Lymph Disorders   282
82 Cancer   286
83 Allergic, Immune and Autoimmune Disorders   290
84 HIV and AIDS   294
85 Respiratory Disorders   298
86 Oxygen Therapy and Respiratory Care   308
87 Digestive Disorders   311
88 Urinary Disorders   315
89 Male Reproductive Disorders   320
90 Female Reproductive Disorders   324

UNIT XIII
GERONTOLOGICAL NURSING

91 Gerontology: The Aging Adult   328
92 Dementias and Related Disorders   331

UNIT XIV
MENTAL HEALTH NURSING

93 Psychiatric Nursing   334
94 Substance Abuse   338

UNIT XV
NURSING IN A VARIETY OF SETTINGS

95 Extended Care   341
96 Rehabilitation Nursing   343
97 Ambulatory Nursing   346
98 Home Care Nursing   348
99 Hospice Nursing   350

PART D
Your Career

UNIT XVI
THE TRANSITION TO PRACTICING NURSE

100 From Student to Graduate Nurse   353
101 Career Opportunities and Job-Seeking Skills   356
102 Advancement and Leadership in Nursing   359

Answers   361

CHAPTER 1

The Origins of Nursing

■ Terminology Review

Write the meaning or definition for the following abbreviations or words. Practice pronouncing each abbreviation or word and its meaning.

1. _____ National Student Nurses' Association
2. _____ oath that physicians repeat based on Hippocrates' philosophy
3. _____ caring for the whole person
4. _____ the medical symbol of a winged staff wrapped with two serpents
5. _____ Acquired Immunodeficiency Syndrome
6. _____ National Council Licensing Examination
7. _____ distinguishing badge of authority or honor
8. _____ given at graduation and symbolizes your school of nursing
9. _____ American Medical Association
10. _____ insignia of nursing and nursing education
11. _____ Diagnosis Related Groups
12. _____ American Nurses Association

a. AIDS
b. AMA
c. ANA
d. Caduceus
e. DRGs
f. Hippocratic oath
g. Holistic healthcare
h. insignia
i. NCLEX
j. Nightingale Lamp
k. NSNA
l. school nursing pin

■ FILL IN THE BLANKS

Fill in the correct answer for the following questions.

1. The word *nurse* derives from the Latin word meaning to _____.

2. During ancient times, a _____ _____ performed rituals to heal the sick.

3. Before 500 BC, people believed disease was caused by punishment by God or _____ _____.

4. _____ is considered to be the Father of Medicine.

5. Beginning in the first century, _____ _____ consisting of both men and women were established to provide care for the sick.

6. European female religious orders were nearly eliminated during the _____.

7. _____ _____ _____ established one of the first schools of nursing in the world in Kaiserswerth, Germany.

8. The first nursing school in the United States was the _____ _____, established in 1849.

9. The first college-based nursing program was established at Teachers College of Columbia

University by Isabel Robb and _____

_____ _____.

10. Formal education in practical nursing became

available in _____.

11. The _____-_____ _____

provided funding for vocational school–based

programs outside the hospital setting.

12. _____ _____ wrote the

curriculum for the first emergency training of

nurses.

13. During World War II, _____

_____ prevented nurses from being

drafted by expanding enrollment of nurses at

the University of Minnesota.

14. A _____ _____ is required

whenever you provide nursing care so that the

patient can easily identify you.

■ Short Answers

*Complete the following questions by providing the
correct answer in your own words.*

1. Describe how Hippocrates influenced modern
   nursing.

2. List three Roman matrons and describe how each
   influenced contemporary nursing.

3. Why was the European Reformation considered
   the dark ages of nursing?

4. Why is Florence Nightingale described as the
   lady with the lamp?

5. List at least five of Florence Nightingale's nursing principles that are still practiced today.

6. List four curricula areas that were taught in
   early practical nursing schools.

7. List three pioneer schools of practical nursing.

8. List the current nursing trends and how they
   influence nursing care.

9. List three common symbols used on nursing
   school pins.

10. Complete the following table.

Historical Timeline	Role of the Nurse
Ancient times	
500 BC, advanced Greek civilization	
First century	
Crusades (1096–1291)	
Reformation (1500s)	
1800s	
1900s	

■ Matching

Match the following American nurses with the appropriate contribution to the development of nursing.

1. _____ The first trained nurse in the United States

2. _____ Founded organization that became the American Nurses Association

3. _____ Cofounded the American Society of Superintendents of Training Schools of Nursing

4. _____ Founder of American public health nursing

5. _____ Campaigned against the inhumane treatment of the mentally ill

6. _____ First African American graduate nurse

7. _____ Pioneer visiting nurse-midwife

8. _____ Founded the American Red Cross

a. Dorthea Lynde Dix
b. Clara Barton
c. Mary Breckinridge
d. Lavinia Lloyd Dock
e. Mary E. Mahoney
f. Melinda Ann Richards
g. Lillian Wald
h. Isabel Hampton Robb

■ Multiple Choice

1. Which school was one of the first formally established schools of nursing in the world?
   a. Ballard School
   b. Kaiserswerth School of Nursing
   c. Nightingale School
   d. Thompson Practical Nursing School

2. Florence Nightingale greatly improved the quality of care during:
   a. the Crimean War
   b. the Korean War
   c. the Vietnam Conflict
   d. World War I

3. Currently, there are more than _____ practical nursing schools in the United States.
   a. 36
   b. 260
   c. 1,300
   d. 2,000

4. Which state was the first to license practical nurses?
   a. Minnesota
   b. Mississippi
   c. New York
   d. Pennsylvania

5. During which war were men actively recruited into nursing?
   a. Desert Storm
   b. Spanish-American War
   c. World War I
   d. World War II

CHAPTER 2

Beginning Your Nursing Career

■ Terminology Review

Match the following definitions with their correct terms and acronyms.

1. _____ laws that establish the minimum level of requirements for competence and practice

2. _____ certified nursing assistant

3. _____ also known as vocational nurses and care for the sick, injured, convalescent, and handicapped under the direction of physicians and registered nurses (RNs)

4. _____ RN, usually with a master's degree, who has specialized in a particular field

5. _____ provides a basis for forming a personal philosophy of nursing, developing problem-solving skills, and providing a reason and purpose for nursing actions

6. _____ mandatory or required of a school for its graduates to be licensed

7. _____ protect the public from unqualified workers and establish standards for the profession or occupation

8. _____ receive 2 to 4 years of education, care for acutely ill persons, teach, direct others in healthcare, and are in charge of various settings

9. _____ voluntary and does not specifically concern graduates; an agency other than the state has reviewed the nursing program in detail

10. _____ when a state doesn't forbid practicing nursing without a license, but does forbid using the title or RN or licensed practical nurse (LPN)

11. _____ dictates that a nurse must have a license to practice nursing

a. accreditation
b. advanced practice nurse
c. approval
d. CNA
e. licensure
f. mandatory licensure
g. nurse practice act
h. permissive licensure
i. practical nurses
j. RNs
k. theoretical framework

■ Short Answers

Complete the following questions with the appropriate answer.

1. Describe the three types of education that lead to the RN license.

2. Describe practical nursing education.

3. Describe the similarities and differences in practice between RNs and LPNs.

4. Review Box 2-2: Nursing standards for the LPN/licensed vocational nurse (LVN). Identify the standards of practice for each of the following categories.

   Education _____

   _____

   Legal/Ethical Status _____

   _____

   Practice _____

   _____

5. Identify three similarities between the Florence Nightingale Pledge and the Practical Nurse's Pledge.

6. Why is it necessary for nursing students and nurses to project a professional image?

7. Review Box 2-4: Projecting the Image of a Nurse. List measures that you already possess that project a positive nursing image. Identify areas in which you need to improve.

8. List the primary roles of the nurse and provide example of each.

3. A _____ _____ program permits LPNs to write the RN licensure examination after completing prerequisite courses and one additional year of education.

4. A program can be _____ by the state's board of nursing without being _____ by a national organization such as National League for Nursing (NLN).

5. The nurse's pledge serves as a guide for _____ _____.

6. The type of nurse assigned to a patient usually depends on the degree of the individual's _____.

7. LPNs may supervise _____ _____ and _____.

8. Nurses must always practice _____.

9. Nursing theories are often expressed in relationship to factors such as mind, body, spirit, emotions, and _____.

10. Many of today's nursing students have the additional responsibilities of a _____, _____, and _____.

■ Fill in the Blanks

Fill in each blank with the correct answer.

1. An associate's degree (AD)-RN is educated primarily as a bedside nurse and is sometimes called a _____ _____.

2. _____ and _____ use the term *vocational nurse* instead of *practical nurse*.

MATCHING

Match the following nurse theorists with their appropriate model and concept.

1. _____ Dorthea Orem

2. _____ Florence Nightingale

3. _____ Betty Neuman

4. _____ Virginia Henderson

5. _____ Sister Callista Roy

a. nature-healing; nature along cures

b. self-care; nursing assists patients to meet self-care needs

c. independent-functioning; mind and body are one

d. adaptation; nursing focuses on holistic care rather than curing

e. systems; goal of the whole person is stability and harmony

■ Multiple Choice

Circle the correct answer.

1. Which of the following was the first national nursing organization to concentrate its efforts on the development and improvement of practical nursing education, together with advancing the interests of PNs?

   a. American Association of Licensed Practical Nurses (AALPN)

   b. Health Occupations Students of America (HOSA)

   c. National Association for Practical Nurse Education and Service (NAPNES)

   d. National League for Nursing and Community Health Accreditation Program (NLN-CHAP)

2. National organizations whose membership include the LPN/LVN include all of the following *except* the:

   a. American Nurses Association (ANA)

   b. American Association of Licensed Practical Nurses (AALPN)

   c. National Association for Practical Nurse Education and Service (NAPNES)

   d. National League for Nursing and Community Health Accreditation Program (NLN-CHAP)

3. Which organization is responsible for the voluntary accreditation of nursing programs?

   a. ANA

   b. AALPN

   c. HOSA

   d. NLN-CHAP

4. A primary benefit of the HOSA is to:

   a. further the cause and image of practical nursing

   b. improve students' knowledge and skills

   c. provide a number of tests to nursing schools

   d. support the accreditation serves of the NLN

5. Nursing practice standards for the LPN/LVN include which of the following?

   a. Education standards stating that the LPN/LVN must complete an accredited nursing program

   b. Practice standards stating that the LPN/LVN may function independently in caring for patients.

   c. Legal/ethical standards stating that the LPN/LVN shall take responsible actions in situations wherein there is unprofessional conduct by a peer or other healthcare provider

   d. Continuing education standards stating that LPNs/LVNs should attend a program preparing for RN practice within 1 year of being licensed.

CHAPTER 3

The Healthcare Delivery System

■ Terminology Review

Match the following definitions with their correct terms and acronyms.

1. _____ system that helps families with limited funds to pay for the care of seriously ill persons

2. _____ fee or premium paid for HMO health services

3. _____ preferred provider organizations

4. _____ units designed to care for the critically ill and are found in acute care facilities

5. _____ point-of-service plan

6. _____ federal health insurance program available to nearly everyone aged 65 years and older

7. _____ health maintenance organizations

8. _____ Social Security Disability Insurance

9. _____ financial obligation charged to the patient at the time of each visit to an HMO

10. _____ federal and state aid for people aged 65 years and older, those who are blind or disabled, or those who are members of families receiving Aid to Families with Dependent Children

11. _____ unlicensed assistive personnel

12. _____ reimbursement system in which a predetermined amount is allocated for treating individuals with specific diagnoses

13. _____ provides 24-hour care under supervision of a registered nurse (RN)

14. _____ diagnosis-related groups

15. _____ National League for Nursing

16. _____ contiguous quality improvement

17. _____ Occupational Safety and Health Administration

18. _____ resource utilization groups

19. _____ Joint Commission for Accreditation of Healthcare Organizations

20. _____ extended care facilities

21. _____ alternative healthcare

22. _____ care that specializes in the care of the terminally ill

23. _____ comprehensive and total care of a person by meeting his or her needs in all areas

24. _____ programs by employees that rewards them for practicing healthy habits

25. _____ concept that started in the 1980s to halt rapidly rising medical costs and to increase efficiency in care delivery

26. _____ person who makes decisions regarding health and has active participation in the choice of the healthcare service

27. _____ organizational reporting system

28. _____ pledge to the public that healthcare services will provide optimal achievable goals and maintain standards excellence in the services rendered

29. _____ minimum level or need for healthcare services

30. _____ same as managed care

31. _____ gives 24-hour services from nursing assistants under supervision of an licensed practical nurse (LPN)/licensed vocational nurse (LVN), with an RN as a consultant

32. _____ when individuals have family or friends assist in their care and is less expensive than hospitalization

33. _____ ability to access a nurse or physician via telephone or computer audio/video link

34. _____ person who is relatively passive in acceptance of health services and providers or when the individual is unable to make decisions about his or her own care

35. _____ care in which outcome relates to the results

a. acuity
b. capitation fee
c. case management
d. chain of command
e. client
f. complementary healthcare
g. copay
h. holistic healthcare
i. home healthcare
j. hospice
k. incentive programs
l. managed care
m. Medicaid
n. Medicare
o. outcome-based care
p. patient
q. prospective payment
r. quality assurance
s. telehealth
t. third-party payment
u. CQI
v. DRG
w. ECF
x. HMO
y. ICF
z. ICU
aa. JCAHO
bb. NLN
cc. OSHA
dd. POS
ee. PPO
ff. RUG
gg. SNF
hh. SSDI
ii. UAP

■ Short Answers

Complete the following questions.

1. List the commonalities between the following pairs listed.
   a. DRGs/RUGs
   b. Medicare/Medicaid
   c. SNF/ICF

2. List three trends or challenges for healthcare in the 21st century. Discuss how each of the trends affects nurses and patients.

TREND	EFFECT ON NURSES	EFFECT ON PATIENTS

3. Outline at least three areas in which you would instruct patients and families to prevent consumer fraud in healthcare.

■ Correct the False Statements

Circle the word True or False that follows the statement. If the word False has been circled, change the underlined word/words to make the statement true. Place your answer in the space provided.

1. The NLN has identified 10 trends for this century, which include an emphasis on <u>treating illness</u>.

   True   False   _____

2. <u>Managed care</u> was implemented to halt rapidly rising medical costs and to increase efficiency in care delivery.

   True   False   _____

3. Medicaid is a <u>state</u>-run program.

   True   False   _____

4. Medicare is available to persons under 65 years of age if they are <u>receiving SSDI</u>.

   True   False   _____

5. The prospective payment system provides a <u>set reimbursement</u> for specific diagnosis.

   True   False   _____

6. Prospective payment for nursing homes based on categories is called <u>diagnosis-related groups</u>.

   True   False   _____

7. <u>Physical therapy</u> is important in teaching skills that will enable people to return to work, manage their homes, or care for themselves again.

   True   False   _____

8. Wellness means the <u>absence of disease</u>.

   True   False   _____

9. <u>Herbalists</u> promote health through the use of herbs and other plants.

   True   False   _____

10. Acupuncture <u>is based on "Chi"</u>, which is believed to be the energy of life.

    True   False   _____

CHAPTER 4

Legal and Ethical Aspects of Nursing

■ Terminology Review

Match the following definitions with the correct terms.

1. _____ injury that occurred because of another person's intentional or unintentional actions or failure to act

2. _____ physical contact with another person without that person's consent

3. _____ tests, treatments, and medications have been explained to the person, as well as the outcomes, the possible complications, and alternative procedures

4. _____ serious crime

5. _____ written statement or photograph that is false or damaging

6. _____ harm done to a patient as a result of neglecting duties, procedures, or ordinary precautions

7. _____ malicious verbal statements that are false or injurious

8. _____ crime that is considered not to be as serious as a felony

9. _____ obtaining license in another state without having to retake the NCLEX examination

10. _____ cessation of brain function

11. _____ wrong committed against a person or property or public good

12. _____ law that protects you from liability if you give emergency care within the limits of first aid and if you act in a reasonable and prudent manner

13. _____ improper, injurious, or faulty treatment of a patient that results in illness or injury

14. _____ threat or the attempt to do bodily harm

15. _____ mercy killing

16. _____ moral principles and values that guide human behaviors

17. _____ controversial issue in which laws concerning it differ among states

18. _____ legal document in which a person either states choices for medial treatment or names someone to make treatment choices if he or she loses decision-making ability

19. _____ law that defines and regulates the practice of nursing the United States

20. _____ legal responsibility for one's actions or failure to act appropriately

a. advance directive

b. assault

c. assisted suicide

d. battery

e. brain death

f. crime

g. ethics

h. endorsement

i. euthanasia

j. felony

k. Good Samaritan Act

l. informed consent

m. liability

n. libel

o. malpractice

p. misdemeanor

q. negligence

r. Nurse Practice Act

s. slander

t. tort

■ Acronym Review

Match the following terms or definitions with the correct acronym.

1. _____ computerized NCLEX

2. _____ National Council of State Boards of Nursing

3. _____ national examination that must be taken and passed to practice as a registered nurse

4. _____ law that requires all healthcare institutions to comply with this act or to forfeit reimbursement form Medicare and other types of funding

5. _____ licensed practical or vocational nurses

6. _____ registered nurse

7. _____ National Council Licensing Examination for practical nurses

8. _____ ensures fairness in the receipt of donated organs

9. _____ American Hospital Association

10. _____ when a person leaves a healthcare facility against medical advice

11. _____ National Association for Home Care

12. _____ basic life-saving technique you will be required to know

13. _____ number of units/hours dictated by state board of nursing needed for licensure renewal

a. AHA
b. AMA
c. CAT
d. CPR
e. CEU/CEH
f. LPN/LVN
g. NAHC
h. NCLEX-PN
i. NCLEX-RN
j. NCSBN
k. PSDA
l. RN
m. UNOS

■ Short Answers

1. A nurse is caring for an 88-year-old male with pneumonia. The client had medication ordered for a fever. The patient developed a fever, but the nurse failed to administer the medication. What type of liability would the nurse have in this situation?

2. List who defines standards of practice for nurses.

3. Two nurses were discussing the incompetence of a patient's physician. The patient overhead the conversation. The nurses could be liable for what type of crime?

4. You have to leave during your scheduled shift to deal with a family emergency. You informed a coworker that you were leaving. During the rest of the shift, a patient fell out of bed and sustained a fractured hip. You are being sued for abandonment of care. What could you have done to prevent this lawsuit?

5. What is the purpose of the Nurse Practice Act?

6. What aspects of nursing schools does the Nurse Practice Act regulate?

7. A patient you are caring for states that your care is the best he has received. He presents you with a gift certificate to a local restaurant. How would you handle this situation?

8. List and discuss the three major types of advance directives.

9. Review Box 4-3: The Code of Ethics for LPNs/LVNs. Site examples of ways that you are adhering to the code.

■ Correct the False Statements

Circle the word True *or* False *that follows the statement. If the word* false *has been circled, change the underlined word/words to make the statement true. Place your answer in the space provided.*

1. Restraining a patient using chemicals without the patient's permission is <u>false imprisonment</u>.

   True   False   _____

2. A person's ability to pay <u>determines</u> whether he or she receives care.

   True   False   _____

3. When a person is expected to die, the pronouncement of death <u>is the same as in a hospital</u>.

   True   False   _____

4. Only individuals who are <u>regulated by the Nurse Practice Acts</u> can legally be called nurses.

   True   False   _____

5. The three functions of the state board of nursing are to <u>initiate, regulate, and enforce the provisions of the Nurse Practice Act</u>.

   True   False   _____

6. <u>Individual hospitals</u> regulate issuing and renewing nursing licenses.

   True   False   _____

7. The purpose of the NCLEX-PN is to determine who <u>can pass the examination with entry-level knowledge.</u>

   True   False   _____

8. <u>Only nurses who are just starting their nursing career</u> should carry malpractice insurance.

   True   False   _____

9. <u>The Good Samaritan Act</u> protects the nurse form liability if the nurse gives emergency care within the limits of first aid and acts in a reasonable and prudent manner.

   True   False   _____

10. The nurse should maintain <u>professional boundaries</u>.

    True   False   _____

■ Multiple Choice

Circle the best answer.

1. Two nurses at a long-term care facility are discussing the condition of a resident. Another resident overhears the conversation. This is an example of:
   a. abandonment of care.
   b. breach of confidentiality.
   c. false imprisonment.
   d. professional accountability.

2. An LVN stops to render assistance to persons involved in a motor vehicle accident. The Good Samaritan Act with protect the LVN as long as he or she provides emergency care:
   a. as efficiently as possible.
   b. focusing on only one person.
   c. in a reasonable and prudent manner.
   d. using only CPR.

3. To protect a patient's confidentiality, the student nurse should gather information about the patient using:
   a. code numbers.
   b. only the patient's first name.
   c. the patient's initials.
   d. the patient's full name.

4. A patient is refusing treatment and leaves the hospital. The nurse would document this as the patient:
   a. believed his or her current care was inadequate.
   b. left against medical advice.
   c. used poor judgment.
   d. was not thinking clearly.

5. Many states require LPNs/LVNs to document currency in nursing by:
   a. completing continuing education units.
   b. periodically taking college courses.
   c. submitting evidence of employment.
   d. writing a letter verifying their current practice.

6. A patient threatens to file a lawsuit and name you in the suit. What action would be prudent?
   a. Ask the patient why you are being named in the suit.
   b. Ask your supervisor to speak with the patient.
   c. Discuss with the patient that you are really a good nurse.
   d. Obtain the services of a lawyer specializing in malpractice.

CHAPTER 5

Basic Human Needs

■ Terminology Review

Match the following terms and definitions.

1. _____ Maslow's definition of basic needs of all people progressing from simple to complex

2. _____ Balance in the body

3. _____ Maslow's third level of needs, which includes need for love, affection, and belonging

4. _____ A person who has reached his or her full potential

5. _____ Focusing on a lower level need that has already been fulfilled

6. _____ Complex needs

7. _____ Synonymous with primary needs

8. _____ First-level needs

9. _____ Needs that must be met to sustain life

10. _____ Self-image

11. _____ Needs met to give quality to life

12. _____ Higher level emotional needs

a. aesthetic needs
b. hierarchy of needs
c. homeostasis
d. physiologic needs
e. primary needs
f. psychological needs
g. regression
h. secondary needs
i. self-actualized
j. self-esteem
k. social needs
l. survival needs

■ Short Answers

1. Describe similarities and differences between primary and secondary needs.

2. What is the essential basic physiologic need and explain why is it essential?

3. Describe ways in which the body eliminates waste.

4. List the characteristics of safety.

5. What action should a nurse take if a patient is suspected of being abused?

6. Discuss difficulties of individuals who are homeless at meeting basic physiologic needs.

7. What is the normal oral temperature?

8. Which needs must people meet before they can address social needs?

11. Describe characteristics of an individual who is self-actualized.

9. Describe nursing activities that will assist the patient to meet love, affection, and belonging needs.

12. List the basic needs of communities that concern the welfare of all its residents.

10. List nursing actions that will help an individual obtain self-esteem.

Complete the following table of basic physiologic needs.

Basic Physiologic Need	Description of Need	Nursing Interventions Used to Meet Need
Oxygen		
Water and fluids		
Food and nutrients		
Elimination of waste products		
Sleep and rest		
Activity and exercise		
Sexual gratification		

■ Matching

Indicate on which level of the Hierarchy of Needs pyramid the following needs are found.

1. _____ Need to be well thought of by others

2. _____ Freedom from harm

3. _____ Spiritual needs

4. _____ Water and fluids

5. _____ Experience one's potential

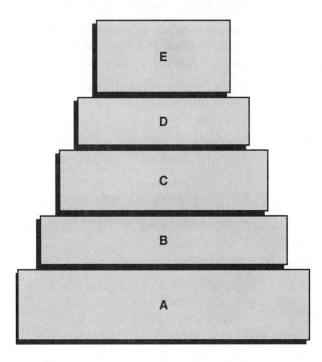

■ Multiple Choice

Circle the best answer.

1. Which of the following is a nursing activity that will help meet basic human needs?
   a. Assist patient to attend worship service
   b. Encourage family members to visit patient
   c. Give immunizations
   d. Provide supplemental oxygen

2. Which of the following nursing interventions will assist a patient to get adequate sleep and rest?
   a. Acknowledge accomplishments of the individual
   b. Be sensitive to patient's societal roles
   c. Provide a safe and quiet environment
   d. Report abuse

3. Which nursing action would assist the patient to feel safe?
   a. Assist with feeding
   b. Explain surgical procedures
   c. Insert urinary catheter
   d. Provide a warm environment

4. A person who is self-actualized may reach this level of Maslow's hierarchy:
   a. many times throughout life.
   b. only during old age.
   c. only during youth.
   d. rarely in a lifetime.

5. Relationships with others are higher level needs that can be addressed only after:
   a. basic physiologic needs are met.
   b. community needs are met.
   c. psychologic needs are met.
   d. self-actualization.

CHAPTER 6

Health and Wellness

■ Terminology Review

Match the following definitions with the correct terms and acronyms.

1. _____ person cannot perform usual activities

2. _____ composed of good physical self-care, prevention of illness/injury, using full intellectual potential, expressing emotions, managing stress appropriately, comfortable and congenial interpersonal relationships, concern about one's environment

3. _____ factors that may or may not be preventable that predispose us to disease

4. _____ physical and mental wear and tear of life

5. _____ coronary artery disease, one of the five leading causes of morbidity and mortality in the United States

6. _____ sexually transmitted diseases

7. _____ established by the United Nations in 1948 to improve worldwide health

8. _____ prostate specific antigen test that is used as a screening tool and to determine the effectiveness of treatment after cancer is diagnosed

9. _____ most prevalent bone disease in the world and causes more that one million fractures in the United States

10. _____ short-term illnesses

11. _____ change in the structure or function of body tissues, biologic systems, or the human mind

12. _____ response to disease that involves a change in function

13. _____ long-term illnesses

14. _____ change in the structure and function of body tissues caused by invasion from harmful microorganisms

15. _____ born early, before the expected due date

16. _____ cause of a disease

17. _____ disorder in which a detectable structural change has occurred in one or more organs that also alter usual function

18. _____ cerebrovascular accident, one of the five leading causes of morbidity and mortality in the United States

19. _____ disorder in which a structural cause cannot be identified

20. _____ number of people with an illness or disorder relative to a specific population

21. _____ genetic transmission of disease from one or both parents

22. _____ chemicals that cause cancer

23. _____ disorders present at birth that may be caused by genetic or unfavorable conditions that affect normal fetus development

24. _____ chances of death associated with a particular illness or disorder

25. _____ sudden infant death syndrome

26. _____ infection that invades one area or organ

27. _____ patterns of living that we choose to follow

28. _____ infections that involve the whole body

29. _____ chronic obstructive pulmonary disease, one of the five leading causes of morbidity and mortality in the United States

30. _____ elevated blood pressure

31. _____ growth of abnormal tissue or tumors

32. _____ coronary heart disease

33. _____ state of complete physical, mental, and social well-being and not merely the absence of disease or infirmity

34. _____ motor vehicle accidents are the leading cause of morbidity and mortality for ages 10 to 24

35. _____ tumor often surrounded by a capsule that usually does not grow back after it is removed

36. _____ form of abuse that occurs to the dependent, often frail, elderly

37. _____ internal stress reducers, even though they may or not be truthful or effective ways of adapting to a stressful situation

38. _____ wild and disorderly growth of cells that is unlike the tissue from which it arises

39. _____ process by which malignant cells spread to other parts of the body

40. _____ balance of all the components of the human organism

41. _____ myocardial infarction

42. _____ violence that occurs in the home

43. _____ another name for a heart attack

44. _____ infection can be spread or transferred from one person to another

a. acute illness
b. benign
c. CAD
d. carcinogenic
e. CHD
f. chronic illness
g. congenital disorders
h. contagious
i. COPD
j. CVA
k. defense mechanisms
l. disease
m. domestic violence
n. dysfunctional
o. elder abuse
p. etiology
q. functional disease
r. health

s. hereditary
t. homeostasis
u. hypertension
v. illness
w. infection
x. lifestyle factor
y. local
z. malignant
aa. metastasis
bb. MI
cc. morbidity
dd. MVA
ee. mortality
ff. myocardial infarction
gg. neoplastic
hh. organic disease
ii. osteoporosis
jj. preterm birth
kk. PSA
ll. risk factor
mm. SIDS
nn. STD
oo. stress
pp. systemic
qq. wellness

■ Correct the False Statements

Circle the word True *or* False *that follows the statement. If the word* false *has been circled, change the underlined word/words to make the statement true. Place your answer in the space provided.*

1. Health is composed of five components: physical health, emotional health, psychological health, social health, and spiritual health.

   True   False   _____

2. An example of morbidity is the rate of women dying from lung cancer that has increased 400% from 1960-1990.

   True   False   _____

3. Many morbidity and mortality rates could be decreased with effective screening measures.

   True   False   _____

4. Preventive services have had <u>positive effects on healthcare issues</u> such as prenatal care for mothers and infants, antismoking campaigns, and mammography of women.

   True   False   _____

5. The top three leading health indications are <u>substance abuse, mental health, and immunizations</u>.

   True   False   _____

6. Smoking <u>three packs of cigarettes</u> per day doubles a person's risk of heart attack and increases the risk of death from heart attack by 70%.

   True   False   _____

7. Recommendations for every American include <u>30 minutes or more of moderate-intensity physical activity most days of the week</u>.

   True   False   _____

8. Children <u>generally engage in adequate</u> amounts of exercise.

   True   False   _____

9. Major components of a healthy diet include <u>reduced fat and sodium intake, adequate calcium intake, and increased fiber and natural carbohydrates intake</u>.

   True   False   _____

10. <u>Lack of adequate exercise</u> is the leading cause of preventable death in the United States.

    True   False   _____

11. <u>Secondhand smoke</u> also causes cardiovascular diseases, heart attacks, and numerous respiratory problems.

    True   False   _____

12. Low-tar, filtered, and menthol cigarettes are <u>safer than</u> plain cigarettes.

    True   False   _____

13. <u>Substance abuse</u> contributes to family strife, domestic violence, work absenteeism, and unemployment.

    True   False   _____

14. <u>Abuse by a male partner</u> is the single largest cause of injury to women in the United States.

    True   False   _____

15. Elder abuse commonly occurs in families <u>where personal and financial resources have been exhausted</u>.

    True   False   _____

■ Case Studies

For each of the following case studies, indicate nursing education that should be done to promote health.

1. A 19-year-old single, unemployed female has just found out she is pregnant.

2. A mother brings her 8-year-old child into the clinic for treatment of cold symptoms. The nurse assess that the child is overweight.

3. A teenage boy shares with you that he is sexually active.

4. A middle-aged man is seen in the clinic for occasional heartburn and chest pain. The man smokes, is overweight, leads a sedentary lifestyle, and frequently eats meals at fast-food restaurants.

■ Multiple Choice

Circle the best answer.

1. A 19-year-old patient is admitted to the hospital for repair of a heart condition that he was born with because his mother contracted German measles during her pregnancy. The heart condition would be considered:
   a. congenital disorder causing an organic disease.
   b. hereditary disorder causing a functional disease.
   c. metabolic disorder causing a functional disease.
   d. traumatic disorder causing an organic disease.

2. The body adapts to change to:
   a. establish high-level wellness.
   b. maintain homeostasis.
   c. maintain optimal health.
   d. maintain self-actualization.

3. Which of the following statements is true regarding lifestyle factors?
   a. Laws regulating substance use are effectively enforced to decrease drug use.
   b. Physical activity is not effective for managing chronic illnesses such as arthritis.
   c. Poor nutrition contributes to congestive heart failure, cancer, and obesity.
   d. Rape and other sexual crimes are reported less frequently today than in the past.

4. Tobacco use:
   a. causes dilatation of the arteries and a decreased heart rate.
   b. has a lifelong effect that cannot be reversed by smoking cessation.
   c. is not dangerous if the smokeless form is used.
   d. may aggravate conditions such as periodontal disease or osteoporosis.

CHAPTER 7

Community Health

■ Terminology Review

Match the following definitions with the correct terms and acronyms.

1. _____ National Institutes of Health

2. _____ Department of Agriculture

3. _____ United States Department of Agriculture

4. _____ American Public Health Association

5. _____ Social Security Administration

6. _____ World Health Organization

7. _____ Visiting Nurse Association

8. _____ National Association of Health Care Centers

9. _____ Food and Drug Administration

10. _____ family-focused healthcare that emphasizes health education and healthy lifestyles

11. _____ group of individuals who interact with each other for the mutual benefit of their common interests to support a sense of unity or belonging

12. _____ subgroups in a community with unique or special healthcare needs

13. _____ Federally Qualified Healthcare

14. _____ United Nations Children's Fund

15. _____ medically underserved areas

16. _____ Office of Public Health and Science, which provides leadership and coordination across agencies of the USPHS and HHA

17. _____ Health and Human Services

18. _____ study of mutual relationships between living beings and their environment

19. _____ contamination and impurity

20. _____ aggregate health of a population

21. _____ chemical element that occurs in nature as a by-product of the disintegration of radium

22. _____ lead poisoning

23. _____ United Nations

24. _____ radioactive energy

25. _____ wastes that are infectious or harmful to humans or animals

26. _____ Department of Labor

27. _____ National Institute for Nursing Research

28. _____ another name for ecology

29. _____ United States Public Health Service

30. _____ Department of Commerce

31. _____ Centers for Disease Control and Prevention

32. _____ study of populations

33. _____ Environmental Protection Agency

34. _____ National Health Information Center

a. APHA

b. biohazardous

c. bionomics

d. CDC

e. community

f. community health

g. demography

h. DOA

i. DOC

j. DOL

k. ecology

l. EPA

m. FDA

n. FQHC

o. HHS

p. MUA

q. NAHCC

r. NHIC

s. NIH

t. NIHR

u. OPHS

v. plumbism

w. pollution

x. primary healthcare

y. radiation

z. radon

aa. SSA

bb. target population

cc. UN

dd. UNICEF

ee. USDA

ff. USPHS

gg. VNA

hh. WHO

ii. WIC

jj. worker's compensation

■ Short Answers

Complete the fo llowing questions.

1. List examples of four types of communities.

2. Describe goals of the United Nations Children's Fund.

3. Identify at least six achievements in public health that have increased life expectancy.

4. Identify four roles of the CDC.

5. Identify four functions of the FDA.

6. List three functions of the SSA.

7. Describe two functions of the Red Cross.

8. Identify organizations that are common to state healthcare services.

9. List causes of pollution for the following areas:

   AIR

   WATER

   LAND

   NOISE

■ Correct the False Statements

Circle the word True *or* False *that follows the statement. If the word* false *has been circled, change the underlined word/words to make the statement true. Place your answer in the space provided.*

1. The OPHS is an office that provides leadership and coordination across agencies of the USPHS and HHA.

   True   False   _____

2. The NIH provides for the safety of foods and cosmetics and the safety and effectiveness of pharmaceuticals, biological products, and medical devices.

   True   False   _____

3. The mission of the CDC is to <u>promote health and quality of life by preventing and controlling disease, injury, and disability</u>.

   True   False   _____

4. The mission of the NIH <u>supports research and establishes a scientific basis for the care of individuals throughout their lifespan</u>.

   True   False   _____

5. <u>The mission of the HHS</u> is to send every worker home whole and healthy every day.

   True   False   _____

6. The nurse would refer a pregnant mother who needs financial help with buying groceries <u>to WIC</u>.

   True   False   _____

7. The goal of the APHA is <u>to provide leadership, influence policies, and establish public health priorities</u>.

   True   False   _____

8. <u>The national and state councils</u> promote safety by analyzing causes of accidents and suggesting preventative measures.

   True   False   _____

9. Direct care services of the <u>Red Cross</u> include skilled nursing, pain management, and hospice.

   True   False   _____

10. The American Cancer Society is an organization that is related <u>to promoting specific health goals</u>.

   True   False   _____

CHAPTER 8

Transcultural Healthcare

■ Terminology Review

Match the following definitions with the correct terms and acronyms.

1. _____ understanding and tolerance of all cultures and lifestyles

2. _____ groups within dominant cultures

3. _____ concepts that members of an ethnic or a cultural group believe to be true

4. _____ shape how an individual perceives right or wrong and what is desirable or valuable

5. _____ belief based on preconceived notions of certain groups of people

6. _____ rules for behavior in a group

7. _____ subculture with physical and cultural characteristics of a group that differ from the predominant group of a particular region

8. _____ rules that members of a culture cannot violate without discomfort and risk of separation from the group

9. _____ members are often required to practice for comfort, acceptance, and inclusion

10. _____ belief that one's own culture is the best and only acceptable way

11. _____ accumulated learning for generational groups of individuals within structured or nonstructured societies

12. _____ Native American medicine man

13. _____ traditional Latino lay person who assists a patient with herbs and counseling

14. _____ theory that illness develops when life forces are out of balance

15. _____ large groups of humankind that share common physical characteristics

16. _____ state in which the soul no longer lives in a body and is free from desire and pain

17. _____ common heritage shared by a specific culture

18. _____ rebirth depends on behavior in life

19. _____ classifying or categorizing people, believing that all those belonging to a certain group are alike

20. _____ caring for patients while taking into consideration their religious and sociocultural backgrounds

21. _____ interweaving and blending of cultures so that identification of cultural groups is difficult

22. _____ ethnic-sensitive nursing care

a. beliefs
b. cultural diversity
c. cultural sensitivity
d. culture
e. curandero
f. ethnocentrism
g. ethnicity
h. ethnonursing
i. karma
j. minority
k. nirvana
l. norms
m. prejudice
n. race
o. rituals
p. stereotype
q. subculture

r.   shaman

s.   taboos

t.   transcultural nursing

u.   values

v.   Yin-Yang

■ Short Answers

Complete the following questions.

1. List three barriers to providing culturally competent nursing care.

2. List nursing considerations that should be included as part of a cultural assessment.

3. Describe qualifications of a professional interpreter.

4. Describe the basic beliefs of the following:

   a. Magicoreligious

   b. Scientific/biomedical

   c. Holistic medicine

   d. Ying-Yang

5. Describe how each of the following would view mental illness:

   a. Magicoreligious

   b. Scientific/biomedical

   c. Holistic medicine

   d. Ying-Yang

■ Case Studies

1. Mr. Littlethunder is a Native American patient on your medical–surgical unit. His infected wound is not improving despite antibiotics and dressing changes.

   a. What cultural information would you obtain during your assessment of Mr. Littlethunder?

   b. Mr. Littlethunder has frequent visits from family and community members. It is discovered that the medicine man has been treating the wound by placing herbs in the wound bed. What action would you take based on this new information?

   c. The patient and medicine man agree to place the herbs outside the wound bed and the wound begins to heal. How could this delay in wound healing have been prevented?

2. You are caring for an East Indian woman who has given durable power of attorney to a family member to make all decisions regarding her care. The patient has been diagnosed with cancer; however, the designated family member does not believe the client should know about the diagnosis.

   a. What information would you want to obtain?

b. What action would you take?

3. A 90-year-old female is admitted to your long-term care unit. The patient has been a practicing Christian Scientist all her life. She has been diagnosed with a painful terminal illness and is currently disoriented and unable to make decisions for herself. Her son has indicated that his mother is to not receive pain medications.

a. How would you handle this situation?

b. The patient's son changes his mind after a few days and allows the patient to have Tylenol for pain. How will you feel about this?

■ Multiple Choice

1. Tashah Michai, age 16, is of East Indian culture. She is scheduled for a physical examination. Dr. Fred Reed asks you to prepare for a pelvic examination and Pap smear. You notice that Tashah is nervous, and her parents state that they must take Tashah home now. The most appropriate action would be:

   a. ask Tashah and her patents if they are uneasy about having a male doctor examine Tashah.

   b. inform Tashah and her parents that a Pap smear should be done because Tashah is now a young woman.

   c. tell Dr. Reed that Tashah and her parents are nervous and uncomfortable and ask him to speak with them.

   d. tell Tashah and her parents to calm down and explain the procedure.

2. Nora Vorna was admitted to your unit last week with end-stage cancer. A new nurse comes to you and complains that the Vorna family is in the room with an electric candelabra. The most appropriate action would be:

   a. encourage the family to remove the candelabra and perform the rituals at home.

   b. determine if the family has received special permission and allow the family members to exercise their cultural practices.

   c. inform the family that candles of any sort are forbidden in the hospital setting.

   d. wait until the family leaves the room and then remove the candelabra.

3. A 40-year-old Chinese American patient is being admitted to your unit. He has lived in this country for 20 years with his family. What action is most appropriate regarding communication with this patient?

   a. Encourage the patient to speak English, and use a writing board to communicate with the patient if necessary.

   b. Instruct the family members that they will need to stay in the hospital to act as interpreters.

   c. Make arrangements for the possibility of an interpreter because even if the patient previously communicated well, he may regress when ill.

   d. No action is needed because a professional interpreter is not needed if the patient has been in the United States for more than 10 years.

4. You discover that a postoperative patient is eating only fruits and bread on the food tray. The patient practices Orthodox Judaism. The most appropriate action would be:

   a. explore the patient's preference and ask dietary to place meat and dairy products in separate dishes.

   b. insist that the patient eat his pork chops because the protein will help him heal.

   c. stress the importance of nutritional intake with the patient and his family.

   d. tell dietary to provide larger portions of fruit and bread.

CHAPTER 9

The Family

■ Terminology Review

Match the following definitions with the correct terms and acronyms.

1. _____ an adult head of the house with dependent children

2. _____ adults who live alone in apartments or houses with no children involved

3. _____ separation or divorce of the adult partners occurs, but both parents continue to assume a high level of childrearing responsibilities

4. _____ married couple that lives together without children

5. _____ blended family

6. _____ brothers and sisters

7. _____ unmarried individuals in a committed partnership living together, with or without children

8. _____ one professional adult member of a family is transferred to another city, and partners must commute a long distance to be together

9. _____ intimate partners of the same sex living together or owning property together

10. _____ nuclear families in which both parents work outside the home

11. _____ children living in temporary arrangements with paid caregivers

12. _____ families that are able to develop socially acceptable means of dealing with stress

13. _____ two or more people who are joined together by bonds of sharing and emotional closeness

14. _____ acquired immunodeficiency syndrome

15. _____ several people live together striving to be self-sufficient and minimize contact with the outside society

16. _____ families in which coping systems disintegrate as stressors build

17. _____ two-generation unit consisting of a husband, wife, and their immediate children (biologic, adopted, or both) living within one household

18. _____ nuclear family and other related people who may live together or in proximity to one another

a. AIDS
b. binuclear family
c. cohabitation
d. communal family
e. commuter family
f. dual-career/dual-worker family
g. dysfunctional family
h. extended family
i. family
j. foster family
k. functional family
l. gay or lesbian family
m. nuclear family
n. nuclear dyad
o. reconstituted family
p. siblings
q. single adult household
r. single-parent family

■ Assessment Review

Indicate if the following findings are effective (E) or ineffective (I) coping patterns.

1. _____ Recognizes that stress is temporary and may be positive

2. _____ Feeling a sense of accomplishment in dealing with stress

3. _____ Focusing on family problems rather than strengths

4. _____ Developing new rules for changing situations

5. _____ Growing to dislike family life as a result of accumulation of stress

6. _____ Increased use of alcohol by family members

7. _____ Gambling to the point of inadequate money available for food

8. _____ Asking professional counselor for guidance with child who is acting inappropriately since parent divorce

9. _____ Seeking medical assistance for ill family member

10. _____ Finalizing will for terminally ill family member

■ Correct the False Statements

Circle the word True *or* False *that follows the statement. If the word* false *has been circled, change the underlined word/words to make the statement true. Place your answer in the space provided.*

1. A <u>transitional stage</u> refers to the period when single young adults are financially independent from their family or origin and live outside the family home.

   True   False   _____

2. During the <u>childbearing phase</u>, socialization of children is a major task.

   True   False   _____

3. <u>All family members</u> are responsible for providing children with food, shelter, and safety.

   True   False   _____

4. <u>Birth weight</u> often plays a large role in shaping the experiences of siblings.

   True   False   _____

5. Dual-career families are those <u>in which both parents work outside the home</u>.

   True   False   _____

6. Universal characteristics of a family include being a <u>small social system and having its own cultural values</u>.

   True   False   _____

7. <u>Allocation of resources</u> includes assigning workloads, including responsibility for household income and household management.

   True   False   _____

8. Adjustment to retirement may be difficult if careful <u>financial planning is not done or if hobbies and activities</u> were not developed in earlier years.

   True   False   _____

9. A patient's family includes <u>any person that he or she identifies as a family member</u>.

   True   False   _____

10. The contracting family phase includes <u>childbearing, childrearing, and child launching</u>.

    True   False   _____

■ Multiple Choice

1. During the finalization stage of divorce, developmental tasks include which of the following?

   a. Dealing with extended family about the divorce

   b. Developing social network

   c. Restructuring finances

   d. Staying connected with extended family

2. Developmental tasks of the contracting family include:
    a. assisting aging parents.
    b. integrating new child members.
    c. planning for own family.
    d. separating from one's own family of origin.

3. A major issue for dual-career families is:
    a. advancing age.
    b. child-care arrangements.
    c. financial income.
    d. social interaction.

4. Which of the following would stress a family the least?
    a. Divorce
    b. Family member diagnosed with chronic illness
    c. Job promotion with increased income
    d. Remarriage and arrival of stepparent

5. Which of the following would promote a child's self-esteem and independence?
    a. Apologize for fairly punishing the child
    b. Do not allow child to make any decisions
    c. Establish and maintain routines
    d. Vary discipline techniques

CHAPTER 10

Infancy and Childhood

■ Terminology Review

Match the following definitions with the correct terms and acronyms.

1. _____ genetic factors inherited from parents

2. _____ handling and self-stimulation of the genital organs

3. _____ from the center to the outside

4. _____ bed-wetting

5. _____ period of human life from age 1 to 12 months

6. _____ the first four weeks of human life

7. _____ from head to tail

8. _____ knowledge, understanding, or perception

9. _____ knowledge that an object seen in a particular spot but temporarily hidden from view under a blanket continues to exist and will return to view when it is uncovered

10. _____ change in body function

11. _____ stage in human life from ages 1 to 3 years

12. _____ sum of all the conditions and factors surrounding a child

13. _____ clinging to family members and pulling away from unfamiliar people

14. _____ change in body size and structure

15. _____ all aspects of growth and development are influenced by each other

16. _____ return to a former state such as when a child is ill

17. _____ attachment to parents and other family caregivers that is of vital importance to infants

a. bonding
b. cephalocaudal
c. cognitive
d. development
e. environment
f. enuresis
g. growth
h. hereditary
i. infancy
j. interdependent
k. masturbation
l. newborn
m. object permanence
n. proximodistal
o. regression
p. stranger anxiety
q. toddler

■ Theorist Review

1. Summarize Havighurst's theory of developmental tasks.

2. Indicate the appropriate order in which Erikson's stages of psychosocial development occur.

   a. _____ autonomy versus shame and doubt

   b. _____ initiative versus guilt

   c. _____ trust versus mistrust

   d. _____ industry versus inferiority

3. Indicate the virtues for each of Erikson's stages of development.

   a. Infancy _____

   b. Toddlerhood _____

   c. Preschool _____

   d. School Age _____

4. Indicate the appropriate order in which Piaget's stages of cognitive development occur.

   a. _____ formal operations

   b. _____ preoperations

   c. _____ sensorimotor

   d. _____ concrete operations

■ Short Answers

Complete the following.

1. List characteristics of human growth and development.

2. Describe the significance of play in a child's development.

3. Discuss the difference between solitary play and parallel play.

4. A parent of a 7-month-old child expresses concern that the infant cannot sit up by herself for more than a few seconds. The parent is concerned that something is wrong with the infant. What would you do?

5. Complete the following table.

Developmental Stage	Age	Physical Development	Cognitive and Motor Development	Key Areas of Concern
Infancy		Gain 1–2 lbs/month Doubled wt by 6 months Teeth erupt at 6–7 months		
Toddlerhood	1–3 years			
Preschool			Dress and undress by themselves	

Developmental Stage	Age	Physical Development	Cognitive and Motor Development	Key Areas of Concern
Preschool (continued)			3-year-olds desire to be independent 4-year-olds have increased vocabulary, counting, print own name 5-year-olds know address and phone number	
School age				Sibling rivaly may lead to jealousy, trauma, verbal arguments and physical fights Responsibilities in the home Sex education

■ Multiple Choice

1. According to Havighurst, developmental tasks of middle childhood include:
   a. begin to form the conscience.
   b. form concepts and be able to name them.
   c. learning to get along with age mates.
   d. learning sex differences and modesty.

2. Which deciduous teeth erupt first in the infant?
   a. Central incisor
   b. Cuspid
   c. Lateral incisor
   d. Second molar

3. Which instructions to parents would be most important?
   a. Correct placement and use of car seats.
   b. Keep windows closed.
   c. Read labels before using any drugs.
   d. Teach child not to run with objects in the mouth.

4. Which action should be used when a toddler has a temper tantrum?
   a. Allow the child to have what he or she wants.
   b. Firmly reprimand the child.
   c. Physically remove child from public setting.
   d. Provide more attention to the child.

5. During the preschool years, children learn sexual roles through:
   a. fantasies and games.
   b. masturbation.
   c. observation.
   d. sexual experimentation.

6. To help school-age children learn responsibility, parents should:
   a. ask the child what activities he or she would like to complete.
   b. assign simple household chores to the child.
   c. encourage child to model behavior.
   d. encourage the child to be involved in caring for siblings.

CHAPTER 11

Adolescence

■ Terminology Review

Write the meaning or definition for the following words. Practice pronouncing the word and its meaning.

1. _____ period when a person becomes able to reproduce sexually

2. _____ onset of menstruation, usually occurs by age 13

3. _____ marked by eating minimal amounts of food, may emerge during adolescence

4. _____ also known as early adolescence occurring between ages 11 and 14 years

5. _____ characterized by a pattern of binge eating; may emerge during adolescence

6. _____ significant group for the adolescent that is made up of contemporaries, or a group of people with whom one associates

7. _____ development period between puberty and maturity during the ages of 11 and 20 years

8. _____ involuntary discharge of semen when sleeping that occurs during sexual maturity of boys

a. adolescence
b. anorexia
c. bulimia
d. menarche
e. nocturnal emission
f. peer group
g. preadolescence
h. puberty

■ Short Answers

1. According to Havighurst, list factors that will contribute to the adolescent successful growing up.

2. Describe three developmental tasks of adolescence according to Havighurst.

3. Describe methods Erickson suggests to help the adolescent succeed in progressing through adolescence.

4. List activities that can help the adolescent develop skills.

5. Complete the table on the following page.

6. Summarize physical changes that occur between the ages 11 and 20 years.

7. List changes that occur during sexual development of boys and girls

Adolescent Stage	When Stage Occurs	Characteristics of Stage
	11–14 years	
	15–17 years	
	18–20 years	

8. Identify the important characteristics of the following adolescent relationships:

RELATIONSHIP	CHARACTERISTICS OF RELATIONSHIP
a. Family	
b. Siblings	
c. Peers	
d. Friends	
e. Boy/girlfriends	

9. List examples of risk-taking behavior.

10. Discuss consequences of an unhealthy adolescent diet.

■ Fill in the Blanks

1. Rapid growth occurs during adolescence, but _____ needs predominate during this period.

2. The tasks of adolescence ultimately involve achieving independence from _____ domination and accepting _____ _____ for oneself.

3. According to Erickson, the major challenge of adolescence is the achievement of _____.

4. _____ _____ is part of cognitive growth and also helps the adolescent prepare for the future.

5. Thinking _____ and developing skills help the adolescent participate in complex problem solving.

6. Many gays and _____ may first come to realize their sexual orientation during their teenage years.

7. Sexual activity at younger ages and _____ _____ _____ are increasing in adolescents.

8. Only _____ is 100% effective against teenage pregnancy and sexually transmitted diseases.

9. Disciplinary measures for teenagers should be _____ and imposed _____ .

■ Theorist Review

Indicate which theorist proposed which of the following concepts. Use E for Erikson, P for Piaget, and H for Havighurst.

1. _____ The ultimate task of adolescence is to "grow up" and includes such activities as achieving emotional independence.

2. _____ Adolescents face challenges with personal identity versus role confusion and develop virtues that include independence, self-esteem, self-reliance, self-control, devotion, and fidelity.

3. _____ Skill development is part of cognitive growth and also serves as preparation for the future.

4. _____ The adolescent aged 12 to 15 years enters the cognitive development state of formal operations in which one thinks in the abstract and does complex problem solving.

5. _____ Tasks of adolescence include preparation for a career, education, and other pursuits.

■ Multiple Choice

1. A mother has brought her son, age 12 years, to the hospital. She states that he has informed her that he has a crush on his best friend. The mother wants to be understanding and asks for help. The nurse should explain that:

   a. for many adolescents, a same-sex crush may reflect a temporary experimental stage in which questioning of sexual preference may occur but does not affect later heterosexuality.

   b. gays and lesbians realize their sexual orientation during early childhood, so these feelings are meaningless if her son has not shown a previous sexual preference.

   c. sexual identity is usually set by the beginning adolescence and her son is gay.

   d. she should let her son know that a gay lifestyle is unacceptable so he will not choose to assume this lifestyle to prevent rejection form his family.

2. A mother expresses concern that her 12-year-old daughter has been alternating from a rebellious independent child to a playful and silly young woman who needs family guidance. She fears that she may have mental problems. The nurse would explain that:

   a. her daughter may have a split personality and should be committed to a mental institution.

   b. if her daughter begins to show moodiness and seclusion, she will need constant supervision to prevent her from spending time reflecting on herself.

   c. the daughter shows signs of regression and needs to have psychological counseling to help her to control her spiritedness.

   d. young adolescents often fluctuate between testing independence and wanting parental approval.

3. During late adolescence which of the following behaviors would be cause for concern?

   a. The teenager enters the work force or joins the military after finishing school.

   b. A young woman or man dates a variety of individuals.

   c. The teenager chooses friends who are 10 years older and wiser about the world than the teen is.

   d. Parents of the adolescent encourage the adolescent to use the home as a base for friendships and personal activities.

4. Which of the following is a correct statement?

   a. Food and eating habits are a concern because gaining 2 or 3 pounds can make adolescent girls depressed and because anorexia and bulimia may emerge during these years.

   b. Peer pressure is natural; families that attempt to model safe habits and practices could confuse the teenager.

   c. Sex education should be provided to adolescents by peers and older adolescents to prevent rejection of the information by the teenager.

   d. Risk-taking behavior is always a result of the teenager's lack of knowledge of the consequences of the risky actions so peer teaching must be done to ensure proper behavior.

CHAPTER 12

Early and Middle Adulthood

■ Terminology Review

Match the following definitions with the correct terms.

1. _____ establishing relationships with others

2. _____ occurs when middle adults decide to pass on learning and share skills with younger generations

3. _____ period in middle adulthood when they must deal with looking at goals of youth and where their life is currently

4. _____ to remain detached from others

a. generativity
b. intimacy
c. isolation
d. midlife transition

■ Adulthood Review

Indicate if the following tasks or the psychosocial development is associated with early adulthood (E) or middle adulthood (M).

1. _____ The individual assists children to become responsible adults.

2. _____ A focus is on strengthening the relationship with his or her partner.

3. _____ The individual becomes involved with civic and religious group activities.

4. _____ The individual must deal with and assist aging parents.

5. _____ A necessary accomplishment is choosing a relationship style.

6. _____ Intimacy versus isolation is the challenge for this developmental age.

7. _____ The virtues that must be developed include production, caring, and cooperation.

8. _____ Generativity versus self-absorption is the challenge for this group.

9. _____ The virtues of this stage are affiliation and love.

10. _____ Accomplishments of this stage include planning for retirement.

■ Matching

Match the following concepts and definitions.

1. _____ occurs between ages 45 and 65; Levinson indicates the transitions include the balance of choices

2. _____ Sheehy's phase of adulthood in which the individual establishes a new home and focuses on career goals

3. _____ occurs during the 40s and 50s; there is a changing self-image and the individual must face his or her own mortality

4. _____ the time between age 18 and 22 when the person must establish an adult identity and establish personal goals

5. _____ a time from 33 to 39 years of age when the major transitions include a balance of choices

6. _____ according to Havighurst's, this stage includes the selection of a mate and beginning an occupation

7. _____ during this period, Levinson's transition could include marriage or divorce

8. _____ a virtue, according to Sheehy, during this stage includes exploration and experimentation

9. _____ includes Havighurst's developmental task of attaining a satisfying career

10. _____ this phase includes the reappraisal of goals and values

11. _____ Levinson states this is a time of balance of choices

a. early adulthood

b. early adult transition

c. catch 30s

d. getting into the adult world

e. middle adulthood

f. midlife transition

g. payoff years

h. settling down

i. time of renewal

j. trying 20s

k. 30s transition

■ Multiple Choice

1. Sheehy's work focuses on:
   a. adult men.
   b. adult women.
   c. childhood development.
   d. childhood and adolescent development.

2. According to Erikson, the developmental challenge of a 50-year-old is:
   a. balancing personal choices.
   b. experimentation and exploration.
   c. generativity versus self-absorption.
   d. intimacy versus isolation.

3. Havignhurst indicates that developmental tasks of the middle adult focus on:
   a. career choices.
   b. family establishment.
   c. relationships.
   d. self-awareness.

4. Many theorists stress that meeting developmental challenges depends on:
   a. cultural influences.
   b. individual characteristics.
   c. support from society.
   d. all of the above.

5. Adults who are referred to as the sandwich generation are:
   a. adults who have children from at least two marriages.
   b. caught between caring for aging parents and their own children.
   c. interested in their own lives and not concerned with people around them.
   d. personally responsible for the overweight youth.

CHAPTER 13

Older Adulthood and Aging

■ Terminology Review

Match the following definitions with the correct terms and acronyms.

1. _____ death

2. _____ the study of the aging process in all its dimensions, including physical, psychological, economic, sociologic, and spiritual

3. _____ labeling and discriminating against older adults

4. _____ American Association of Retired Persons

a. AARP
b. ageism
c. gerontology
d. mortality

■ Theorist Review

Associate the theorist with the following statements on the development of older adults by indicating H for Havighurst, E for Erikson, L for Levinson, and S for Sheehy.

1. _____ The challenge of this age is ego integrity versus despair.

2. _____ Older adulthood involves the task of adjusting to the death of a spouse or companion.

3. _____ A task of the older adult is to establish social relationships with persons of the same age and with younger persons.

4. _____ Older adults need to feel comfortable with the changes that occur and to attain the dignity that is part of aging.

5. _____ Necessary accomplishments in the older adulthood include the need to balance choices and achieve stability and to accept life choices.

6. _____ Life after age 65 is a time for adults to find a new balance of involvement with society and with the self.

7. _____ Successful transition in older adulthood results in wisdom and stability.

8. _____ Renunciation, wisdom, and dignity are virtues the older adult should develop.

9. _____ A developmental task includes adjusting to retirement and a fixed income.

10. _____ Like Levinson, this theorist stresses that older adults have the opportunity to value themselves apart form the standards and agendas of others.

■ Nursing Actions

Indicate if the following actions by a nurse would be appropriate (A) or inappropriate (I) as discussed in this chapter.

1. _____ The nurse explains to an older adult that the changes related to aging are pathologic and cannot be adapted to, so acceptance of pending disability is important.

2. _____ Care provided to an older adult in the hospital is adjusted, when possible, to allow the patient to watch her morning gospel show as she does every morning at home.

3. _____ Avoid discussing the death of the patient's spouse or peers, or past activities, to prevent morbid thinking or depression.

4. _____ Expect that patients who are older will be more concerned about the opinion of others and will respond to stress more violently because of their age.

5. _____ Limit research in nursing to persons aged 65 to 75 years because this group is the fastest growing segment of the population of the United States.

6. _____ Assist family members to arrange for home assistance for an aging parent to help the parent live at home and retain independence as long as possible.

7. _____ Encourage older adults to choose and plan activities before and after retirement because activity is necessary for life.

8. _____ Discuss exciting trips the older adult should take because his or her finances are better at this time than during their earlier years and they can afford to enjoy life.

9. _____ Refer to the older adult as "gramps" or "honey" to put them at ease.

10. _____ Assist the older adult with walking if he or she has an unsteady gait.

■ Multiple Choice

Circle the correct answer.

1. Which of the following is not a developmental task of the older adult?

   a. Adjusting to changes in physical health

   b. Begin preparation for death by withdrawing from society

   c. Find satisfaction with new roles and relationships

   d. Recognize one's life accomplishments

2. Which of the following attitudes reflects ageism?

   a. Older adults can learn new concepts.

   b. Older adults should be allowed to drive an automobile as long as they can drive safely.

   c. Older adults should be respected for their life experiences.

   d. Older adults should not have the same diagnostic tests as younger adults.

3. According to Erikson, which of the following statements indicates successful mastering of psychosocial development skills?

   a. "I feel like my life has been too short."

   b. "I have lived a full long life."

   c. "I have never been successful in any of my business ventures."

   d. "I wish I would have gotten married and had a family."

4. The fastest growing segment in the older adult population is:

   a. 65 to 70 years

   b. 70 to 75 years

   c. 75 to 85 years

   d. older than 85 years

5. When discussing spirituality with an older adult, the nurse should be aware that:

   a. older adults are more likely to value religion and spirituality.

   b. older adults do not like to openly discuss religion and spirituality.

   c. older adults use spirituality and religion to only deal with physical changes.

   d. older adults rarely need quiet time to pray or reflect.

CHAPTER 14

Death and Dying

■ Terminology Review

Match the following definitions with the correct terms and acronyms.

1. _____ nonverbal stage of depression in which the person realizes the impact of the loss

2. _____ final stage of dying in which an individual gradually separates form the world

3. _____ state in which an individual faces a medical condition that will end in death within a limited period

4. _____ verbal stage of depression in which the individual concentrates on past losses

a. detachment
b. preparatory depression
c. reactive depression
d. terminal illness

■ Correct the False Statements

Circle the word True *or* False *that follows the statement. If the word* false *has been circled, change the underlined word/words to make the statement true. Place your answer in the space provided.*

1. As humans age, every person must face his or her own <u>mortality.</u>

   True   False   _____

2. Death is considered a private matter <u>in all cultures.</u>

   True   False   _____

3. According to Bernard and Schneider, the <u>first level of spiritual support</u> for the dying person is strength generated by prayer.

   True   False   _____

4. One gift you can bring to patients and families is honoring the process of dying through continued <u>interaction, attention, and concern</u>.

   True   False   _____

5. All terminally ill people pass through the <u>stages of dying</u>.

   True   False   _____

6. The <u>first stage</u> of dealing with death is anger and rage.

   True   False   _____

7. The bargaining and developing awareness stage of death <u>tends to be</u> <u>a long drawn-out phase</u>.

   True   False   _____

8. Family members may interpret a dying person's acceptance of death as <u>rejection of life and of them</u>.

   True   False   _____

9. The final stage of dying is when the individual gradually <u>separates from the world</u>.

   True   False   _____

10. The effort of family members to appear hopeful and cheerful <u>is helpful for</u> the dying person.

    True   False   _____

11. Death often forces people to consider profound questions: <u>the meaning of life, existence of the soul, and the possibility of an afterlife.</u>

    True   False   _____

12. The patient who is in the anger stage of dying is rebelling against <u>your actions</u>.

True   False   _____

■ Matching

Match the suggestion for helping a person cope with death with both the stage of dealing with death and the statements found in each stage. Each question will have two answers.

1. _____ Provide physical care, be there, and keep the room lighted.

2. _____ Continue to include the person in conversation.

3. _____ Try to assist in patient's wishes; offer spiritual assistance.

4. _____ Answer questions honestly, do not argue.

5. _____ Listen, do not take the patient's behavior personally.

6. _____ Offer encouragement, allow person to rest.

a. anger
b. depression
c. denial
d. detachment
e. acceptance
f. bargaining
g. "No, not me."
h. "Why me?"
i. "Yes me."
j. "My time is close, and it's OK."
k. "Yes me, but..., If I could just live until..."
l. No communication

■ Multiple Choice

Circle the best answer.

1. During the final stages of death, which religious group would you expect to have a priest perform last rites and chanting rituals?
   a. Amish
   b. Buddhist
   c. Episcopal
   d. Hindu

2. A patient who is Roman Catholic and has a terminal illness is requesting the sacrament of the sick. The most appropriate action would be:
   a. contact the patient's priest.
   b. notify your supervisor of the request.
   c. offer to perform the sacrament for the patient.
   d. refuse to participate with the patient's spiritual needs.

3. To support the patient who is dying and to honor the process of dying, the nurse should:
   a. assume that the patient wants privacy and respect the patient's wishes.
   b. be available to the patient by providing your home telephone number.
   c. continue to interact with the patient and his or her family.
   d. only interact with the patient when he or she asks you to.

4. A family member complains that the dying family member has rejected life and no longer loves him or her. The nurse understands that the dying person is in which stage of dying?
   a. Acceptance
   b. Bargaining
   c. Denial
   d. Detachment

5. During the final stage of dying, nursing care focuses on:
   a. emotional needs.
   b. physical needs.
   c. psychosocial needs.
   d. social needs.

CHAPTER 15

Organization of the Human Body

■ Terminology Review

Match the following definitions with the correct terms.

1. _____ anterior or front

2. _____ study of how the body functions

3. _____ four areas that the abdominal cavity can be divided into

4. _____ vertical plane that passes through the body longitudinally from head to toe, dividing it into front and back parts

5. _____ divides the body into right and left sides

6. _____ body pictured standing erect with arms at sides and palms turned forward

7. _____ muscular partition between the abdomen and thoracic cavities

8. _____ study of body structure

9. _____ space within the body that contains internal organs

10. _____ vocabulary used in the healthcare field

11. _____ structural unit of the body made up of organs

12. _____ posterior or back

13. _____ imaginary flat surface that divides the body into sections

14. _____ structural unit of the body that is made up of tissues

15. _____ study of disorders of functioning

16. _____ dividing the body into superior and inferior parts

17. _____ hairlike threads that sweep materials across the cell

a. anatomic position
b. anatomy
c. body cavity
d. cilia
e. diaphragm
f. dorsal
g. frontal
h. medical terminology
i. organ
j. pathophysiology
k. physiology
l. plane
m. quadrant
n. sagittal
o. system
p. transverse
q. ventral

Match the following definitions with the following chemical terms.

18. _____ physical and emotional equilibrium that a person strives to maintain

19. _____ substances change into other substances that no longer have the same chemical structures as before

20. _____ blend of two or more substances without forming a new compound

21. _____ ability to process, obtain energy from, and create new products using the chemicals found in foods

22. _____ two or more elements react chemically to form a substance

23. _____ pure, simple chemical

24. _____ change in state of a substance but not the chemical structure

25. _____ complex protein structure that speeds up chemical reactions

26. _____ smallest part of any element

a. atom
b. chemical change
c. compound
d. element
e. enzyme
f. homeostasis
g. metabolism
h. mixture
i. physical change

Match the following definitions with the correct terms.

27. _____ cell division into two parts

28. _____ control center of the cell that is responsible for reproduction and coordination of other cellular activities

29. _____ all parts that make up a cell

30. _____ another name for cell membrane

31 _____ structural unit of the body that is made up of cells

32 _____ surround the cell's outer boundary and is capable of selective permeability

33 _____ part of the nucleus that carries genetic factors

34. _____ area of the cell not located in the nucleus

35. _____ basic structural unit found in the body

36. _____ carries information about inherited characteristics

37. _____ cell division to produces eggs or sperms that contain half the number of chromosomes

a. cell
b. cell membrane
c. chromosome
d. cytoplasm
e. gene
f. meiosis
g. mitosis
h. nucleus

i. plasma membrane
j. protoplasm
k. tissue

Match the following definitions with the correct acronyms.

38. _____ is found mostly in the nucleus and contains chromosomes

39. _____ right upper quadrant

40. _____ carry oxygen and carbon dioxide needed for cellular respiration or the formation of energy

41. _____ left lower quadrant

42. _____ destroy pathogens and develop immunity to some diseases

43. _____ left upper quadrant

44. _____ is responsible for taking the genetic message from the DNA molecule and transporting this message to the ribosomes

45. _____ right lower quadrant

a. DNA
b. RNA
c. LUQ
d. RUQ
e. LLQ
f. RLQ
g. RBCs
h. WBCs

■ Correct the False Statements

Circle the word True *or* False *that follows the statement. If the word* false *has been circled, change the underlined word/words to make the statement true. Place your answer in the space provided.*

1. Cholecystitis is the removal of the gall bladder.

    True   False   _____

2. Leukocyte is a red blood cell.

    True   False   _____

3. Encephalopathy is a disease involving the <u>brain.</u>

   True   False   _____

4. <u>Cardiology</u> is the science of the heart.

   True   False   _____

5. Hepatitis it the <u>removal of the intestines.</u>

   True   False   _____

6. Dysphagia is <u>difficulty eating.</u>

   True   False   _____

7. Intravenous means <u>pertaining to within an artery</u>.

   True   False   _____

8. <u>Tracheotomy</u> is the creation of an opening in the trachea.

   True   False   _____

9. <u>Polyuria</u> means a lot of urine.

   True   False   _____

10. Atrophy means <u>a failure of muscular coordination</u>.

    True   False   _____

■ Short Answers

Provide the best answer.

1. Indicate if the following tissues are epithelial (E), connective (C), muscle (M), or nerve (N).

   a. _____ blood

   b. _____ neurons

   c. _____ calluses

   d. _____ bone

   e. _____ cardiac

   f. _____ glands

   g. _____ adipose

   h. _____ skeletal

2. Supply the correct directional terms for the following examples.

   a. the elbow is _____ to the shoulder

   b. the knee is _____ to the toes

   c. the _____ membranes cover the walls of body cavities

   d. the heart is _____ within the thoracic cavity

   e. the skin is _____ from the muscles

   f. the chest is _____ to the spine

   g. the kidneys are _____ to the spine

3. What contents are contained in the dorsal cavity?

4. What organs are in the thoracic cavity?

5. What organs are found in the LUQ of the abdomen?

6. List the structural levels of the body from smallest to largest.

7. List the three types of soft connective tissue.

8. Describe the functions of membranes.

9. Describe the difference between mitosis and meiosis.

10. Explain how systems function.

■ Multiple Choice

Circle the best answer.

1. The powerhouse of the cell is the:
   a. centrosome
   b. endoplasmic reticulum
   c. golgi apparatus
   d. mitochondria

2. During the first stage of mitosis the:
   a. cell begins to elongate and thin at the middle.
   b. centrosomes separate and are drawn to opposite ends of the cell.
   c. chromosomes split and move toward each centrosome
   d. cytoplasm splits in half.

3. The two phases of metabolism are:
   a. anabolism and catabolism.
   b. contractility and conductivity.
   c. irritability and reproduction.
   d. physical and chemical.

4. Which of the following is a function of epithelial tissues?
   a. Absorb and secrete substances from the digestive tract.
   b. Anchor and support body structures.
   c. Conduct impulses to and from all parts of the body.
   d. Provide movement of the body.

5. Components of the hematologic system include:
   a. blood
   b. blood vessels
   c. heart
   d. skin

6. Which type of plane describes dividing the body into top and bottom sections?
   a. Coronal
   b. Fontal
   c. Midsagittal
   d. Transverse

7. Which type of soft connective tissue is important to cell nutrition?
   a. Adipose
   b. Areolar
   c. Elastic
   d. Fibrous

CHAPTER 16

The Integumentary System

■ Terminology Review

Match the following definitions with the correct terms.

1. _____ patches of melanin clustered together

2. _____ excessive perspiration

3. _____ ear wax

4. _____ yellowish pigment found in parts of the epidermis and dermis, it is a precursor to vitamin A

5. _____ transfer of heat from one object to another by direct contact

6. _____ process of the dead outer layer of skin being rubbed off through washing and friction

7. _____ baldness

8. _____ return of water in the air through vapor

9. _____ the outermost protective layer of the skin, which is composed of squamous epithelium stratified into layers

10. _____ subcutaneous tissue

11. _____ glands that produce ear wax

12. _____ another name for the dermis

13. _____ transfer of heat from one surface to the surrounding gases

14. _____ true skin

15. _____ tough, resistant, and flexible fibrous protein

a. alopecia
b. carotene
c. cerumen
d. ceruminal glands
e. collagen
f. conduction
g. convection
h. corium
i. dermis
j. desquamation
k. diaphoresis
l. epidermis
m. evaporation
n. freckles
o. hypodermis

Match the following definitions with the correct terms and acronyms.

16. _____ skin tone

17. _____ oily secretion from oil glands

18. _____ creates a waterproof barrier on the outer skin

19. _____ process of maintaining the body's internal temperature

20. _____ dissemination of heat by electromagnetic waves

21. _____ condition in which the melanocytes stop making melanin, causing localized areas of distinct white spots

22. _____ covering

23. _____ layer beneath the dermis and on top of the layer of muscle

24. _____ applying medications through the skin

25. _____ oil glands

26. _____ ultraviolet light

27. _____ scaly

28. _____ sun protection factor

29. _____ brown–black pigment found mostly in the basal layer of the epidermis, which gives skin its color

30. _____ sweat glands

31. _____ hemoglobin

a. integument
b. keratin
c. melanin
d. radiation

e. sebaceous glands
f. sebum
g. skin turgor
h. squamous
i. subcutaneous tissue
j. sudoriferous glands
k. thermoregulation
l. transdermally
m. vitiligo
n. UV light
o. Hgb or Hb
p. SPF

■ Anatomy Review

Identify the parts of the skin in the following diagram. Complete this exercise without referring to your textbook using the following list.

epidermis
subcutaneous layer
hair follicle
artery
nerve endings
adipose cells
fibrous connective tissue
pore of sweat gland
stratum corneum
stratum germinativum
sebaceous gland
papilla
arrector pili muscle
pressure receptor
vein
dermis
nerve
sudoriferous gland

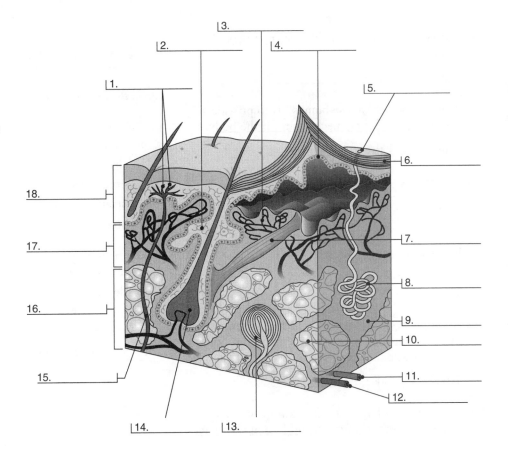

■ Correct the False Statements

Circle the word True *or* False *that follows the statement. If the word* false *has been circled, change the underlined word/words to make the statement true. Place your answer in the space provided.*

1. <u>Langerhans cells in the dermis</u> provide an immune response.

   True   False   _____

2. Mitosis of the nail occurs in the <u>lunula</u>.

   True   False   _____

3. The skin protects against <u>water loss or gain</u>.

   True   False   _____

4. The <u>sensation function</u> of skin is to detect heat, cold, pain, pressure, and touch.

   True   False   _____

5. People of all races have <u>different numbers</u> of melanocytes.

   True   False   _____

6. The purpose of "goose bumps" is to provide a <u>protective insulating mechanism for the body</u>.

   True   False   _____

7. Sunscreens should have an SPF <u>of at least 5</u>.

   True   False   _____

8. Hair can reveal <u>environmental exposure to heavy metals</u> more accurately than a blood specimen.

   True   False   _____

9. <u>Apocrine sweat glands</u> are widely distributed over the body, especially on the upper lip, forehead, back, palms, and soles.

   True   False   _____

10. Some effects of aging on the skin include <u>wrinkling, reduced skin turgor, and lose of elasticity</u>.

    True   False   _____

11. The integumentary system is composed of the skin and its <u>accessory structures: hair, nails, and glands</u>.

    True   False   _____

12. Decreased exposure to the sun and decreased intake of irradiated milk put the older adult at risk for <u>vitamin C deficiency</u>.

    True   False   _____

13. Native Americans usually have <u>dark brown, moist, and sticky cerumen</u>.

    True   False   _____

14. Graying of hair is due to a decrease in <u>keratin production</u>.

    True   False   _____

15. Very young infants do not have the ability to <u>shiver to produce heat</u>.

    True   False   _____

■ Multiple Choice

Circle the best answer.

1. The part of the skin that is the thin outermost protective layer is:
   a. dermis.
   b. epidermis.
   c. stratum basale.
   d. stratum corneum.

2. The stratum germinativum is constantly producing new cells to replace the:
   a. dermis.
   b. hypodermis.
   c. stratum basale.
   d. stratum corneum.

3. Which of the following nursing actions would be appropriate for the older adult who has lost subcutaneous fat due to aging?

   a. Advise patient to bathe daily

   b. Encourage the use of makeup

   c. Place a fan in the room

   d. Provide extra blankets

4. During hot weather, which instruction should be given to the older adult to prevent heat stroke?

   a. Change position frequently when sitting

   b. Encourage an adequate amount of sunshine each day

   c. Increase fluid intake

   d. Wear warm clothing to cover the arms

5. The body's first line of defense against infection is:

   a. adequate hydration.

   b. thermoregulation.

   c. the skin.

   d. vitamin D.

6. Which of the following actions can assist in keeping the skin healthy?

   a. Avoid the use of sunscreen products

   b. Eating a healthy diet

   c. Smoking cigarettes

   d. Stay in the sun

7. The medical term for hair loss is:

   a. alopecia.

   b. corium.

   c. desquamation.

   d. vitiligo.

8. The yellowish pigment that is a precursor to vitamin A is:

   a. carotene.

   b. collagen.

   c. keratin.

   d. melanin.

CHAPTER 17

Fluid and Electrolyte Balance

■ Terminology Review

Match the following definitions with the correct terms and acronyms.

1. _____ dynamic process through which the body maintains balance by constantly adjusting to internal and external stimuli

2. _____ ability of a membrane to allow molecules to pass through it

3. _____ solution with a high solute number

4. _____ atom that has lost or gained one or more electrons

5. _____ inside the blood vessels

6. _____ substance dissolved in a solvent

7. _____ an electrolyte that is made up of a cation other than a hydrogen ion and an anion other than a hydroxyl ion

8. _____ dilute solution that has less solutes

9. _____ solution that dissolves solutes

10. _____ between the cells

11. _____ diffusion of water across a semipermeable membrane

12. _____ nonvisible water loss

13. _____ same NaCl concentration as normal body fluids

14. _____ compound that contains the hydrogen ion

15. _____ positively charged ion

16. _____ relay of information about a given condition to the appropriate organ or system

17. _____ fluid accumulation in the peritoneal cavity

18. _____ negatively charged ion

19. _____ compound that contains the hydroxyl ion

20. _____ solutes that generate an electrical charge when dissolved in water

21. _____ severe generalized edema

22. _____ excessive loss of water from the body

23. _____ transport of water and dissolved materials through a membrane from an area of higher pressure to an area of lower pressure

24. _____ random movement of molecules from an area of higher concentration to an area of lower concentration

25. _____ accumulation of water in the interstitial fluid compartment of the body

26. _____ chemical system set up to resist changes, particularly in the level of hydrogen ions

a. acid
b. anasarca
c. anion
d. ascites
e. base
f. buffer
g. cation
h. dehydration
i. diffusion
j. edema
k. electrolyte
l. feedback
m. filtration
n. homeostatsis
o. hypertonic
p. hypotonic
q. insensible
r. interstitial
s. intravascular
t. ion

u. isotonic

v. osmosis

w. permeability

x. salt

y. solute

z. solvent

l. K+

m. Na+

n. NaCl

o. NS

p. OH-

■ Matching

Match the following definitions with the acronyms.

1. _____ milliequivalents

2. _____ sodium

3. _____ calcium

4. _____ intracellular fluid

5. _____ sodium chloride

6. _____ arterial blood gas

7. _____ potassium

8. _____ extracellular fluid

9. _____ chloride

10. _____ milliliters

11. _____ water

12. _____ normal saline

13. _____ cerebral spinal fluid

14. _____ hydrogen ion

15. _____ potential of hydrogen or power of hydrogen

16. _____ hydroxyl ion

a. ABGs

b. CSF

c. H$_2$O

d. ICF

e. ECF

f. mEq

g. mL or ml

h. pH

i. Ca++

j. Cl-

k. H+

■ Short Answers

Complete the following questions by writing in the best answer.

1. List the three primary regulators of ECF fluid volume and discuss the mechanism of action of each.

2. Describe the term third-spacing.

3. List the four ways in which edema can occur and provide an example of each.

4. List the four functions of water.

5. List the major electrolytes responsible for normal functioning of neurons and muscle cells.

6. Describe two nursing actions that would be appropriate to maintain appropriate levels of the electrolytes in the preceding question.

7. Contrast the transportation of diffusion, filtration, osmosis, and active transport.

8. Describe how heat can speed up the process of diffusion.

9. Explain the significance of monitoring arterial blood gases when caring for patients.

10. Explain why infants are at risk for fluid and electrolyte imbalances.

▪ Multiple Choice

Circle the best answer.

1. Dehydration results from the excessive loss of:
   a. H^+.
   b. H_2O.
   c. H_2O_2.
   d. OH.

2. Negative feedback occurs:
   a. only during times of illness.
   b. only at the time of death.
   c. when the original signal is intensified.
   d. when the original signal is reversed.

3. ICF is located:
   a. inside the cells.
   b. inside the blood vessels.
   c. outside the brain and spinal cord.
   d. outside the cells.

4. Large or specialized molecules that need assistance are transported by:
   a. active transport.
   b. diffusion.
   c. filtration.
   d. osmosis.

5. Filtration requires:
   a. diffusion.
   b. mechanical pressure.
   c. osmosis.
   d. a sodium and potassium pump.

6. A primary regulator of the acid in the body is the:
   a. cardiovascular system.
   b. nervous system.
   c. respiratory system.
   d. urinary system.

7. Normal blood pH is:
   a. 6.75–7.0
   b. 7.25–7.35
   c. 7.35–7.45
   d. 7.75–7.85

8. Most of the body's fluids are located:
   a. inside the cells.
   b. in the plasma.
   c. in the ECF.
   d. in the lymph system.

9. An increase in aldosterone will result in reabsorption of sodium and:
   a. acids.
   b. magnesium.
   c. potassium.
   d. water.

10. The most important cation in the extracellular fluid is:
    a. chloride.
    b. phosphate.
    c. potassium.
    d. sodium.

11. The most important anion in the intracellular fluid is:
    a. chloride.
    b. phosphate.
    c. potassium.
    d. sodium.

12. The body has a greater tendency toward acidosis and so has a greater need for:

    a. carbon dioxide.

    b. carbonic acid.

    c. hydrogen.

    d. sodium bicarbonate.

13. Which of the following would help maintain normal fluid and electrolyte balance in the older adult?

    a. Encourage fluids

    b. Encourage decreased activity

    c. Encourage increased sodium intake

    d. Encourage sips of water with medication

CHAPTER 18

The Musculoskeletal System

■ Terminology Review

Match the following definitions with the correct terms.

1. _____ deterioration in size and function of cells

2. _____ last four vertebrae that are small and incomplete and fuse in adults

3. _____ sponge-like end of long bones

4. _____ increasing the angle between two bones

5. _____ ability to stretch

6. _____ another name for a joint

7. _____ ability to return to normal length after stretching

8. _____ small flat sacs lined with synovial membrane and filled with synovial fluid

9. _____ manner of walking

10. _____ decreasing the angle between two bones

11. _____ shaft of the long bone

12. _____ ability to shorten and become thicker

13. _____ depression of a joint

14. _____ type of connective tissue organized into a system of fibers

15. _____ heel bone

a. acetabulum
b. articulation
c. atrophy
d. bursae
e. calcaneous
f. cartilage
g. coccyx
h. contractility
i. diaphysis
j. elasticity
k. epiphysis
l. extensibility
m. extension
n. flexion
o. gait

Match the following definitions with the correct terms.

16. _____ upper jaw bone

17. _____ hunchback

18. _____ a muscle's state of slight contraction and the ability to spring into action

19. _____ swayback

20. _____ points at which bones attach to each other

21. _____ outer aspect of the ankle bone

22. _____ shortening and thickening of the muscle, which causes movement

23. _____ blood formation

24. _____ increase in muscle tension but not muscle length

25. _____ located between ribs

26. _____ ability to respond to a stimulus

27. _____ strong fibrous bands that hold bones together

28. _____ soft substance in the hollow inner part of bones

29. _____ formation of bone by osteoblasts and is the process by which bones become hardened through an increase in calcified tissue

30. _____ inner aspect of the ankle bone

a. hematopoiesis

b. intercostals muscles

c. irritability

d. isometric

e. isotonic

f. joint

g. kyphosis

h. lateral malleolus

i. ligaments

j. lordosis

k. marrow

l. maxilla

m. medial malleolus

n. muscle tone

o. ossification

Match the following definitions with the correct terms.

31. _____ act of removal by absorption

32. _____ juncture where pubic bones meet in front and are joined by a pad of cartilage

33. _____ spine

34. _____ bone-building cells

35. _____ range of motion

36. _____ attach muscle to bones

37. _____ angle of the pelvic opening

38. _____ cells that assist in the resorption or breakdown of bone

39. _____ hard fibrous connective tissue membrane that covers most of the outside of bones

40. _____ hardened mature bone cell

a. osteoblast

b. osteoclast

c. osteocyte

d. periosteum

e. pubic arch

f. ROM

g. resorption

h. symphysis pubis

i. tendons

j. vertebral column

■ Anatomy and Physiology Review

Indicate whether the terms or phrases listed below involve structure/anatomy (S) or function/physiology (F).

1. _____ masseter

2. _____ joints

3. _____ osteoclasts

4. _____ xiphoid process

5. _____ ATP

6. _____ manubrium

7. _____ tibia

8. _____ hormones

9. _____ gives shape to the body

10. _____ rectus femoris

11. _____ provides locomotion

12. _____ stores calcium

13. _____ anterior superior iliac spine

14. _____ gluteus maximus

15. _____ produce heat

■ Numbers Game

Choose from the following numbers to correctly complete the sentences. Some numbers may be used more than once or not at all.

0, 3, 5, 7, 12, 25, 40, 90, 28, 204, 250, and 1,000

1. More than _____% of the total bones in the human body are found in the hands and wrists.

2. Skeletal muscle comprises _____ % of total body weight.

3. Each muscle fiber is about the size of a human hair and can hold approximately _____ times its own weight.

4. The angle of the pelvic opening is less than _____% in men and greater than _____% in women.

5. The skull is made up of _____ bones.

6. There are _____ thoracic vertebrae.

7. The human body has _____ bones.

8. There _____ different types of muscles.

9. The first _____ ribs are true ribs and attach directly to the sternum.

10. The auditory ossicles are composed of _____ bones in each ear.

■ Anatomy Identification

Label the parts of the skeleton using the following list.

humerus
metacarpals
ilium
phalanges
clavicle
metatarsals
vertebral column
mandible
tarsals
ulna
scapula
radius
calcaneius
costal cartilage
femur
cranium
ribs
patella
tibia
pelvis
sternum
fibula
carpals
sacrum
facial bones

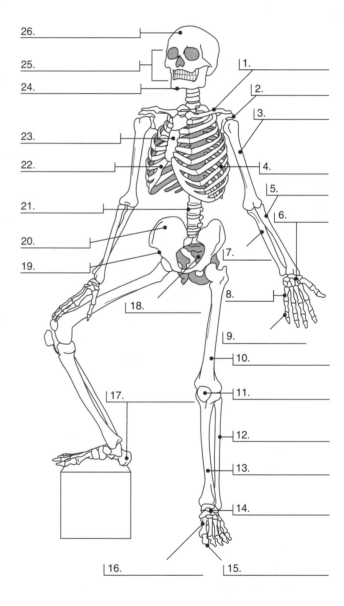

26. _____
25. _____
24. _____
23. _____
22. _____
21. _____
20. _____
19. _____
18. _____
1. _____
2. _____
3. _____
4. _____
5. _____
6. _____
7. _____
8. _____
9. _____
10. _____
11. _____
12. _____
13. _____
14. _____
17. _____
16. _____
15. _____

■ Multiple Choice

Circle the best answer.

1. Red bone marrow is responsible for:
   a. cushioning the bone with fat.
   b. manufacturing RBCs, WBCs, and platelets.
   c. ossification.
   d. weight bearing.

2. Synarthroses joint's action is to provide:
   a. motion like a door on hinges.
   b. motion like turning a doorknob.
   c. no motion.
   d. a slight degree of motion.

3. An example of a hinge joint is:
   a. bones of the skull.
   b. finger.
   c. thumb.
   d. wrist.

4. Which of the following is part of the axial skeletal system?
   a. Fibula
   b. Humerus
   c. Pelvic girdle
   d. Ribs

5. The function of fontanels in an infant are to:
   a. allow for growth of the infant's head.
   b. ensure the skull keeps its shape.
   c. give the infant his or her individual appearance.
   d. provide a framework for muscles to attach.

6. Which of the following is a function of skeletal muscles?
   a. dilating the eyes.
   b. locomotion.
   c. moving food along the gastrointestinal tract.
   d. propel blood through vessels.

7. In which muscle could an intramuscular injection be given?
   a. Bicep
   b. External oblique
   c. Gluteus medius
   d. Vastus medialis

8. Which of the following factors affects the rate of bone growth?
   a. Exercise
   b. Heredity
   c. Hormones
   d. Nutrition

9. Moving an extremity in circles is an example of:
   a. circumduction.
   b. eversion.
   c. pronation.
   d. rotation.

CHAPTER 19

The Nervous System

■ Terminology Review

Match the following definitions with the correct terms and acronyms.

1. _____ also called glial cells

2. _____ peripheral nervous system

3. _____ type of neuron that transmits messages from the CNS to all parts of the body

4. _____ central nervous system

5. _____ nerve cell

6. _____ type of neuron that which carries messages between sensory and motor pathways

7. _____ carries impulses away from the neuron cell body

8. _____ autonomic nervous system

9. _____ fatty covering

10. _____ study of the nervous system

11. _____ tiny space that separates the neurons from each other

12. _____ receive impulses and transmit these impulses toward the neuron cell body

13. _____ type of neuron that receives messages from all parts of the body and transmit to the CNS

14. _____ chemical that an axon releases to allow nerve impulses to cross the synapse and reach the dendrites

a. afferent
b. axon
c. dendrites
d. efferent
e. interneurons
f. myelin sheath
g. neuron
h. neuroglia
i. neurology
j. neurotransmitter
k. synapse
l. ANS
m. CNS
n. PNS

Match the following definitions with the correct terms.

15. _____ includes the midbrain, pons, and medulla

16. _____ has reflex control of heart rate, sneezing, hunger, secretions from glands in the stomach, and constrictions within the respiratory tract

17. _____ largely responsible for maintaining a person's level of awareness

18. _____ group of spinal nerves

19. _____ functions as an important reflex center

20 _____ comprises 80% of the brain's volume

21 _____ cerebrospinal fluid

22. _____ functions directly or indirectly to the regulation of visceral activities

23. _____ stimulus causes an organized rapid exchange of sodium and potassium ions across the cell membrane, which spreads like an electric current

24. _____ protective membranes covering the brain and spinal cord

25. _____ crossing

26. _____ end organs that initially receive stimuli from outside and within the body

27. _____ reflex center in the cord receives and sends messages through the nerve fibers

28. _____ located between the hemispheres and brain stem

29. _____ automatic or involuntary response to a stimulus

a. action potential
b. brain stem
c. cerebrum
d. decussation
e. hypothalamus
f. limbic system
g. meninges
h. midbrain

i. plexus
j. receptor
k. reflex
l. reflex arc
m. thalamus
n. vagus nerve
o. CSF

■ Anatomy Review

Label the following diagram with the correct term and indicate the function of each.

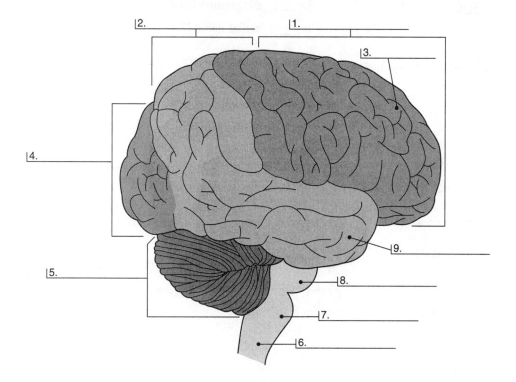

■ Correct the False Statements

Circle the word True *or* False *that follows the statement. If the word* false *has been circled, change the underlined word/words to make the statement true. Place your answer in the space provided.*

1. <u>Sensory receptors</u> receive information, such as pain or cold, and afferent cell bodies transmit the information to the CNS.

   True   False   _____

2. Cerebrospinal fluid forms a protective cushion around and within the CNS, <u>letting the brain float within the cranial vault</u>.

   True   False   _____

3. <u>The parasympathetic nervous system</u> is activated during times of stress or emergency.

   True   False   _____

4. People who have had a cerebrovascular accident affecting one brain hemisphere will exhibit symptoms such as paralysis <u>on the same side of the body</u>.

   True   False   _____

5. An action potential takes <u>only seconds</u>.

   True   False   _____

6. Peristalsis is an example of <u>voluntary control</u>.

   True   False   _____

7. The frontal lobe is responsible <u>for higher mental processes</u>.

   True   False   _____

8. Generally, nerve cells <u>cannot reproduce themselves</u>.

   True   False   _____

9. The <u>dura mater</u>, which is thin and vascular, lies closely over the brain and spinal cord.

   True   ·   False   _____

10. The "all or none" law describes how impulses <u>can be</u> partially transmitted.

    True   False   _____

■ Matching

Match the terms in Part A as they relate to another term in Part B.

PART A

1. _____ sensory
2. _____ cranial nerve VII
3. _____ parasympathetic
4. _____ ranial nerve II
5. _____ motor
6. _____ cranial nerve X
7. _____ sympathetic
8 _____ lexus
9. _____ brain and spinal cord
10. _____ neurotransmitter
11. _____ pons
12. _____ ventricles

PART B

a. optic
b. vagus
c. cavity
d. acetylcholine
e. afferent
f. group of spinal nerves
g. homeostasis
h. facial
i. bridge
j. efferent
k. emergency
l. central nervous system

■ Multiple Choice

Circle the best answer.

1. The trigeminal nerve, cranial nerve V, is responsible for:
   a. hearing.
   b. controlling swallowing.
   c. sensations of head and face.
   d. smell.

2. The parasympathetic nervous system would have which of the following responses?
   a. Increased heart rate
   b. Constriction of pupil
   c. Relaxation of urinary bladder
   d. Stimulation of sweat glands

3. The fight-or-flight response of the sympathetic nervous system would have which of the following effects?
   a. Decreased strength of heart beat
   b. Dilation of bronchi of lungs
   c. Dilation of digestive organ blood vessels
   d. Emptying of the urinary bladder

4. The middle layer of the meninges, which is a delicate web of tissue, is the:
   a. arachnoid.
   b. dura mater.
   c. pia mater.
   d. white matter.

5. The function of the olfactory nerve or cranial nerve I is:
   a. eye movements.
   b. hearing.
   c. smell.
   d. vision.

CHAPTER 20

The Endocrine System

■ Terminology Review

Match the following definitions with the correct terms.

1. _____ chemical regulators that integrate and coordinate body activities

2. _____ raises blood sugar

3. _____ secreted by the adrenal cortex and they regulate the amount of electrolytes in the body

4. _____ secrete substances into ducts that open into the body's external or internal surface

5. _____ stored sugar

6. _____ another name for the anterior lobe of the pituitary

7. _____ produced in the beta cells whose primary function is to control blood's glucose level

8. _____ consist of mineralcorticoids, glucocorticoids, and the sex hormones

9. _____ hormone produced in the kidneys that stimulates RBC production

10. _____ glands that secrete hormones directly into the bloodstream

11. _____ hormone-like substances that share characteristics with hormones and neurotransmitters

12. _____ another name for the posterior lobe of the pituitary

13. _____ the master controller

14. _____ group of specialized cells that secrete a substance in response to signals

15. _____ influence the synthesis of glucose, amino acids, and fats during metabolism

a. adenohypophysis
b. corticosteroids
c. endocrine glands
d. erythropoietin
e. exocrine glands
f. gland
g. glucagon
h. glucocorticoids
i. glycogen
j. hormones
k. hypothalamus
l. insulin
m. mineralcorticoids
n. neurohypophysis
o. prostaglandins

■ Acronym Review

Match the following definitions with the acronyms.

1. _____ secreted by the placenta to help maintain pregnancy

2. _____ stimulates ovulation and formulation of the corpus luteum in women

3. _____ increases blood calcium

4. _____ hormones involved in the body's inflammatory process

5. _____ stimulates growth and secretion of ovarian follicles and the production of sperm

6. _____ regulates body metabolism

7. _____ stimulates milk production in women

8. _____ stimulates growth in all body tissues

9. _____ triiodothyronine

10. _____ produced by the heart to help maintain fluid homeostasis and regulate blood pressure

11. _____ released by anterior pituitary to stimulate the thyroid gland

12. _____ stimulates the adrenal cortex to produce glucocorticoids

13. _____ melanocyte-inhibiting factor

a. ACTH
b. ANP

c. FSH
d. GH
e. HCG
f. LH
g. LT
h. MIF
i. PRL
j. PTH
k. T₃
l. T₄
m. TSH

■ Anatomy and Physiology Review

Identify the following structures and briefly indicate the function of each structure.

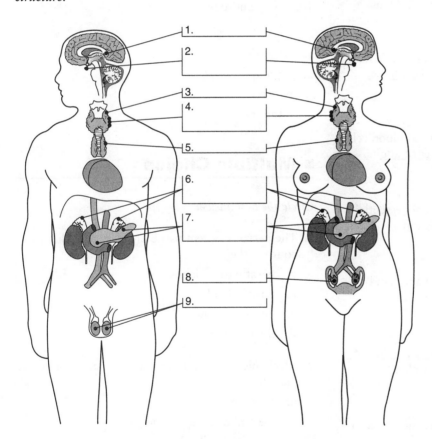

■ Correct the False Statements

Circle the word True *or* False *that follows the statement. If the word* false *has been circled, change the underlined word/words to make the statement true. Place your answer in the space provided.*

1. Renin is a hormone this is produced by the juxtaglomerular apparatus that <u>assists in the control of blood pressure</u>.

   True   False   _____

2. Prostaglandins are <u>hormones</u> whose effects are localized to the area in which they are produced.

   True   False   _____

3. It is possible for an organ, under certain conditions<u>, to temporarily be an endocrine gland</u>.

   True   False   _____

4. Epinephrine and norepinephrine are made from amino acids and <u>are secreted by the adrenal medulla</u>.

   True   False   _____

5. Erythropoietin, which stimulates red blood cell formation, is produced in the <u>liver of adults</u>.

   True   False   _____

6. The parathyroid glands are small <u>nonessential glands involved in calcium regulation</u>.

   True   False   _____

7. The neurohypophysis of the pituitary gland releases <u>oxytocin and vasopressin</u>.

   True   False   _____

8. The hypothalamus is a <u>large simple portion</u> of the brain attached to the pituitary gland.

   True   False   _____

9. <u>Exocrine glands</u> secrete hormones directly into the bloodstream.

   True   False   _____

10. Alpha cells in the pancreas secrete the hormone <u>glucagon</u>.

   True   False   _____

■ Matching

Match the following hormones with the gland that secretes the hormone. Some answers may be used more than once.

1. _____ growth hormone

2. _____ insulin

3. _____ catecholamines

4. _____ calcitonin

5. _____ oxytocin

6. _____ glucocorticoids

7. _____ thyroid-stimulating hormone

8. _____ glucagon

9. _____ vasopressin

10. _____ androgens

a. adrenals
b. thyroid
c. pancreas
d. pituitary

■ Multiple Choice

Circle the best answer.

1. The nervous system tissue of the hypothalamus controls the:
   a. parathyroid glands.
   b. pineal gland.
   c. pituitary gland.
   d. thymus gland.

2. Mechanisms that influence hormonal blood levels include:
   a. action potential.
   b. the "all or none" principle.
   c. negative feedback.
   d. positive feedback.

3. The gland responsible for controlling the body's rate of metabolism is the:
   a. pancreas.
   b. parathyroid.
   c. thymus.
   d. thyroid.

4. This gland secretes hormones that play a role in cellular immunity.
   a. Adrenal
   b. Parathyroid
   c. Pineal
   d. Thymus

5. Which of the following hormones are released during stressful situation?
   a. Androgens
   b. Norepinephrine
   c. Oxytocin
   d. PTH

6. Which hormone is responsible for lowering blood calcium levels?
   a. Testosterone
   b. Growth hormone
   c. Vasopressin
   d. Calcitonin

7. Which of the following is a significant finding for a patient who is taking glucocorticoids?
   a. Elevated temperature
   b. Normal blood pressure
   c. Slight elevation in heart rate
   d. Regular respirations

8. What symptoms would be seen in a patient who lacks adequate insulin production?
   a. Elevated blood glucose levels
   b. Fractures
   c. Lowered blood pressure
   d. Moon face

CHAPTER 21

The Sensory System

■ Terminology Review

Match the following definitions with the correct terms.

1. _____ farsightedness

2. _____ another name for membranous labyrinth

3. _____ receptors that help the body know its location or position

4. _____ tunnels and chambers that fill the bony labyrinth of the ear

5. _____ sensation that either you or the room is spinning

6. _____ part of the retina that receives color and adds to visual acuity

7. _____ smell

8. _____ part of the retina that helps us with night vision

9. _____ ear wax

10. _____ adjustment by the lens to make a sharp clear image

11. _____ small and intricate structure located within the cochlea

12. _____ gradual loss of the function of accommodation

13. _____ ball-shaped cavity of the skull that holds the eye

14. _____ nearsightedness

15. _____ produce tears that keep the eye's surface moist and lubricated

16. _____ degenerative loss of hearing

a. accommodation
b. cerumen
c. cones
d. hyperopia
e. labyrinth
f. lacrimal glands
g. membranous labyrinth
h. myopia
i. olfaction
j. orbit
k. organ of Corti
l. presbycusis
m. presbyopia
n. proprioceptors
o. rods
p. vertigo

ANATOMY REVIEW OF THE EYE

Label the following parts of the eye.

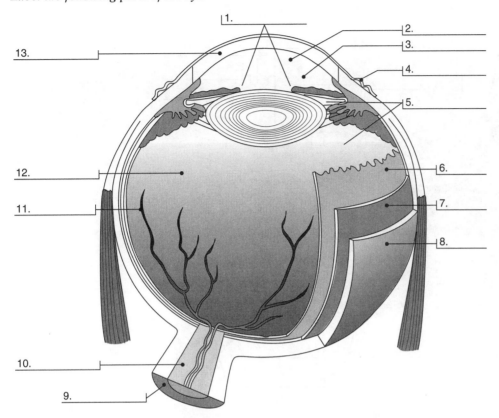

Draw a line indicating the path of light entering the eye and focusing on the retina and optic disc. List the structures that this ray of light passes through in the eye.

■ Anatomy Review of the Ear

Label the following parts of the ear.

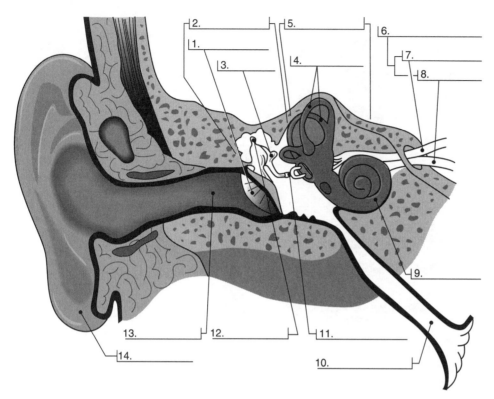

Indicate the structures that a sound wave is transmitted through.

■ Anatomy and Physiology Review

Indicate whether the following terms or phrases involve structure/anatomy (S) or function/physiology (F) or effects of aging (A).

1. _____ blink reflex

2. _____ lacrimal gland

3. _____ tears

4. _____ decreased efficiency of receptors

5. _____ constricting pupil

6. _____ retina

7. _____ cranial nerve III

8. _____ cerumen

9. _____ equalize pressure in middle ear

10. _____ refraction

11. _____ amplify sound waves

12. _____ presbyopia

13. _____ diminished taste

14. _____ stapes

15. _____ smell

16. _____ decreased appetite

17. _____ maintain intraocular pressure

■ Multiple Choice

Circle the best answer.

1. The pinna, or external ear, is also know as the:
   a. auricle.
   b. abducens.
   c. incus.
   d. ossicle.

2. The organ of Corti is located inside the:
   a. auricle.
   b. cochlea.
   c. malleus.
   d. stapes.

3. The clinical term that describes a sensation that the room is spinning is called:
   a. presbycusis.
   b. tinnitus.
   c. tympanic.
   d. vertigo.

4. The "white of the eye" is also known as the:
   a. cornea.
   b. iris.
   c. retina.
   d. sclera.

5. Aqueous humor is located in:
   a. anterior and posterior chambers.
   b. cochlea.
   c. semicircular canals.
   d. vitreous body.

6. Which of the following controls pupil accommodation?
   a. Cranial nerve I
   b. Cranial nerve II
   c. Cranial nerve III
   d. Cranial nerve IV

7. Which of the following separates the middle ear from the inner ear?
   a. Oval window
   b. Membranous labyrinth
   c. Organ of Corti
   d. Tympanic membrane

8. The eustachian tube protects the middle ear by:
   a. allowing fluid into the middle ear.
   b. protecting the ear from foreign particles.
   c. opening during swallowing or yawning.
   d. stopping vibration of the ossicles.

9. Which of the following is a basic taste perceived by the taste buds?
   a. Rancid
   b. Pungent
   c. Sour
   d. Spicy

10. A nursing implication for a patient with a loss of sense of taste would include:
    a. allow for adequate lighting.
    b. encourage to eat, even when not hungry.
    c. speak in low tones.
    d. increase salt intake.

CHAPTER 22

The Cardiovascular System

■ Terminology Review

Match the following definitions with the correct terms.

1. _____ outer layer of the cardiac wall

2. _____ reversible cell injury due to decreased blood and oxygen supply

3. _____ blood flow through capillaries

4. _____ middle and thickest layer of the heart

5. _____ valve between the left atrium and the left ventricle

6. _____ area in the right atrium where blood leaves the coronary arteries

7. _____ membrane lining the heart's interior wall

8. _____ another name for the mitral valve

9. _____ upper two chambers of the heart

10. _____ amount of pressure the ventricles must overcome to empty their contents

11. _____ largest artery in the body

12. _____ inferior part of the heart formed by the tip of the left ventricle

13. _____ valve between the left ventricle and the aorta

14. _____ atrial relaxation followed by ventricular relaxation

15. _____ occurs when two vessels that nourish the same area connect

a. afterload
b. aorta
c. aortic valve
d. apex
e. atria
f. bicuspid valve
g. collateral circulation
h. coronary sinus
i. diastole
j. endocardium
k. epicardium
l. ischemia
m. microcirculation
n. mitral valve
o. myocardium

Match the following definitions with the correct terms.

16. _____ mount of blood that the ventricles pump out in one minute

17. _____ valves that each ventricle empties through

18. _____ atrioventricular node

19. _____ valves located between the atria and ventricles

20. _____ three-layer sac that surrounds and protects the heart

21. _____ difference between systolic and diastolic pressure

22. _____ valve between the right ventricle and pulmonary artery

23. _____ valve between the right atrium and right ventricle

24. _____ divides the heart into right and left halves

25. _____ fluid between the visceral and parietal layers that acts as a lubricant and reduces friction

26. _____ amount of pressure against the ventricle wall at the end of diastole

27. _____ two lower chambers of the heart

28. _____ sequence of dual contractions, the atria followed by the ventricles

29. _____ function of cardiac output and systemic vascular resistance

30. _____ rhythmic expansion of the arteries

a. pericardial fluid
b. pericardium
c. preload
d. pulmonic valve
e. pulse
f. pulse pressure
g. semilunar valves
h. septum
i. systole
j. tricuspid valve
k. ventricles
l. AV node
m. AV valves
n. BP
o. CO

a. CO2
b. dBP
c. HR
d. IVC
e. LAD
f. LCA
g. MI
h. PDA
i. S1
j. S2
k. SA node
l. sBP
m. SV
n. SVC
o. SVR

Match the following definitions with the correct terms.

31. _____ first heart sound produced by the closure of the AV valves

32. _____ carbon dioxide

33. _____ large vein that returns blood from the head, neck, and arms

34. _____ force opposing the movement of blood through the blood vessels

35. _____ pressure exerted against the vessel walls during ventricular systole

36. _____ large vein that returns blood from the lower body

37. _____ second heart sound produced by the closure of the semilunar valves

38. _____ heart's pacemaker

39. _____ localized area of dead tissue caused by lack of blood supply

40. _____ volume of blood ejected with each heartbeat

41. _____ left anterior descending artery

42. _____ pressure exerted during ventricular diastole

43. _____ posterior descending artery

44. _____ number of heart beats per minute

45. _____ left coronary artery

■ Correct the False Statements

Circle the word True *or* False *that follows the statement. If the word* false *has been circled, change the underlined word/words to make the statement true. Place your answer in the space provided.*

1. Heart valves allow for underline{multidirectional} flow through the heart.

   True   False   _____

2. A cardiac output of underline{4 to 6 LPM} is normal.

   True   False   _____

3. The principle arteries that supple heart muscle are the underline{superior and inferior arteries}.

   True   False   _____

4. The underline{septum} divides the heart into left and right halves.

   True   False   _____

5. The heart lies between the lungs in the underline{pericardium}.

   True   False   _____

6. The apical pulse is counted at the underline{base of the heart}.

   True   False   _____

7. <u>Chordae tendineae</u> are strands anchored to pap-
illary muscles.

True _____ False _____ _____

8. The purpose of valves is to <u>prevent backflow of
blood</u>.

True _____ False _____ _____

9. <u>Veins</u> carry blood away from the heart and
<u>arteries</u> carry blood to the heart.

True _____ False _____ _____

10. Heart sounds are produced due to <u>closure of
valves</u>.

True _____ False _____ _____

■ Short Answers

*Complete the following by providing brief and specific
answers.*

1. How did coronary arteries receive their name?

2. Describe why the semilunar valves were so
named.

3. Describe two changes in the conduction system of
the heart as a result of aging.

4. Name the atrioventricular valves and describe
their anatomic location.

5. Define Starling's Law.

6. Describe the relationship between the autonomic
nerves in the medulla of the brain and the heart.

7. You have recorded a patient's blood pressure and
she nervously asks, "Is it all right? The doctor
says I have high blood pressure, what does that
mean?" You would explain:

■ Anatomy Review

Label the structures of the heart on the following diagram.

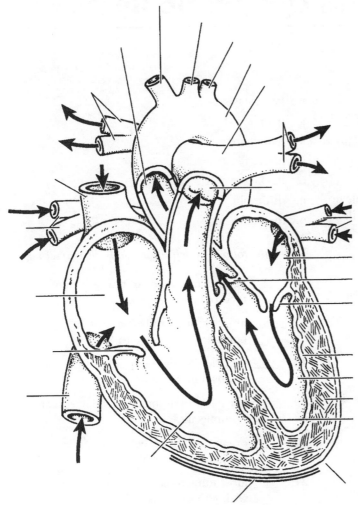

CHAPTER 23

The Hematologic and Lymphatic Systems

■ Terminology Review

Match the following definitions with the correct terms.

1. _____ loss of considerable amount of blood

2. _____ type of cells that play an important role in the immune response; B cells and T cells are two types

3. _____ laboratory test of donor and recipient cells to check for agglutination

4. _____ smallest of blood's formed elements that are essential for blood clotting

5. _____ converts soluble fibrinogen into insoluble threads of fibrin

6. _____ inherited antigens

7. _____ plasma protein that is essential for blood clotting

8. _____ joining together

9. _____ insoluble threads that entrap red blood cells (RBCs) and platelets to form a clot

10. _____ clot that circulates

11. _____ process in which neutrophils engulf and devour invaders

12. _____ stationary clot

13. _____ production and maturation of blood cells

14. _____ cessation of bleeding

15. _____ thin, watery, colorless liquid

a. anastomose
b. cross-matching
c. embolus
d. endocytosis
e. fibrin
f. fibrinogen
g. hematopoiesis
h. hemorrhage

i. hemostasis
j. lymph
k. lymphocyte
l. platelet
m. Rh factor
n. thrombin
o. thrombus

Match the following definitions with the correct terms.

16. _____ agranular leukocytes that are changed to macrophages

17. _____ argest group of plasma protein; approximately 60% to 80%

18. _____ they defend the body against disease, toxins, and irritants

19. _____ plasma protein made in the liver; carries fat molecules

20. _____ organ containing lymphoid tissue designed to filter blood

21. _____ most numerous of the blood cell; disks without a nucleus

22. _____ blood clotting

23. _____ clumping of cells; cross-matching checks for this

24. _____ contained in each RBC and composed of pigment and protein

25. _____ ring of lymphatic tissue around the pharynx

26. _____ smallest of the blood's formed elements; platelets

27. _____ fluid portion of circulating blood

28. _____ engulfing and destroying invaders; action of some white blood cells (WBCs)

29. _____ plasma protein essential for clotting

30. _____ small bundles of special lymphoid situated in clusters along lymphatic vessels

a. thrombocytes
b. erythrocytes
c. albumin
d. hemoglobin
e. phagocytosis
f. plasma
g. lymph nodes
h. leukocytes
i. spleen
j. monocytes
k. prothrombin
l. agglutination
m. globulin
n. coagulation
o. tonsils

Match the following definitions with the correct acronyms.

31. _____ person's blood does not contain D factor

32. _____ white blood cells

33. _____ person's blood contains D factor

34. _____ red blood cells

35. _____ specialized cells in brain capillaries only allow certain substances from the blood to enter the brain

36. _____ hemoglobin

37. _____ mean arterial blood pressure

a. BBB
b. Hgb or Hb
c. MABP
d. RBC
e. Rh+
f. Rh-
g. WBC

■ Correct the False Statements

Circle the word True *or* False *that follows the statement. If the word* false *has been circled, change the underlined word/words to make the statement true. Place your answer in the space provided.*

1. Hematopoiesis originates in the <u>red bone marrow</u>.

   True   False   _____

2. All white blood cells <u>fight infections</u>.

   True   False   _____

3. Lymph is a thin, <u>waterless, colorless fluid</u>.

   True   False   _____

4. In the aging adult, stem cells and marrow reserves tend to <u>increase</u>.

   True   False   _____

5. Lymph drains in the <u>lymphatic vessels</u> and then back to veins.

   True   False   _____

6. <u>Compatible blood</u> can lead to fatal transfusion reactions.

   True   False   _____

7. The <u>tonsils</u> are an organ of the lymphatic system.

   True   False   _____

8. Peyer's patches are located in the <u>large intestine</u>.

   True   False   _____

9. A <u>stationary clot</u> is called a thrombus.

   True   False   _____

10. The hepatic vein leads to the <u>superior vena cava</u>.

    True   False   _____

11. The <u>spleen</u> can be removed without ill effects.

    True   False   _____

12. Blood is considered a <u>connective tissue</u>.

    True   False   _____

13. Lymph on carries fluid <u>away</u> from tissues.

    True   False   _____

14. The hepatic portal circulation is unique because it begins and ends with <u>arterioles</u>.

    True   False   _____

15. <u>Globulin </u>is one of the plasma proteins.

    True   False   _____

■ Numbers Game

Choose from the following numbers to make each of the following statements correct.

0	55
80	120
45	1
10	6
4	3
25	500

1. Plasma is _____% of the blood volume.

2. The liver and spleen destroy red blood cells in about _____ days.

3. Approximately _____trillion red blood cells are found in the body.

4. Approximately _____% of the population belongs to blood group AB.

5. Eosinophils can survive up to _____ days.

6. Approximately _____% of Asians and Native Americans are Rh negative.

7. Formed elements comprise _____% of the blood volume

8. _____% of the population is of the blood group B.

9. The spleen is approximately _____ inches long.

10. Albumin accounts for up to _____% of the plasma proteins

■ Multiple Choice

Circle the best answer.

1. The primary objective of the connective tissue known as blood is to:
   a. filter waste products.
   b. maintain a constant environment for the rest of the body tissues.
   c. participate in antibody production to fight foreign invaders.
   d. produce and bring red blood cells to maturity.

2. Which of the following is a lymphatic organ?
   a. Spleen
   b. Tongue
   c. Vertebrae
   d. White blood cells

3. The pulmonary veins are the only veins that:
   a. are not unidirectional.
   b. carry blood to the lungs.
   c. carry nonoxygenated blood.
   d. carry oxygenated blood.

4. When tissue is injured, platelets break down and cause the release of a chemical called:
   a. D factor.
   b. fibrinogen.
   c. prothrombin.
   d. thromboplastin.

5. The most numerous of the white blood cells are the:
   a. eosinophils.
   b. lymphocytes.
   c. neutrophils.
   d. platelets.

CHAPTER 24

The Immune System

■ Terminology Review

Match the following definitions with the correct terms.

1. _____ immunity that is inherited or genetic

2. _____ type of immunity in which macrophages engulf and destroy antigens after antibodies have identified them for destruction

3. _____ body's ability to recognize and destroy specific pathogens and to prevent infectious diseases

4. _____ artificial type of acquired immunity by injecting an antigen into a person's system

5. _____ type of immunity produced by T cells

6. _____ person is deliberately exposed to a causative agent

7. _____ develop into cells that produce antibodies

8. _____ form of antigen destruction

9. _____ large cells

10. _____ proteins that act as messengers to help regulate some of the functions of the lymphocytes and macrophages during the process of the immune response

11. _____ portion of the blood plasma that contains all antibodies

12. _____ attained through natural or artificial sources

13. _____ changes the antigen, rendering it harmless to the body

a. acquired immunity
b. antibody-mediated immunity
c. artificial acquired immunity
d. B cells/B lymphocytes
e. cell-mediated immunity
f. complement fixation
g. cytokine

h. gamma globulin
i. humoral immunity
j. immunity
k. immunization
l. inborn immunity
m. macrophage

Match the following definitions with the correct terms.

14. _____ gland in which T cells mature

15. _____ specific defense mechanisms that are able to recognize and to respond to specific substances

16. _____ protein substance the body produces in response to an antigen

17. _____ foreign substance or molecule entering the body that stimulates an immune response

18. _____ person is not deliberately exposed to a causative agent

19. _____ gamma globulins

20. _____ help protect against viral infections and can detect and destroy some cancer cells

21. _____ defense mechanisms that fight against a variety of foreign invaders

22. _____ immunoglobulins

23. _____ substance injected with an inoculation

a. natural acquired immunity
b. nonspecific immunity
c. specific immunity
d. T cells/T lymphocytes
e. thymus
f. vaccine
g. Ab
h. Ag
i. Ig
j. IgG

■ Correct the False Statements

Circle the word True *or* False *that follows the statement. If the word* false *has been circled, change the underlined word/words to make the statement true. Place your answer in the space provided.*

1. <u>T cells</u> mature in the bone marrow.

   True   False   _____

2. Antibodies <u>do not</u> destroy antigens but label them for destruction.

   True   False   _____

3. <u>Cell-mediated immunity</u> refers to the destruction of antigens by T cells.

   True   False   _____

4. <u>Radial immunity</u> refers to destruction of antigens by antibodies.

   True   False   _____

5. T lymphocytes are responsible for <u>tissue acceptance</u> after organ transplantation.

   True   False   _____

6. Bone marrow and the thymus are considered <u>primary</u> lymphoid organs.

   True   False   _____

7. Dust cells are located in the <u>liver</u>.

   True   False   _____

8. <u>Interleukins</u> stimulate T cell growth.

   True   False   _____

9. <u>Antibodies</u> are substances the immune system recognizes as foreign.

   True   False   _____

10. The thymus gland begins to <u>enlarge</u> at puberty.

    True   False   _____

■ Completion

Complete the sentence by filling in the blank.

1. _____ is a protein made by several types of cells that inhibits virus production and infection.

2. _____ are also called antibodies and gamma globulins.

3. Bone marrow is responsible for the production and maturation of _____ lymphocytes.

4. Nonspecific immunity is one of the body's _____ systems.

5. Autoimmune disease can occur if the immune system is _____.

■ Case Study

A patient has just given birth to her first child. She asks you the advantages of breast milk over formula. Strictly from an immunologic viewpoint you explain the role of breast milk in relation to her infant's immune system. What would you tell her?

■ Multiple Choice

Circle the correct answer.

1. A complement is a group of proteins normally present but inactive in the:
   a. blood.
   b. bone marrow.
   c. lymph.
   d. thymus.

2. IgE is one of the immunoglobulins that:
   a. is responsible for allergic reactions.
   b. protects mucosal surfaces.
   c. protects the fetus before birth.
   d. stimulates complement activity.

3. Respiratory tract cilia and mucous membranes are examples of:
   a. Antigen–antibody reaction.
   b. antibody-mediated immunity.
   c. cell-mediated immunity.
   d. nonspecific immunity.

4. The thymus is located in the:
   a. marrow.
   b. mediastinum.
   c. medulla.
   d. mid pons.

5. Macrophages destroy:
   a. antibodies.
   b. antigens.
   c. B cells.
   d. T cells.

6. Monocytes are agranular and so are:
   a. basophils.
   b. eosinophils.
   c. lymphocytes.
   d. neutrophils

CHAPTER 25

The Respiratory System

■ Terminology Review

Match the following definitions with the correct terms.

1. _____ breathing air into the lungs

2. _____ cell breathing

3. _____ cover of cartilage that guards the larynx

4. _____ normal respiration

5. _____ smaller than bronchi with thinner walls and decreased amount of cartilage

6. _____ exchange of gases within the alveoli of the lungs

7. _____ tiny hair-like projections

8. _____ clusters at the end of alveolar ducts

9. _____ breathing out

10. _____ trachea divides into these smaller tubes

11. _____ eustachian tubes

12. _____ difficulty breathing

13. _____ bronchioles branch into these

14. _____ connects the nasopharynx with the middle ear

15. _____ dome-shaped muscle separating the thoracic and abdominal cavities

a. alveolar duct
b. alveolar sac
c. auditory tube
d. bronchi
e. bronchiole
f. cellular respiration
g. cilia
h. diaphragm
i. dyspnea

j. epiglottis
k. eupnea
l. Eustachian tube
m. expiration
n. external respiration
o. inspiration

Match the following definitions with the correct terms.

16. _____ area lying between the lungs in the thorax

17. _____ membrane that lines the chest cavity

18. _____ double-layered sac of serous membrane

19. _____ part of the pharynx that extends from the uvula to the epiglottis

20. _____ exchange of gases within the cells

21. _____ tube-shaped passage for air and food

22. _____ lowest portion of the pharynx

23. _____ cone-shaped organs for gas exchange

24. _____ exchange of gases between a person's external environment and the body's internal cells

25. _____ part of the pharynx that extends from the nares to the uvula

26. _____ located between the ribs

27. _____ space between the two layers of pleura

28. _____ nostrils

29. _____ another name for pleural space

30. _____ boxlike structure made of cartilages held together by ligaments

a. intercostals muscles
b. internal respiration
c. laryngopharynx
d. larynx

e. lung

f. mediastinum

g. nares

h. nasopharynx

i. orophyarynx

j. parietal pleura

k. pharynx

l. pleura

m. pleural cavity

n. pleural space

o. respiration

f. vocal cord

g. ERV

h. FRV

i. IC

j. IRV

k. RV

l. TLC

m. VC

n. V_T

Match the following definitions with the correct terms.

31. _____ maximum volume of air inhaled and exhaled with each breath

32. _____ volume of air remaining in the lungs after a maximum exhalation

33. _____ membrane layer covering the lungs

34. _____ volume of air in the lungs after a maximum inspiration

35. _____ chemical that helps that alveoli from collapsing

36. _____ volume of air inhaled and exhaled with each breath

37. _____ two triangle-shaped membranous folds that vibrate to produce sound

38. _____ breathing

39. _____ functional residue volume

40. _____ windpipe

41. _____ maximum volume of air inhaled after a normal expiration

42. _____ expiratory reserve volume

43. _____ volume of air exhaled from the point of maximum inspiration

44. _____ four cavities found on each side of the nasal area

a. sinus

b. surfactant

c. trachea

d. ventilation

e. visceral pleura

■ Correct the False Statements

Circle the word True *or* False *that follows the statement. If the word false has been circled, change the underlined word/words to make the statement true. Place your answer in the space provided.*

1. The pleura has <u>three layers</u>.

    True   False   _____

2. Smoking can <u>increase</u> the efficiency of the respiratory function.

    True   False   _____

3. <u>Sneezing and coughing</u> are protective reflexes of the respiratory system.

    True   False   _____

4. <u>Internal respiration</u> is the exchange of gases between the environment and the lung.

    True   False   _____

5. The turbinates in the nasal cavity <u>help to warm, filter, and moisten air</u> before it enters the lungs.

    True   False   _____

6. <u>The pharynx</u> helps to lighten the skull and provide resonance for the voice.

    True   False   _____

7. The trachea's <u>cartilaginous rings'</u> functions keep the airway open at all times.

    True   False   _____

8. The alveoli are composed of <u>several layers of cells</u>, which enhance gas exchange.

   True   False   _____

9. Surfactant in the lungs <u>works to break up surface tension</u>.

   True   False   _____

10. The right lung has <u>three</u> lobes and the left lung has <u>two</u> lobes.

    True   False   _____

11. Expiration <u>requires energy for the process</u>.

    True   False   _____

12. The <u>pons</u> work to automatically control the depth and rate of respiration.

    True   False   _____

13. The exchange of gases at the cellular level occurs by the process of <u>active transport</u>.

    True   False   _____

14. Oxygen is transported <u>by hemoglobin</u>.

    True   False   _____

15. An important function of the respiratory system is the <u>regulation of the pH of body fluids</u>.

    True   False   _____

■ Multiple Choice

Circle the best answer.

1. Which of the following is not a natural effect of aging?
   a. Alveoli may collapse due to insufficient surfactant.
   b. Chest walls become stiffer.
   c. Lungs become less elastic.
   d. Mucous secretion in the lining of the respiratory tract decreases.

2. The exchange of gas at the cellular level is called:
   a. external respiration.
   b. internal respiration.
   c. inspiration.
   d. ventilation.

3. The primary function of the respiratory system is:
   a. gas exchange.
   b. mucous production.
   c. production of sound from vocal cords.
   d. regulation of body pH.

4. The sinuses drain directly into the:
   a. bronchi.
   b. nasal cavities.
   c. throat.
   d. trachea.

5. Normal respiration is called:
   a. apnea.
   b. dyspnea.
   c. eupnea.
   d. tachypnea.

■ Anatomy Review

Label the following diagram.

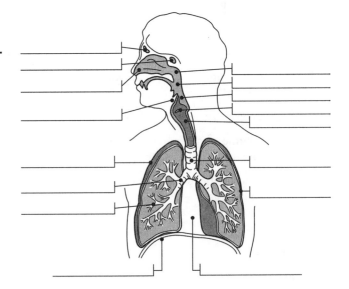

CHAPTER 26

The Digestive System

■ Terminology Review

Match the following definitions with the correct terms.

1. _____ muscle located between the esophagus and the stomach

2. _____ difficulty in swallowing

3. _____ digestive tract

4. _____ finger-like projection of the cecum that has no known function

5. _____ first portion of the small intestine, which is 10 to 12 inches long

6. _____ process of transferring food elements into circulation for transportation

7. _____ semiliquid that is formed in the stomach when food mixes with gastric juices

8. _____ first portion of the large intestine

9. _____ ball of food mixed with saliva

10. _____ process of eliminating solid intestinal wastes from the colon

11. _____ breakdown of food into usable materials for energy

12. _____ longest portion of the large intestine

13. _____ swallowing process

14. _____ vomiting

15. _____ greenish-brown liquid manufactured by the liver

a. absorption
b. alimentary canal
c. appendix
d. bile
e. bolus
f. cardiac sphincter
g. cecum
h. chyme
i. colon
j. defecation
k. deglutition
l. digestion
m. duodenum
n. dysphagia
o. emesis

Match the following definitions with the correct terms.

16. _____ extends from the pharynx to the stomach

17. _____ large sheet of serous membrane that covers many abdominal organs

18. _____ secretions that digest food

19. _____ portion of the small intestine that is about 11 feet long

20. _____ controls the opening between the stomach and the duodenal portion of the small intestine

21. _____ dead-end lymph capillaries within each villus that absorb fat-soluble nutrients

22. _____ to take in

23. _____ stores and releases bile as needed

24. _____ act of chewing

25. _____ middle section of the small intestine

26. _____ mouth

27. _____ gum

28. _____ body's largest glandular organ located in the right upper abdominal cavity

29. _____ waves of contractions in the gastrointestinal (GI) tract that move food along

30. _____ colloid particles that transport digested fats to the intestinal villi for absorption

a. enzyme
b. esophagus
c. gallbladder
d. gingiva
e. ileum
f. ingestion
g. jejunum
h. lacteal
i. liver
j. mastication
k. micelle
l. oral cavity
m. peristalsis
n. peritoneum
o. pyloric sphincter

Match the following definitions with the correct terms.

31. _____ folds in the stomach
32. _____ tough skeletal muscle covered with mucous membrane
33. _____ finger-like projections of the intestine
34. _____ gastrointestinal
35. _____ lower narrow portion of the stomach
36. _____ secretion of salvia, controlled by nervous system
37. _____ carbohydrates
38. _____ lower esophageal sphincter
39. _____ thin watery fluid that contains ptyalin
40. _____ adenosine triphosphate
41. _____ terminates at the anal canal

a. pylorus
b. rectum
c. rugae
d. saliva
e. salivation
f. tongue
g. villi
h. ATP
i. CHO
j. GI
k. LES

■ Short Answers

Indicate the best answer for the following questions.

1. List three functions of the liver.

2. How long does it take to process food?

3. List the functions of saliva.

4. Describe the main types of flavors.

5. Describe the function of rugae.

6. What is the main function of the large intestine?

7. Describe the liver's role regarding vitamins.

8. Describe the endocrine and exocrine functions of the pancreas.

9. Explain the difference between mechanical and chemical digestion.

10. Explain the purpose of villi and microvilli in the small intestine.

■ Multiple Choice

Circle the best answer.

1. The conversion of food into substances that can be easily absorbed is:
   a. chemical digestion.
   b. deglutition.
   c. mastication.
   d. mechanical digestion.

2. The last portion of the small intestine is the:
   a. cecum.
   b. duodenum.
   c. ileum.
   d. jejunum.

3. The digestive process begins in the:
   a. anus.
   b. esophagus.
   c. large intestine.
   d. mouth.

4. The substance in dead-end lymph capillaries within each villus is:
   a. amylase.
   b. chyle.
   c. lipase.
   d. trypsin.

5. Basil metabolism refers to:
   a. the amount of calories the body uses at rest.
   b. the breakdown of the chemical bonds in food.
   c. the breakdown of larger molecules into smaller ones.
   d. the transfer of food into the circulation for transport.

■ Anatomy Review

Label the following diagram.

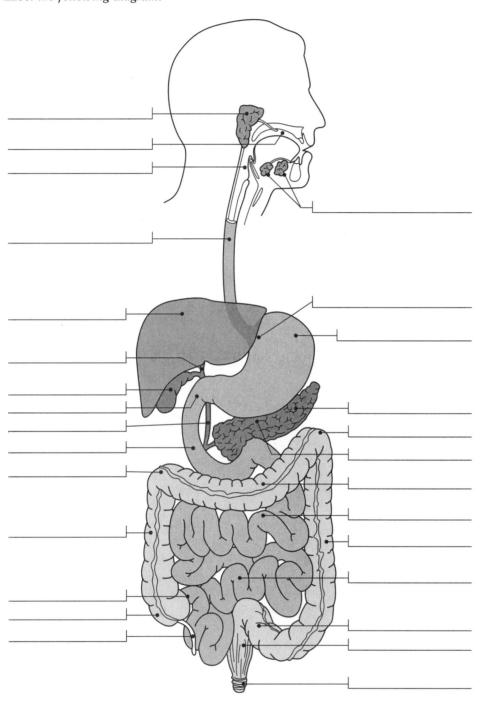

CHAPTER 27

The Urinary System

■ Terminology Review

Match the following definitions with the correct terms.

1. _____ cluster of capillaries at one end of each nephron

2. _____ functional unit of the kidney

3. _____ process of removing particles from a solution by allowing the liquid solvent to pass across a barrier, much like a sieve

4. _____ outer reddish part of the kidney

5. _____ reservoir for urine

6. _____ funnel-shaped structure that partially encloses the glomerulus

7. _____ middle portion of the convoluted tube

8. _____ contains part of the renal tubules, the loops of Henle, and the collecting tubules

9. _____ waking up to void at night

10. _____ cup-like extensions of the renal pelvis

11. _____ secreted by the juxtaglomerular apparatus to help regulate blood pressure

12. _____ long twisted tube extending from Bowman's capsule

13. _____ release of urine from the body

14. _____ bean-shaped organ that extracts wastes from the blood, balances body fluids, and forms urine

15. _____ maximum amount of a substance excreted from the kidneys

a. bladder
b. Bowman's capsule
c. calyx
d. convoluted tubule
e. filtration
f. glomerulus
g. kidney
h. loop of Henle
i. micturition
j. nephron
k. nocturia
l. renal cortex
m. renal medulla
n. renal threshold
o. renin

Match the following definitions with the correct terms or acronyms.

16. _____ tube through which urine passes to outside the body

17. _____ amount of filtrate formed in all glomeruli of both kidneys per minute

18. _____ produced by the kidneys to stimulate red bone marrow to increase red blood cell (RBC) production

19. _____ renin-angiotensin-aldosterone mechanism

20. _____ upper limit of a substance excreted is reached within a given time period

21. _____ increases the reabsorption of water by the kidney tubules, which decreases the amount of urine excreted

22. _____ first portion of the convoluted tube

23. _____ another name for urination

24. _____ consists of specialized glandular cells responsible for maintaining blood pressure

25. _____ narrow tubes that carry urine from the kidneys to the bladder

26. _____ final portion of the convoluted tubule that is the end of the nephron unit

27. _____ release of urine

28. _____ hormone secreted by the cells of the atria of the heart, which increases kidney filtration and blood flow then blood volume is low

a. ureter

b. urethra

c. urination

d. voiding

e. ADH

f. ANP

g. DCT

h. EPO

i. GFR

j. JGA

k. PCT

l. RAA

m. TM

▪ Completion

Using the list of the following numbers, complete the statements. (Not all numbers will be used.)

1	6	95
2	8	100
3	16	250
4	40	400
5	75	500

1. The average length of the urethra in men is _____ inches.

2. A bladder can hold more than _____ liter(s) of fluid.

3. The kidneys are approximately_____ inches long.

4. Urine is approximately_____% solutes.

5. The average female urethra is fewer than_____ inches long.

6. Urine is normally _____% water.

7. Most adults experience a need to void when the bladder fills to about _____ to _____ mL.

▪ Case Study

Before you empty a patient's urinal you note several things before discarding it. State what you would take note of and why.

▪ Sequencing

Number the following structures in the correct order for the formation of urine. The first structure involved in urine formation should be number 1. Continue to number the items.

_____ distal convoluted tubule

_____ proximal convoluted tubule

_____ glomerulus

_____ collecting tubule

_____ afferent arteriole

_____ loop of Henle

_____ Bowman's capsule

▪ Correct the False Statements

Circle the word True *or* False *that follows the statement. If the word* false *has been circled, change the underlined word/words to make the statement true. Place your answer in the space provided.*

1. Urine is <u>less acidic</u> than blood.

    True   False   _____

2. Human beings <u>can</u> survive using only one third of their nephrons.

    True   False   _____

3. The <u>Bowman's capsule</u> has three layers: endothe-
lium, basement membrane, and epithelium.

   True   False   _____

4. The <u>afferent arteriole</u> carries away the remaining
blood from the glomerulus.

   True   False   _____

5. When blood pressure <u>or blood volume</u> falls too
low, renin is secreted.

   True   False   _____

6. The RAA mechanism <u>raises blood pressure</u>.

   True   False   _____

7. Aldosterone promotes sodium and water retention to <u>decrease blood volume</u>.

   True   False   _____

8. <u>Erythropoietin</u> stimulates red bone marrow to
increase formation of red blood cells.

   True   False   _____

9. The glomeruli <u>have a lower blood pressure</u> than
most body capillaries.

   True   False   _____

10. <u>Resorption</u> is the process by which substances
move from the blood into the urine.

   True   False   _____

CHAPTER 28

The Male Reproductive System

■ Terminology Review

Match the following definitions with the correct terms.

1. _____ fold of loose skin that forms a hood-like covering on the glans penis

2. _____ accumulation of sperm cells and secretions in the urethra

3. _____ when the penis becomes firm during sexual excitement

4. _____ physical and emotional pleasurable sensation that occurs at the climax of sexual intercourse

5. _____ sex cells

6. _____ smooth cap of the penis

7. _____ sexual intercourse

8. _____ located below the prostate gland and secrete alkaline mucus to coat the urethra and neutralize the pH of urine

9. _____ transports sperm from the epididymis to the ejaculatory duct

10. _____ forceful expulsion of semen from the ejaculatory ducts through the urethra

11. _____ male hormone

12. _____ surgical removal of the foreskin

13. _____ specialized endocrine cells between seminiferous tubules

14. _____ andropause

a. androgen
b. bulbourethral gland
c. circumcision
d. climacteric
e. copulation
f. ductus deferens
g. ejaculation
h. emission
i. erection
j. foreskin
k. glans penis
l. gonad
m. interstitial cells
n. orgasm

Match the following definitions with the correct terms.

15. _____ saclike structure that encloses the testes

16. _____ interstitial cell-stimulating hormone

17. _____ sperm cells

18. _____ sticky alkaline yellowish substance that serves as a fluid medium for sperm

19. _____ cylindrical organ located immediately in front of the scrotum

20. _____ produce spermatozoa and secrete sex hormones

21. _____ major androgen that produces secondary sexual characteristics

22. _____ area within the testes where sperm cells are produced and mature

23. _____ secrete semen

24. _____ follicle-stimulating hormone

25. _____ area between the scrotum and the anus

26. _____ stage of life during which the reproductive organs become fully functional

27. _____ glandular tissue that adds an alkaline secretion to semen

a. penis
b. perineum
c. prostate
d. puberty
e. scrotum
f. semen
g. seminal vesicle
h. seminiferous tubule
i. spermatozoa
j. testes
k. testosterone
l. FSH
m. ICSH

■ Correct the False Statements

Circle the word True *or* False *that follows the statement. If the word* false *has been circled, change the underlined word/words to make the statement true. Place your answer in the space provided.*

1. The underline{epididymis} is tightly coiled and is approximately 20 feet long.

   True   False   _____

2. The temperature of the <u>testes is higher</u> than the internal body to facilitate sperm production.

   True   False   _____

3. The urethra in the male serves as a passageway for <u>urine only</u>.

   True   False   _____

4. <u>Seminal vesicles</u> secrete semen, which contains nutrients, citric acid, coagulation proteins, and prostaglandins.

   True   False   _____

5. Sperm survive better in an <u>acid</u> environment than in an <u>alkaline</u> environment.

   True   False   _____

6. <u>FSH</u> is the major androgen responsible for secondary sexual characteristics.

   True   False   _____

7. Normal spermatogenesis does not occur if the testes are <u>too warm or too cold</u>.

   True   False   _____

8. It takes about <u>4</u> months for sperm cells to mature until they are stored in the ductus deferens.

   True   False   _____

9. Once ejaculated into the woman's vagina, a sperm can survive <u>up to 3 days</u>.

   True   False   _____

10. As men age, they may experience <u>enlarging of the prostate gland</u>.

   True   False   _____

■ Case Study

You are assigned to care for a 36-year-old patient immediately after outpatient surgery for bilateral inguinal hernia repair. Although you do not know the patient's name or gender, you are aware that men are more likely to experience this type of hernia because:

■ Multiple Choice

Circle the best answer.

1. Male hormones are called:
   a. androgens.
   b. estrogens.
   c. gonads.
   d. spermatozoa.

2. The sac that supports and protects the testes is the:
   a. ductus deferens.
   b. epididymis.
   c. prostate.
   d. scrotum.

3. The main male androgen is:
   a. estrogen.
   b. progesterone.
   c. spermatozoa.
   d. testosterone.

4. Sperm cells are stored in the:
   a. bulbourethral gland.
   b. ductus deferens.
   c. epididymis.
   d. prostate.

5. This organ serves as the common passageway for both the urinary and reproductive systems.
   a. genitals.
   b. gonads.
   c. penis.
   d. testes.

CHAPTER 29

The Female Reproductive System

■ Terminology Review

Match the following definitions with the correct terms.

1. _____ inner mucous layer of the uterus

2. _____ thin pair of skin folds medial to the labia minora

3. _____ flow of blood and other materials from the uterus through the vagina if fertilization does not take place

4. _____ thin mucous membrane over the vaginal opening

5. _____ time menstruation ceases

6. _____ female sex hormones

7. _____ first menstrual period

8. _____ includes luteinizing hormone and follicle-stimulating hormone

9. _____ two rounded folds of skin posterior to the mons pubis

10. _____ fringe-like ends of the oviducts

11. _____ produce lubricant for the vagina

12. _____ passageway for the ovum from the ovary to the uterus

13. _____ narrow lower end of the uterus that opens into the vagina

14. _____ modified sweat glands that produce milk

15. _____ small erectile structure that responds to sexual stimulation

a. Bartholin gland
b. cervix
c. clitoris
d. endometrium
e. estrogen
f. fallopian tube
g. fimbriae
h. gonadotropic hormones
i. hymen
j. labia majora
k. labia minora
l. mammary gland
m. menarche
n. menopause
o. menstruation

Match the following definitions with the correct terms.

16. _____ when the ovum bursts through the ovary

17. _____ immature egg cell

18. _____ muscular canal

19. _____ estrogen replacement therapy

20. _____ hollow, muscular, upside-down, pear-shaped organ

21. _____ external genitallia

22. _____ egg cells

23. _____ female sex organ

24. _____ follicle-stimulating hormone

25. _____ produced by the corpus luteum

26. _____ fatty pad over the symphysis pubis

27. _____ fertilized ovum

28. _____ another name for fallopian tubes

29. _____ area between the vaginal orifice and the anus

30. _____ luteinizing hormone

a. mons pubis
b. oocyte
c. ova
d. ovary
e. oviduct
f. ovulation

g. perineum

h. progesterone

i. uterus

j. vagina

k. vulva

l. zygote

m. FSH

n. LH

o. ERT

■ Completion

Fill in each of the following statements with the correct answer.

1. If the ovum is not fertilized, secretion of _____ decreases and the corpus luteum begins to decline.

2. Each _____ develops in different stages throughout a woman's life.

3. Luteinizing and follicle-stimulating hormones stimulated by the hypothalamus are considered _____ _____.

4. During pregnancy, the uterus increases its size about _____ times.

5. A(n) _____ _____ occurs when the ovum becomes fertilized and enters the abdominal cavity or becomes lodged in the oviduct.

6. Menses occurs about every _____ days.

7. The three layers of the uterus are _____, _____, and _____.

8. Ovulation occurs around day _____ of the menstrual cycle.

9. Engorgement of the _____ with blood leads to orgasm in women.

10. A(n) _____ is a cut in the perineum to prevent tearing during childbirth.

■ Correct the False Statements

Circle the word True *or* False *that follows the statement. If the word* false *has been circled, change the underlined word/words to make the statement true. Place your answer in the space provided.*

1. The purpose of the fimbriae is to <u>move the ovum toward the uterus</u>.

    True   False   _____

2. The <u>vagina's functions</u> are to receive sperm, provide exit for menstrual flow, and serve as the birth canal.

    True   False   _____

3. <u>Estrogens and testosterone</u> cause breast enlargement in girls with the onset of puberty.

    True   False   _____

4. <u>Prolactin and oxytocin</u> stimulate the mammary glands to produce and release milk after childbirth.

    True   False   _____

5. Estrogens include <u>estradiol, estriol, and follicle-stimulating hormone (FSH)</u>.

    True   False   _____

6. During the life of a woman, approximately <u>2 million primary oocytes</u> will develop into mature egg cells.

    True   False   _____

7. Headaches, insomnia, anxiety, or depression can occur during <u>menopause</u>.

    True   False   _____

8. The <u>uterine cycle</u> consists of the follicular, ovulation, and luteal phases.

    True   False   _____

9. The woman <u>continues to ovulate</u> during menopause.

   True   False   _____

10. During the <u>ovulation phase,</u> FSH stimulates follicles to begin to ripen.

    True   False   _____

■ Anatomy Review

Label the following diagram.

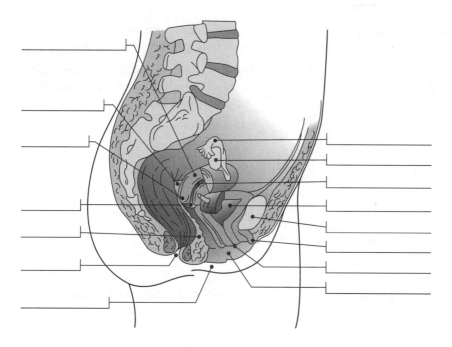

CHAPTER 30

Basic Nutrition

■ Terminology Review

Match the following definitions with the correct terms and acronyms.

1. _____ study of nutrients and how they are handled by the body, as well as the impact of human behavior and environment on the process of nourishment

2. _____ body's storage form of carbohydrate

3. _____ foundation of every body cell and is the only nutrient that builds and repairs tissue

4. _____ contain two sugar molecules

5. _____ disease due to vitamin D deficiency in which the bones do not harden

6. _____ person must obtain these through food because the body cannot make them in sufficient quantities to meet its needs

7. _____ classic disease of vitamin C deficiency

8. _____ is found only in animal tissues and is a member of the sterols group

9. _____ substances needed for growth, maintenance, and repair of the body

10. _____ disease of the nervous system that leads to paralysis and death from heart failure and is caused by deficiency of thiamine

11. _____ hydrogen is added to liquid oils to make them more stable and decrease the chance of rancidity

12. _____ abnormally low blood sugar

13. _____ contain one sugar molecule such as glucose

14. _____ disease caused from niacin deficiency

15. _____ building-blocks of protein

16. _____ carbohydrates, fats, and proteins

17. _____ foods that provide significant amounts of key nutrients per volume consumed

18. _____ composed of three fatty acids and one glycerol

19. _____ naturally occurring chemicals in plant foods that may help prevent disease

20. _____ foods that are solid at room temperature because they already contain their full complement of hydrogen

21. _____ bad nutrition

22. _____ fats

23. _____ vitamins and minerals

24. _____ micronutrients that are vital for building bones, teeth, maintaining muscle tone, and other body functions

25. _____ abnormally high blood sugar

26. _____ complex carbohydrates made of long chains of many sugar molecules

a. amino acid
b. beriberi
c. cholesterol
d. disaccharide
e. essential nutrient
f. glycogen
g. hydrogenated
h. hyperglycemia
i. hypoglycemia
j. lipid
k. macronutrients
l. malnutrition
m. micronutrient
n. mineral
o. monosaccharide
p. nutrient
q. nutrient density
r. nutrition
s. pellagra

t. phytochemical

u. polysaccharide

v. protein

w. rickets

x. saturated fat

y. scurvy

z. triglyceride

■ Acronym Review

Match the following definitions with the correct acronyms.

1. _____ good cholesterol

2. _____ amount of heat required to raise the temperature of 1 kg of water 1° Centigrade

3. _____ carries oxygen

4. _____ standards set by the Food and Nutrition Board of the National Academy of Sciences in 1941 for the intake of specific nutrients to meet the needs of healthy Americans

5. _____ hydrochloric acid

6. _____ total calories needed to keep body processes going

7. _____ vitamins are guaranteed to meet set purity and solubility standards if the have the seal by this agency

8. _____ four standards that list reference intake levels of essential nutrients for most healthy population groups

9. _____ agency that requires cereals and breads to be fortified with folic acid

10. _____ bad cholesterol

11. _____ daily nutrient intake value that is estimated to meet the requirement of half of the healthy individuals in the life stage and gender group

12. _____ commercial forms of fructose used in sweetened processed foods and drinks

13. _____ agency that introduced the Food Guide Pyramid

14. _____ Centers for Disease Control

15. _____ recommended nutrient intake that is assumed to be adequate

16. _____ was used to describe optimal weight for optimal health

17. _____ made of carbon, hydrogen, and oxygen and are classified as either simple of complex

18. _____ measures weight in relation to height

19. _____ highest level of daily nutrient intake that is likely to pose no risk of adverse health effects

20. _____ protein–calorie malnutrition

21. _____ disorder that can occur in pregnant women, especially if they have a family history of diabetes

22. _____ metabolic disorder that can occur in premature infants and infants

a. AI

b. BMI

c. CDC

d. CHO

e. DRIs

f. EAR

g. FDA

h. GDM

i. HCL

j. HDL

k. HFCS

l. IBW

m. kcal or C

n. LDL

o. PCM

p. PKU

q. RBC

r. RDA

s. REE

t. UL

u. USDA

v. USP

■ Lifespan Nutrition Review

Indicate if the following actions would be appropriate (A) or inappropriate (I) to promote good nutrition.

1. _____ Encourage the pregnant woman to consume 50% more calories during the second and third trimesters than before her pregnancy.

2. _____ Instruct new mothers to feed infants every 3 hours to promote a routine and improve digestion.

3. _____ Inform women who wish to become pregnant that intake of folic acid, protein, iron, calcium, and vitamin D are especially important.

4. _____ Teach parents of toddlers that children should be allowed to eat to satisfy hunger because appetite fluctuates widely with growth patterns.

5. _____ Adolescents should be provided specific foods at meals and for snacks to prevent snacking and meals with empty calories such as junk foods.

6. _____ Inform early and middle adulthood patients that caloric requirements may decrease because the individual is no longer growing.

7. _____ Assess individuals in older adulthood for economic difficulties or poor dental status that may result in poor nutritional intake.

8. _____ Encourage all individuals to eat more protein and fewer carbohydrates to decrease calorie intake.

9. _____ During the first trimester of pregnancy, calorie needs do not increase.

10. _____ Teenagers need extra food to meet the needs of growth and body development.

■ Short Answers

Complete the following questions.

1. Using the text on page 365, determine the body mass index (BMI) for a patient who weighs 190 pounds and is 5 feet, 9 inches tall.

   Outline teaching for this patient based on the information you have obtained.

2. Describe the difference between complete and incomplete proteins. Give an example of each type of protein.

3. Indicate the caloric value for each of the following:
   a. carbohydrate _____
   b. fat _____
   c. protein _____

   Calculate the total calories in each of the following:
   d. 15 g carbohydrate _____
   e. 4 g fat _____
   f. 10 g protein _____

4. Describe what is meant by empty calories.

5. Explain why it is important to have adequate amounts of carbohydrates in the diet.

6. List the four functions of water.

7. List four of the top leading causes of death that are associated with dietary excesses and imbalances.

■ Food Pyramid

Label the following illustration by placing the correct letter by the titles provided. Indicate the number of servings that are recommended each day in each category.

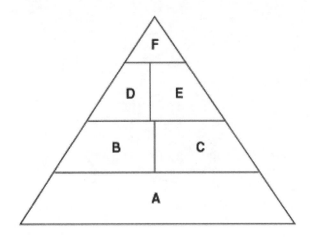

1. Fruits _____

2. Vegetables _____

3. Meat _____

4. Milk _____

5. Grain_____

6. Fats, oils, and sweets_____

■ Multiple Choice

Circle the best answer.

1. Water-soluble vitamins include:
   a. A, D, E, and K.
   b. B complex, D, and K.
   c. C and B complex.
   a. K, C, and thiamine.

2. Which of the following is a good source of protein?
   a. Butter and cream
   b. Salad oils and dressings
   c. Fish and eggs
   d. Pasta and rice

3. Which of the following minerals plays a part in bone formation?
   a. Copper
   b. Fluorine
   c. Iron
   d. Magnesium

4. A female patient is 30 years old and 5 feet, 6 inches tall with an average body frame. Calculate her ideal body weight.
   a. 115 pounds
   b. 120 pounds
   c. 125 pounds
   d. 130 pounds

5. While teaching a 12th-grade class about nutrition and healthy eating, you would be sure to include that:
   a. overnutrition contributes to such conditions as hypertension and osteoporosis.
   b. overnutrition is not possible in teenage years because energy expenditure is so high.
   c. teenagers do not get atherosclerosis so they should not worry about saturated fats.
   d. the nutritional problems of most Americans are due to deficiencies of proteins.

6. A mother of a 2-year-old states, "I know she needs to eat more." You should suggest to the mother to:
   a. fill the child's plate at each meal then encourage seconds.
   b. insist that the child "clean her plate" each meal.
   c. not worry as long as the child has reasonable intake from each major food group.
   d. provide the child with privacy during meals.

7. Which of the following is a necessary trace mineral?
   a. Calcium
   b. Iron
   c. Potassium
   d. Sodium

8. Which of the following is one of the major minerals needed in the human diet?

   a. Copper

   b. Chromium

   c. Fluoride

   d. Magnesium

9. A major function of vitamin A (retinol) is:

   a. formation and maintenance of mucosal epithelium.

   b. promotes normal appetite.

   c. stimulates calcium reabsorption form the kidneys.

   d. synthesis of blood clotting proteins.

10. What percentage of the American population is considered overweight?

    a. 10%

    b. 29%

    c. 51%

    d. 66%

CHAPTER 31

Transcultural and Social Aspects of Nutrition

■ Terminology Review

Match the following definitions with the correct terms.

1. _____ are made from corn or flour and are served with meals, along with rice and refried beans

2. _____ concept of balancing intake of cold and hot foods

3. _____ a good source of calcium and protein made of soybean curd

4. _____ separate dishes are used to prepare and serve meat and dairy foods; pork, shellfish, and rabbit are not allowed

5. _____ diet that excludes all animal products such as meat, fish, poultry, eggs, milk, and dairy products

6. _____ diet based mainly on plant foods

7. _____ refers to cooking style and particular foods that blacks and whites in the southeastern United States commonly eat

a. kosher
b. soul food
c. tofu
d. tortillas
e. vegan
f. vegetarian
g. Yin-Yang

■ Nutritional Needs Review

Indicate if the following action would be appropriate (A) or inappropriate (I) to help patient with transcultural or social food pattern influences meet nutritional needs.

1. _____ Encouraging intake of dairy products by persons who have lactose intolerance to meet their calcium needs

2. _____ Instructing patients to boil vegetables for long periods of time to improve texture and vitamin content

3. _____ Assisting African American patients in planning meals to reduce sodium, fat, and sugar to prevent chronic diseases

4. _____ Discussing the need for lacto-ovo vegetarians to eat the same plant proteins from day to day to maintain protein levels

5. _____ Placing patients in rooms or areas with other patients at mealtime to encourage intake

6. _____ Serving ham and shellfish to a patient who is an Orthodox Jew

7. _____ Serving tea or coffee with the meal for a patient who is Islamic or Muslim

8. _____ Stressing adequate nutrient intake over a low-fat or low-calorie diet when nutritional needs are increased because of illness or injury

9. _____ Requesting a diet with no meat for the meals on Friday for a patient who is Roman Catholic

10. _____ Initiating a referral to social services for a patient who does not have money for food

11. _____ Encouraging a patient to change his or her beliefs about food to alter eating habits

12. _____ Encouraging patients living in the North to eat more fruits and vegetables

■ Matching

Match the dietary practices and concern with the appropriate ethnic group. Answers may be used more than once.

1. _____ limited use of meats; malt beer may be given to children

2. _____ believes in the Yin (cold)-Yang (hot) concept of balancing intake

3. _____ milk is rarely used after childhood

4. _____ calcium and protein intake may be inadequate

5. _____ food has great religious and social significance; milk is seldom used

6. _____ raw vegetables are rarely served

7. _____ diet provides essential nutrients but may be low in calcium

8. _____ high rate of obesity

9. _____ raw vegetables are rarely served; diet is high in fiber.

10. _____ familiar fruits and vegetables may not be available or affordable in the United States

a. Asian American—Chinese
b. Native Americans
c. Puerto Rican
d. South Asian
e. Middle Eastern

■ Multiple Choice

Circle the best answer.

1. Limiting sodium in the Japanese American's diet is difficult because of the extensive use of:
   a. soy sauce.
   b. tea.
   c. tofu.
   d. Vegetables.

2. A lacto-vegetarian diet includes:
   a. plant foods plus dairy products.
   b. plant foods plus eggs.
   c. plant foods plus dairy products and eggs.
   d. only plant-based foods.

3. The main entrée for Middle Eastern Americans usually consists of:
   a. chicken and rice.
   b. pork and rice.
   c. rice and vegetables.
   d. vegetables and legumes.

4. To meet protein needs in the diet, the nurse would instruct the lacto-ovo vegetarian to:
   a. eat meat once a day.
   b. eat adequate calorie and varied plant proteins each day.
   c. eat only dairy products for one meal each day.
   d. pay special attention to combining proteins.

5. Which of the following offers protection against food frauds?
   a. A diet that consists of a rigid daily menu
   b. A diet that can be followed for a short period of time only
   c. A diet that compares the servings recommended in the Food Pyramid
   d. A diet that promotes rapid weight loss

CHAPTER 32

Diet Therapy and Special Diets

■ Terminology Review

Match the following definitions with the correct terms.

1. _____ drinks excessive amounts of water

2. _____ diet used to help treat individuals with elevated blood lipids

3. _____ diet composed of foods that the body can absorb completely so that little residue is left for the formation of feces

4. _____ diet that is prescribed as part of the treatment of more than one disease or condition

5. _____ loss of appetite or refusal to eat

6. _____ diet that consists entirely of liquids

7. _____ opening through the skin

8. _____ swallowing disorder

9. _____ diet extremely low in carbohydrates and that is sometimes as high as 80% to 90% fat

10. _____ diet used to help control blood sugar and weight in persons with diabetes mellitus

11. _____ goal of this diet is to limit foods that stimulate the production of gastric acid

12. _____ providing liquid nourishment through a tube into the gastrointestinal (GI) tract

13. _____ special diet that considers the disease process and the patient's general condition

14. _____ when given peripherally, these must be hypotonic or isotonic

15. _____ diet that can be either a digestive soft or a mechanical soft

16. _____ elevated blood lipids

a. anorexia
b. bland diet
c. carbohydrate-controlled diet
d. dysphpagia
e. fat-controlled diet
f. hyperlipidemia
g. infusion
h. ketogenic diet
i. liquid diet
j. low-residue diet
k. modified diet
l. polydipsia
m. soft diet
n. stoma
o. therapeutic diet
p. tube feeding

■ Acronym Review

Match the following definitions with the correct acronyms.

1. _____ feeding tube that is inserted into the small intestine through the abdominal wall

2. _____ tube that is passed through the patient's nose and into the stomach

3. _____ a variety of sterile solutions that the body needs that are injected directly into the vein

4. _____ percutaneous endoscopic gastrostomy

5. _____ specifically formulated solution that is nutritionally complete to meet a specific individual's needs when the GI tract is not functioning properly

6. _____ gastroesophageal reflux disease

7. _____ feeding tube that is placed directly into the stomach through the abdominal wall

8. _____ contains lesser concentrations of the same ingredients in total parenteral nutrition (TPN) that are administered into a peripheral vein

a. G tube
b. J tube
c. IV
d. NG tube
e. GERD
f. PEG
g. PPN
h. TPN

■ Correct the False Statements

Circle the word True *or* False *that follows the statement. If the word* false *has been circled, change the underlined word/words to make the statement true. Place your answer in the space provided.*

1. Nutritional supplements are given on time so that they <u>do not ruin the patient's appetite for the next meal</u>.

   True   False   _____

2. Diet counseling is generally most effective when <u>verbal instructions</u> are provided.

   True   False   _____

3. The nurse should <u>elevate the head of the bed</u> when feeding a patient with a swallowing disorder.

   True   False   _____

4. Low-residue diets may be ordered for <u>postsurgical patients</u>.

   True   False   _____

5. <u>Carbohydrate-counting diets</u> may be inadequate in iron, calcium, and some vitamins and minerals.

   True   False   _____

6. Bland diets are often prescribed for patients with <u>GERD</u>.

   True   False   _____

7. Whole grain breads and nuts <u>are encouraged</u> on a low-residue diet.

   True   False   _____

8. The carbohydrate-controlled diet uses the <u>carbohydrate and fat exchange groups</u>.

   True   False   _____

9. Carbohydrate counting is based upon <u>counting grams of carbohydrates in all foods and beverages consumed</u>.

   True   False   _____

10. Ketogenic diets are low in carbohydrates and <u>as high as 80% to 90% fat</u>.

    True   False   _____

11. Simple intravenous (IV) therapy <u>can be used for several weeks</u> without supplemental nutrition.

■ Matching

Match the list of diet types with the classification of diet modifications.

1. _____ liquid, soft, high-fiber, low-residue, and bland diets

2. _____ high calorie, low calorie

3. _____ high and low fat; protein, sodium, calcium, or potassium controlled

4. _____ six small feedings per day

5. _____ "no eggs or no milk on trays"

a. nutrients
b. specific allergens
c. consistency and texture
d. energy value
e. amount

■ Skill Drill

Order the following steps in administering an intermittent tube feeding.

1. _____ wash hands before putting on gloves

2. _____ prepare formula

3. _____ clamp the tube and disconnect the feeding set-up

4. _____ position patient with head of bed elevated at least 30 to 40 degrees

5. _____ hang the feeding bag set-up 12 to 18 inches above stomach

6. _____ fill bag and prime tubing

7. _____ gather equipment and supplies

8. _____ adjust the flow according to order

9. _____ determine placement of feeding tube

10. _____ explain procedure to the patient

11. _____ clamp the tubing

12. _____ add 30–60 mL of water to bag and run into basin

■ Multiple Choice

Circle the best answer.

1. Fluid restrictions may be prescribed for a patient who has:
   a. anorexia.
   b. dysphagia.
   c. hyperlipidemia.
   d. polydipsia.

2. When helping the patient with a swallowing disorder eat his/her meal, which action would be appropriate?
   a. Encourage the patient to lie flat after eating.
   b. Encourage swallowing after each portion of food.
   c. Follow each bite with a drink of water.
   d. Provide only IV nutrition.

3. A clear liquid diet should not be used for more than:
   a. one day
   b. two days
   c. three days
   d. four days

4. Which action should be taken if a full liquid diet is going to be used long-term?
   a. Add a thickening agent for texture
   b. Add nutritional supplements
   c. Encourage six meals per day
   d. Encourage increased water

5. Which type of diet would be ordered for a post-surgical patient, which acts as a transition between liquid and general diet?
   a. Digestive soft
   b. High fiber
   c. Mechanical soft
   d. Therapeutic

6. A Step One Diet for hyperlipidemia is comprised of what percentage of fat?
   a. 10%
   b. 30%
   c. 50%
   d. 55%

7. On a protein-restricted diet, protein should be:
   a. combined with a low-calorie diet.
   b. spread evenly throughout the day.
   c. followed only for several days.
   d. plant based.

8. Which of the following is an example of a high-quality protein?
   a. Eggs
   b. Fortified cereal
   c. Nuts
   d. Peanut butter

9. Which of the following would be appropriate for a patient on a sodium-restricted diet?

    a. Encourage the use of soy sauce to season food

    b. Instruct the patient to drink at least a quart of milk each day

    c. Recommend potassium salt replacement for all patients

    d. Use blends of herbs and spices to season food

CHAPTER 33

Introduction to the Nursing Process

■ Terminology Review

Match the following definitions with the appropriate terms.

1. _____ fifth step in the nursing process, which includes the measurement of the effectiveness of nursing care

2. _____ framework for thinking and acting that combines critical-thinking skills and scientific problem solving; is a systematic method that directs the nurse and patient as they together determine the need for nursing care, plan and implement the care, and evaluate the results

3. _____ guidelines that are developed for each patient using the nursing process to ensure consistency of care among nursing staff

4. _____ when applying the nursing process, the patient is a partner in determining the goals of care; nursing focusing on the patient, not the task

5. _____ precise method to investigate problems and to arrive at solutions

6. _____ first step of the nursing process, which includes the systematic and continuous collection of data

7. _____ experimental problem solving that tests ideas to decide which methods work and which do not

8. _____ is a complicated mix of inquiry, knowledge, intuition, logic, experience, and common sense used to arrive at answers when faced with a problem

9. _____ third step in the nursing process, which is the development of goals for care and possible activities to meet them

10. _____ fourth step of the nursing process, which includes providing actual nursing care

11. _____ second step in the nursing process, which is the statement of the patient's actual or potential problem

a. patient oriented
b. critical thinking
c. evaluation
d. implementation
e. nursing assessment
f. nursing diagnosis
g. nursing care plans
h. nursing process
i. planning
j. scientific problem solving
k. trial and error

■ Short Answers

1. Explain how trial and error has been used in healthcare.

2. Describe characteristics an individual would possess when thinking critically.

3. Explain how critical thinking relates to problem solving.

4. Describe benefits of using the nursing process.

5. Identify the steps in the nursing process.

6. List characteristics of the nursing process.

■ Matching

Match the specific step of the nursing process in which the nurse would perform the identified acts. Each item may be used more than once.

1. _____ write a nursing care plan (NCP)

2. _____ plan for future nursing care; revise plan as needed

3. _____ identify assessment priorities; collect data

4. _____ put NCP into action; continue collecting data

5. _____ recognize significant data; recognize patterns or clusters

6. _____ complete an initial patient interview

7. _____ set a goal for the patient to ambulate 20 feet

8. _____ bathe a patient

9. _____ review the patient's past medical records

10. _____ decide if the plan of care was effective

a. nursing assessment
b. nursing diagnosis
c. planning
d. implementation
e. evaluation

■ Fill in the Blanks

Complete each sentence with the correct word.

1. Trial and error is used carefully when working with _____ because of the possible harmful results.

2. Scientific problem solving requires both _____ _____ and imagination.

3. The nursing process allows the nurse to identify _____and _____ problems.

4. The nursing process is an important tool for providing _____ and _____ effectiveness of nursing care given in any setting.

■ Matching

Match the steps of scientific problem solving with the related steps in the nursing process.

1. _____ formulate tentative solution; choose preferred solutions

2. _____ evaluate the result; formulate another tentative solution

3. _____ gather information relative to the problem

4. _____ identify the problem

5. _____ test solutions

a. nursing assessment
b. nursing diagnosis
c. planning
d. implementation
e. evaluation

CHAPTER 34

Nursing Assessment

■ Terminology Review

Match the following definitions with the appropriate terms and abbreviations.

1. _____ draw conclusions regarding the patient's health problems

2. _____ way to solicit information from the patient

3. _____ systematic and continuous collection and analysis of information about the patient.

4. _____ activities of daily living

5. _____ interview also know as a health interview

6. _____ measurable and observable pieces of information

7. _____ assessment tool that relies on the use of the five senses

8. _____ patient's opinions or feelings about what is happening

9. _____ chief complaint

10. _____ complete and accurate information about the patient

a. health interview
b. ADLs
c. objective data
d. data analysis
e. observation
f. CC
g. nursing assessment
h. subjective data
i. nursing history
j. data

■ Short Answers

Complete the following short-answer questions.

1. List the three methods used to collect data.

2. Describe the four types of observation and give an example of each.

3. Describe the difference between an admission interview and a medical history.

4. List characteristics of nursing assessment.

5. What are the best sources for obtaining information about a patient?

6. What are two questions you can use when concluding an initial patient interview.

7. Briefly list and describe the steps in data analysis.

■ Data Collection Matching

Indicate if the following are subjective or objective data. Use an S for subjective and O for objective.

1. _____ weight of 150 lbs
2. _____ respirations 14/minute
3. _____ dislikes bananas
4. _____ urine output
5. _____ allergic to penicillin
6. _____ history of seizures
7. _____ smokes 1 pack of cigarettes/day
8. _____ blood chemistry values
9. _____ results of chest radiograph
10. _____ came to the hospital because of chest pain
11. _____ odor of alcohol on breath
12. _____ temperature is 37° Centigrade
13. _____ complains of difficulty sleeping before hospitalization
14. _____ light-brown skin
15. _____ states she suffers from menstrual cramps

Multiple Choice

Circle the most appropriate answer.

1. A patient is admitted to the hospital with complaints of numbness in her legs alternating with weakness. Which of the following questions would be a priority for the nurse to ask?
   a. "Are you sexually active and do you have any sexual concerns?"
   b. "Do you have any problems walking by yourself or do you need assistance?"
   c. "Do you have any speech problems?"
   d. "Do you need to see someone from social services?"

2. Which of the following in an example of subjective data?
   a. Patient has blue coloring at the fingertips and under fingernails.
   b. Patient states pain is at an intensity of 8 out of 10.
   c. The patient's blood pressure is 130/58.
   d. The patient's respirations are shallow and nonlabored.

3. During a nursing history, the patient refuses to answer a personal question. The most appropriate response by the nurse would be to:
   a. emphasize how important it is for the patient to answer the question.
   b. instruct the patient that he or she must answer the question to receive care.
   c. rephrase the question to try to trick the patient into answering.
   d. respect the patient's right to refuse to answer personal questions.

4. Biographic data during the nursing history includes:
   a. patient's address.
   b. chief complaint.
   c. family relationships.
   d. medical relationships.

5. Which skill does the nurse use throughout assessment to guide thoughts and actions?
   a. Critical thinking
   b. Interview
   c. Observation
   d. Validation

CHAPTER 35

Diagnosis and Planning

■ Terminology Review

Match the following definitions with the appropriate terms and abbreviations.

1. _____ statement about a patient's actual or potential health concerns that can be managed by independent nursing interventions

2. _____ physicians identify the disease a person has by studying physiologic manifestations

3. _____ association that has maintained a list of acceptable nursing diagnosis since 1973

4. _____ as evidenced by

5. _____ related to

6. _____ situation in which the nurse works with physicians or healthcare providers on a common patient problem

7. _____ development of goals to prevent, reduce, or eliminate problems and to identify nursing interventions that will assist in meeting these goals

8. _____ measurable patient behavior that indicates whether the person has achieved the expected benefit of nursing care

9. _____ goal that can be met in a matter of hours or days

10. _____ flip-file that records patient's background information and medical and nursing treatment

11. _____ outcome that requires more than a few days to achieve

12. _____ formal guideline for directing the nursing staff to provide patient care

13. _____ as needed

14. _____ cause of a problem

a. AEB
b. collaborative problem
c. etiology
d. expected outcome
e. Kardex
f. long-term objective
g. medical diagnosis
h. NANDA
i. nursing care plan
j. nursing diagnosis
k. planning
l. PRN
m. R/T
n. short-term objective

■ Short Answers

Complete the following questions with the correct short answer.

1. Describe the main difference between the application of medical and nursing diagnoses.

2. List two purposes of nursing diagnoses and describe why you believe each is important to nursing.

3. What are the parts of a nursing diagnosis?

4. Using Box 35-1, rewrite the following expected outcomes to be more measurable of patient behavior.

   Patient will move in the hallway

   Patient's lung will sound better

   Patient will know about medications

   Patient will want to quit smoking

   Patient will do dressing change

5. Review the NANDA list in the back of your book. Identify three nursing diagnosis stems that relate to survival needs or imminent life-threatening needs. (Do not use the same examples used in the text.)

6. Describe characteristics of an expected outcome and provide an example for each.

■ Identifying Nursing and Medical Diagnoses

1. Indicate if the following diagnoses are nursing diagnoses (N) or medical diagnoses (M).

   a. _____ Ineffective Airway Clearance
   b. _____ Pneumonia
   c. _____ Hyperthermia
   d. _____ Pain
   e. _____ Diabetes
   f. _____ Urinary Retention
   g. _____ Spiritual Distress
   h. _____ Gastric Ulcer
   i. _____ Seizures
   j. _____ Caregiver Role Strain

2. Using the list of NANDA-approved nursing diagnoses in the back of your textbook, write two nursing diagnoses that might apply to a patient with the following medical diagnoses.

MEDICAL DIAGNOSIS	NURSING DIAGNOSIS
Pneumonia	a. _____
	b. _____
Fracture of the femur	c. _____
	d. _____
Decubitus ulcer	e. _____
	f. _____

■ Multiple Choice

1. Healthcare facilities require nursing care plans (NCPs) to be established within:
   a. 1 hour
   b. 12 to 14 hours
   c. 3 to 4 days
   d. 7 days

2. Which of the following statements regarding NCP is correct?
   a. NCPs are updated when the patient's condition changes.
   b. NCPs address every problem the patient has.
   c. Any NCP can be used for a patient with a similar problem.
   d. NCPs do not become part of a client's record.

3. Which of the following healthcare professionals would write an NCP?
   a. Nursing aide
   b. Physician
   c. Registered nurse
   d. Speech therapist

4. During the planning stage of the nursing process, which activity does the nurse complete first?
   a. Establish expected outcomes
   b. Select nursing interventions
   c. Set priorities
   d. Write a nursing care plan

CHAPTER 36

Implementing and Evaluating Care

■ Terminology Review

Match the following definitions with the correct terms and acronyms.

1. _____ skills used in implementing the nursing care plan (NCP) that involve knowing and understanding information

2. _____ responsibility for one's actions

3. _____ when a patient does not achieve an expected outcome by the designated time

4. _____ careful examination of all aspects of the healthcare organization by the facility and outside accrediting agencies

5. _____ nursing actions that do not require a physician's order

6. _____ evaluation of nursing activities and patient outcomes as they are demonstrated in the nursing documentation

7. _____ method of providing high-quality care while effectively using healthcare resources and controlling costs

8. _____ skills that involve believing, behaving, and relating

9. _____ process by which the patient is prepared for continued care outside the healthcare facility or for independent living at home

10. _____ step of the nursing process that is carrying out the plan

11. _____ as needed

12. _____ quality assurance committee

13. _____ person who plans and directs all necessary activities to coordinate the patient's care

14. _____ clinical care path

15. _____ nursing actions that carry out a physician's orders

16. _____ diagnostic-related group

17. _____ nursing peer review

18. _____ skills that require safe and competent performance

19. _____ quality assurance

20. _____ nursing audit

21. _____ nursing actions performed collaboratively with other care providers

22. _____ evaluation of outcomes of care from the patient's point of view

23. _____ measurement of the effectiveness of assessing, diagnosing, planning, and implementing

24. _____ planning method in which the optimal sequencing and timing of healthcare interventions are identified

a. accountability
b. case management
c. case manager
d. CCP
e. chart audit
f. clinical care path
g. dependent actions
h. DRG
i. discharge planning
j. evaluation
k. implementation
l. independent actions
m. intellectual skills
n. interdependent actions
o. interpersonal skills
p. NA
q. NPR
r. nursing peer review
s. PRN

t. QA

u. QAC

v. quality assurance

w. technical skills

x. variance

■ Short Answers

1. Indicate whether the following are dependent (D), interdependent (ID), or independent (I) nursing actions for the following actions:

    a. _____ administering routine medications

    b. _____ providing a back rub

    c. _____ assisting with oral hygiene

    d. _____ inserting a urinary catheter

    e. _____ administering prn medication

    f. _____ spending time talking with a patient

    g. _____ changing a wound dressing that was ordered as needed

    h. _____ Inserting an IV

    i. _____ documenting care

2. What are the three action phrases of implementation of nursing care?

3. List the three steps in evaluating nursing care?

4. List persons who are involved in discharge planning.

5. Compare and contrast the nursing care plan (NCP) and the clinical care path (CCP).

6. Explain why documentation of a variance from the CCP is important.

7. Describe components of discharge planning.

■ Nursing Process Review

Match the following items with the steps of the nursing process. Each answer may be used more than once.

1. _____ patient will ambulate 50 feet every shift

2. _____ potassium level of 3.4 mEq

3. _____ decreased cardiac output

4. _____ patient was able to self-administer insulin injection

5. _____ teach patient the signs and symptoms of infection

6. _____ patient's pain will remain a 3 or below on pain scale of 1 to 10

7. _____ anxiety

8. _____ patient states, "I feel nauseated."

9. _____ ambulate patient with assistance

10. _____ nausea relieved with medication

a. assessment

b. diagnosis

c. planning

d. implementation

e. evaluation

▪ Multiple Choice

Circle the best answer for the following questions.

1. Discharge planning should be:
   a. completed immediately before discharge.
   b. completed only if the patient requests help.
   c. started after the patient has been in the hospital a few days.
   d. started when the patient is admitted to the facility.

2. Which type of skill is the nurse using when the nurse sits and holds a crying patient's hand?
   a. Intellectual
   b. Interdependent
   c. Interpersonal
   d. Technical

3. A nurse makes a medication error by administering the wrong medication. Who is responsible for this error?
   a. No one
   b. Nurse
   c. Pharmacist
   d. Physician

4. Which of the following is an example of implementation of the nursing process?
   a. Completing a nursing history
   b. Determining if patient outcomes were met
   c. Developing a nursing diagnosis
   d. Providing a backrub

5. Which of the following is an example of evaluation of the nursing process?
   a. Analyzing the response to a medication
   b. Documentation of a treatment
   c. Obtaining vital signs
   d. Performing a dressing change on a wound

6. For which of the following patients would a case manager be most helpful?
   a. Patient who has had minor surgery
   b. Patient who is homeless and needs dialysis
   c. Patient who is seen at a clinic for a cold
   d. Patient who has a broken arm

7. Which accrediting body requires each healthcare facility to have a quality assurance committee?
   a. AMA
   b. ANA
   c. JCAHO
   d. State nursing boards

8. The nurse evaluates a patient's response to the nursing care that has been implemented. The nurse determines that the goals were not met. Which nursing action would be most appropriate?
   a. Encourage the patient to try harder to reach the established goals
   b. Encourage the nursing staff to implement all interventions
   c. Report the findings to the QAC
   d. Revise the nursing care plan

CHAPTER 37

Documenting and Reporting

■ Terminology Review

Match the following definitions with the correct terms and acronyms.

1. _____ medical information system

2. _____ data, assessment, plan, evaluation

3. _____ assessment, plan, intervention, evaluation

4. _____ lists all medications that the physician has ordered for the patient with spaces for the caregiver to mark when medications are given

5. _____ plan, intervention, evaluation

6. _____ electronic health record housed in a computer network

7. _____ conversations with patients, nursing observations, and assessments are shared only with the appropriate caregivers in the proper setting

8. _____ documentation system that uses subjective and objective data, followed by analysis and plan

9. _____ change-of-shift report given by caregivers moving from patient to patient, discussing pertinent information

10. _____ documentation entered at regular intervals to summarize a patient's condition or response to treatment

11. _____ minimum data set

12. _____ exchanging information between outgoing and incoming staff on each shift

13. _____ SOAP note format plus intervention, evaluation, and revision

14. _____ medication administration record

15. _____ recorded in error

16. _____ data, action, response, education

17. _____ manual or electronic account of a patient's relationship with a healthcare facility

18. _____ charting by exception

19. _____ standard form used by long-term care and home care agencies as part of the admitting nursing history

20. _____ graph or form that records large amount of information collected at intervals during a specified period in brief concise entries

a. APIE
b. CBE
c. change-of-shift reporting
d. confidentiality
e. DARE
f. DAPE
g. Flow sheet
h. health record
i. MAR
j. medical information system
k. medication administration recorded
l. minimum data set
m. MIS
n. MDS
o. PIE
p. progress note
q. RIE
r. SOAP
s. SOAPIER
t. walking rounds

■ Documentation Systems Table

Complete the following table.

	Manual Health Record	Electronic Health Record
Benefits		
Disadvantages		

■ Short Answers

Complete the following by providing an appropriate answer.

1. List the four categories of information included in the health record.

2. Describe how you would correct an incorrect entry made into the health record.

3. Translate the following underlined words in the scenario. Write the correct word for each underlined abbreviation.

   Mr. N. is a 70-year-old male with pneumonia and has a <u>hx</u> of frequent respiratory infections. He is admitted to the unit. His orders include:

   <u>Dx</u> - pneumonia

   Normal saline <u>IV</u> to run at 100 <u>mL/hr.</u>

<u>BRP</u>, regular diet, vital signs <u>QID</u>

Alupent 0.3 mL in 3 mL NS <u>per</u> nebulizer

Chest x-ray in <u>AM</u>

Levaquin 500 mg IV <u>qd</u>

4. Read the following scenario and document the information using DAR format in space provided.

   M.W. is a 50-year-old patient with colon cancer. The patient complained of feeling warm at 1800 hours. Her skin was moist, warm to touch and her temperature was 101 degrees F. She had ordered: Tylenol gr X po q 4-6 hours prn fever. The nurse administered the Tylenol and the temperature was 99.4 degrees F at 1900 hours.

   D-

   A-

   R-

5. Describe guidelines to follow for documentation. List an example with each guideline.

6. Explain what information is exchanged during the change-of-shift report.

7. Indicate if the following action would be appropriate (A) or inappropriate (I).

   a. _____ describe exactly what you observe and document what you see.

   b. _____ document medications as you leave the medication area to avoid forgetting to document after leaving the patient's room

   c. _____ use direct quotes and enclose patient statements with quotation marks when charting

   d. _____ when charting by exception, list only abnormalities or unexpected findings in the progress notes using SOAPIER format

   e. _____ leave vacant lines in the health record to allow an opportunity to add information later if necessary

   f. _____ if an error is made during charting, use correction fluid and change incorrect information

   g. _____ introduce the oncoming nurse to the patient to build rapport

■ Matching

Match the following observations to be charted with the specific term. Refer to Table 37-3 for help.

1. _____ excessive perspiration

2. _____ rapid breathing

3. _____ slow heartbeat

4. _____ loss of appetite

5. _____ descriptive terms of skin

6. _____ descriptive terms of pain

7. _____ decay of tissue

8. _____ blood in urine

9. _____ unable to control urination

10. _____ drainage containing pus

11. _____ no evidence of fever

12. _____ bloated, filled with gas

13. _____ vaginal drainage

14. _____ bath for face, neck, arms, back, and genitals

15. _____ expectorating blood in sputum

a. afebrile

b. anorexia

c. bradycardia

d. diaphoresis

e. distention

f. dull, aching, burning

g. hematuria

h. hemoptosis

i. hypernea

j. incontinence

k. lochia

l. necrosis

m. pale, moist, rough

n. partial bath

o. purulent

CHAPTER 38

The Health Facility Environmnet

■ Terminology Review

Match the following definitions with the appropriate term.

1. _____ area where most patient care is provided

2. _____ instrument used to examine inside the ears, nose and throat

3. _____ examination of a body after death

4. _____ portable, lightweight, sturdy toilet

5. _____ enables healthcare providers to communicate with patients in different locations using a telephone and a computer

6. _____ reasons for specific steps in every nursing procedure

7. _____ department that directs efforts toward preventing physical disability

8. _____ allows healthcare providers at the nursing station to communicate to patients' rooms

9. _____ focuses on fine motor skills and activities of daily living

10. _____ where studies and experiments on animals are conducted to understand, cure, or prevent human diseases

11. _____ area containing several patient units

12. _____ place where dead bodies are kept

13. _____ instrument used for examining the eyes

14. _____ assists patients who have certain cardiac and respiratory disorders

15. _____ specific policies outlining standards of care

a. autopsy
b. patient unit
c. commode
d. intercom
e. morgue
f. nursing unit
g. occupational therapy
h. ophthalmoscope
i. otoscope
j. physical therapy
k. protocol
l. rationale
m. research laboratory
n. respiratory therapy
o. telecommunications

■ Fill in the Blanks

Supply the department responsible for the activities provided (abbreviations provide a hint).

1. _____
   (CCU) cares for patients with serious heart disorders

2. _____
   (PEDS) unit responsible for the care of children

3. _____
   (REHAB) provides physical medicine, psychosocial support, and other services to people who have a physical disability to help them regain as much capacity for activity as possible

4. _____
   (ED) gives care to persons whose conditions require immediate attention

5. _____

   (OB) sometimes called the birthing center; provides care to mothers and newborns

6. _____

   (also called palliative care) gives physical and emotional care to individuals who are dying

7. _____

   (CSS) cleans and sterilizes equipment for use throughout the hospital

8. _____

   (also called continuous quality improvement) promotes the organization's efforts toward quality care

9. _____

   department responsible for cleaning units in hospitals and ECFs; help prevent the spread of infection

10. _____

    CDU) provides care for persons who abuse chemical substances

■ Short Answers

Complete the following questions with the appropriate answer in the space provided.

1. List the four components of the basic patient unit in the hospital, ECF, and home care settings. Provide an example of each.

2. Identify housekeeping measures that will help prevent accidents and infections.

3. Review In Practice: Nursing Care Guideline 38-1.

   Summarize in your own words guidelines that you will adhere to during all nursing procedures.

4. Complete the following hospital personnel and services table.

Department Category	Examples and Abbreviations of Department	Function of Each Department
	1. Pathologists 2. Nuclear Medicine 3. Electroencephalography	1. 2. 3.
Direct Client Care Departments	1. 2.	1. Medical-surgical unit for musculoskeletal disorders 2. Care of surgical clients before, during, and after surgery
	1. Intensive care unit (ICU) 2. Dialysis Unit	1. 2.
Support services	1. Dietary department (nutritional therapy) 2. 3.	1. 2. Dispenses medications 3. Processes clients when they enter or leave the facility

5. A patient is admitted to the medical-surgical unit about 6 pm. The patient expresses being frightened because this is the patient's first hospitalization. The patient normally bathes in the evening before going to sleep. Outline teaching and evening care you would provide.

CHAPTER 39

Emergency Preparedness

■ Terminology Review

Match the following definitions with the correct terms and acronyms.

1. _____ disaster outside a facility, but it impairs normal operations of the facility

2. _____ skilled nursing facility

3. _____ Occupational Safety and Health Administration, which enforces employee right-to-know laws

4. _____ process of sorting and classifying injured persons to determine priority of needs

5. _____ rescue, alert/alarm, confine, and extinguish fire

6. _____ laws that state employees have a right to know about dangers associated with hazardous substances or harmful or infectious agents in the workplace

7. _____ system used to identify quickly people who are going to die quickly if they do not receive immediate medical care

8. _____ provides overall direction of a facility's activities during a disaster

9. _____ cardiopulmonary resuscitation

10. _____ material safety data sheet

11. _____ disaster in or impaired function of a facility

12. _____ provides assistance and support in many environments both inside and outside healthcare facilities during a disaster

a. command center
b. CPR
c. disaster medical assistance team
d. employee right-to-know laws
e. external disaster
f. internal disaster
g. MSDS
h. OSHA
i. RACE
j. simple triage and rapid treatment
k. SNF
l. triage

■ Fill in the Blanks

Fill in the correct answer for each of the following questions.

1. Complete the following statements regarding accident prevention:

   a. Keep floors _____ and clean to prevent falls.

   b. _____ medicine carts and do not leave them unattended.

   c. Use a _____ _____ when necessary to move or walk patients.

   d. Keep halls free of _____ .

   e. Raise the _____ of the patient's bed to prevent back strain when you work with a patient.

   f. Make sure _____ packages are unopened and that medications have not _____.

2. A(n) _____ _____ may be used by staff to request emergency assistance.

3. Complete the following statement regarding using and storing hazardous substances:

   a. _____ labels carefully and note emergency information.

   b. Use _____ equipment as recommended.

   c. Do not use hazardous materials in familiar _____ or drink containers.

   d. Keep household _____ in their original containers.

   e. Do not use gasoline _____.

4. The MSDS provides information about a _____ potential dangers and describes the product, its ingredients, physical properties, fire or explosion hazards, and reactivity.

5. Every staff member in a facility should participate in accident _____ and in patient and employee _____.

6. All healthcare providers must learn how to _____ and _____ the code system(s) used in the facility

7. Making good decisions and coping with disruptions are easier when you are prepared for a _____ or _____.

■ Short Answers

Complete the following questions with the appropriate answer.

1. Identify five potentially hazardous materials.

2. When telephone service is disrupted, what other means may be used to communicate with staff and other healthcare providers?

3. You live in an area where frequent power outages occur during the summer months. Describe the steps you would take to prepare for these outages.

4. How would you prepare differently for power outages in the winter months?

■ Matching

Match the class of fire extinguisher with the type of fire it is used to extinguish. More than one answer may be correct for each.

1. _____ pressurized water

2. _____ carbon dioxide

3. _____ dry chemical

4. _____ all purpose

a. Class A fires: wood, paper, etc.
b. Class B fires: flammable liquids, etc.
c. Class C fires: electrical fires

■ Multiple Choice

Circle the best answer to each of the following questions.

1. When developing a personal emergency procedure for a fire, the nurse would instruct the family to:
   a. carry flares in the car.
   b. establish a place to meet outside the home.
   c. keep extra batteries on hand.
   d. plan for child care.

2. The nurse observes a nursing assistant ambulating an unsteady patient. The nurse's best response would be:
   a. assist with ambulating the patient.
   b. instruct the nursing assistant to get help.
   c. instruct the nursing assistant to use a gait belt.
   d. report the nursing assistant.

3. A confused patient is admitted to the nursing unit. To ensure patient safety, the nurse should:
   a. check on the patient frequently to observe how the patient is adjusting.
   b. leave overhead lights on during the night to comfort the patient.
   c. put the patient's bed in a high position to discourage getting out of bed.
   d. use side rails to prevent patient from falling out of bed.

4. The nurse receives a bomb threat over the telephone when working on the nursing unit. Which action by the nurse is appropriate?
   a. Ask a coworker to look out the window for the person
   b. Ask the caller why he or she hates people
   c. Ask the caller where the bomb is
   d. Hang up immediately

5. A bomb threat has occurred on a nursing unit. The nurse observes an unusual package. The nurse's best response would be:
   a. ask coworkers if the package belongs to them.
   b. clear the area.
   c. gently move the package to a safe area.
   d. open the package.

6. What is the first intervention a nurse should complete when a fire occurs in a patient care area?
   a. Alert coworkers
   b. Confine the fire
   c. Extinguish the fire
   d. Rescue the patients

CHAPTER 40

Microbiology and Defense Against Disease

■ Terminology Review

Match the following definitions with the correct terms.

1. _____ microorganisms that cause disease in a person who is susceptible due to compromised immune system or other factors

2. _____ indicates various antibiotics to which the organism is sensitive

3. _____ a growth of microorganisms prepared for laboratory study

4. _____ specific cause of a disease

5. _____ poisons

6. _____ study of bacteria

7. _____ microorganisms that cause disease

8. _____ place where a microorganism can survive before moving to a place where it can multiply

9. _____ organelle that makes bacteria capable of movement

10. _____ toxin within the cell wall that is released when the microorganism dies

11. _____ microorganisms that require oxygen for growth

12. _____ pathogen's strength to cause disease

13. _____ protective capsule around some microorganisms

14. _____ diseases that can be spread from one person to another

15. _____ period from the onset of initial symptoms to more severe symptoms

16. _____ free from microbial contamination

17. _____ round or spherical bacterium

18. _____ living carriers of pathogens

19. _____ spiral-shaped bacterium

20. _____ minute living cells not visible to the naked eye

21. _____ a large number of people in the same area are infected by a disease in a relatively short time

22. _____ group of single-celled organisms that does not have a true nucleus

23. _____ communicable diseases that are transmitted to many individuals quickly and easily

24. _____ microorganisms that live on or within another living being

25. _____ microorganisms smaller than a bacteria that lack most characteristics of living organisms

26. _____ microorganisms that cannot survive in the presence of oxygen

27. _____ toxins manufactured by a microorganism and excreted into the surrounding tissue

28. _____ pus forming

29. _____ time from when the pathogen enters the body to the appearance of the first symptoms of illness

30. _____ organisms that are present all or most of the time in the environment or on the body

31. _____ infection caused by a fungus

32. _____ rod-shaped bacterium

a. aerobe
b. anaerobe
c. bacillus
d. bacteria
e. bacteriology
f. coccus
g. communicable
h. contagious
i. culture
j. endemic
k. endotoxin
l. epidemic
m. etiology
n. exotoxin
o. flagellum
p. incubation period
q. microorganisms
r. mycosis
s. opportunistic
t. parasite
u. pathogen
v. prodromal
w. reservoir
x. sensitivity
y. spirillum
z. spore
aa. sterile
bb. supportive
cc. toxin
dd. vector
ee. virulence
ff. virus

■ Correct the False Statements

Circle the word True *or* False *that follows the statement. If the word* false *has been circled, change the underlined word/words to make the statement true. Place your answer in the space provided.*

1. A key ingredient for microbial growth is the presence of <u>inorganic nutrients</u>.

    True   False   _____

2. A substance's <u>pH level</u> affects a microorganisms' growth.

    True   False   _____

3. Most pathologic organisms flourish at temperatures <u>above normal</u> body temperature.

    True   False   _____

4. All microorganisms require <u>water or moisture</u> to grow.

    True   False   _____

5. A culture and sensitivity test identifies <u>endemic</u> microorganisms.

    True   False   _____

6. Gram staining is a way to rapidly categorize bacteria in two large groups: <u>gram-sensitive or gram-resistant</u>.

    True   False   _____

7. Bacteria are classified according to physical shape, movement, <u>Gram-stain reaction, and relationship to oxygen</u>.

    True   False   _____

8. <u>Aerobic</u> bacteria are the most difficult to destroy.

    True   False   _____

9. Antibiotics should be taken as prescribed to prevent <u>drug-resistant bacteria</u>.

    True   False   _____

10. Antibiotics <u>should be stopped after</u> symptoms of the illness disappear.

    True   False   _____

11. The order of the chain of infection includes: <u>vehicle of transmission, portal of entry, portal of exit, reservoir, and susceptible host</u>.

    True   False   _____

12. <u>Isolation</u> is the single most useful and effective means of breaking the chain of infection.

    True   False   _____

13. Diseases can <u>be transmitted</u> by direct or indirect contact and airborne methods.

    True   False   _____

14. <u>Toxins cause harmful effects</u> by traveling through the circulatory system to damage other body cells.

    True   False   _____

15. The four stages of a normal course of an infection are: <u>incubation period, prodromal stage, full stage of illness, and convalescence stage.</u>

    True   False   _____

■ Microorganisms Classification Table

Complete the following table.

Microorganism	Characteristics	Virulence	Example
Algae			
Fungi a. Yeasts b. Molds			
Protozoa			
Bacteria			
Viruses			

■ Chain of Infection

Draw the chain of infection. Label the five parts of the chain. Indicate at least one method between each chain that may be used to stop the chain of disease spread.

CHAPTER 41

Medical Asepsis

■ Terminology Review

Match the following definitions with the correct terms and acronyms.

1. _____ practice of reducing the number of microorganisms or preventing and reducing transmission of microorganisms from one person to another

2. _____ microorganisms outside the body that cause infection

3. _____ Hospital Infection Control Practices Advisory Committee

4. _____ infections that patients acquire when in a healthcare facility

5. _____ barrier equipment that includes gloves, eye protection, gowns, and masks

6. _____ chemicals that decrease the number of pathogens in an area

7. _____ microorganisms present within the person's body that cause infection

8. _____ Centers for Disease Control

9. _____ practices that minimize or eliminate organisms that can cause infection and disease

10. _____ tuberculosis

11. _____ therapy that invades the body by means other than normal

12. _____ blood-borne pathogens

13. _____ blood infections

a. antimicrobial agent
b. asepsis
c. bacteremia
d. BBP
e. CDC
f. endogenous
g. exogenous
h. HICPAC
i. invasive
j. medical asepsis
k. nosocomial infection
l. personal protective equipment
m. TB

■ Short Answers

1. For the following scenarios, identify factors that would predispose the patient to nosocomial infections.

   a. 89-year-old female with an indwelling urinary catheter. She has had repeated urinary tract infections and has been treated with many antibiotics. She has difficulty eating.

   b. 44-year-old male who is a cross-country truck driver. He has smoked cigarettes for 20 years. He is admitted to the hospital for removal of his gallbladder.

c. 2-year-old male admitted with scald burns to upper body.

d. 70-year-old female on bed rest. Admitted for repair of right hip fracture. She complains of not being able to sleep in the hospital due to the noise level. She has an IV and urinary catheter.

e. 36-year-old male admitted with bipolar disorder. Patient is homeless and has minor scratches on both upper and lower extremities.

2. Review the scenarios in the previous question. Describe measures that the nurse could do to prevent spreading nosocomial infections for these patients.

3. Indicate if the following actions would be appropriate (A) or inappropriate (I).

   a. _____ removing soiled gloves by grasping the inside of one glove first and pulling it off, then grasping the inside of the other glove and pulling it off with the first glove inside

   b. _____ using double-bag technique to remove contaminated refuse and linen from a patient's room

   c. _____ shaking linen to remove loose debris, then placing it on the floor for removal when fresh linen is on the bed

   d. _____ sending items to be sterilized to central supply room in plastic bags

   e. _____ monitoring the compliance of others regarding infection control practices

   f. _____ using nonprescribed medications only if they belong to other family members who had similar symptoms

   g. _____ removing jewelry, except a plain wedding band, before washing hands

   h. _____ when washing hands, wetting your hands and forearms with water, keeping the hands lower than your elbow.

4. List the most common nonsocomial infections.

5. What is the most common nosocomial infection?

6. Describe areas for teaching the spread of infection for patients and their families.

■ Handwashing Sequencing

Number the following actions in the correct order for handwashing. The first action should be number 1. Continue to number the items.

_____ wash with scrubbing motion for a minimum of 10 to 15 seconds

_____ repeat procedure if hands are very soiled

_____ stand in front of sink and avoid leaning against it

_____ use clean paper towel to turn off faucets

_____ wet hands and forearms, keeping the hands lower than your elbows

_____ rinse thoroughly, keeping hands lower than elbows

_____ dry hands thoroughly with a paper towel

_____ remove jewelry

_____ clean fingernails with sweeping motion

_____ turn on water and regulate its flow and temperature

_____ apply antibacterial soap

■ Multiple Choice

Circle the correct answer for each of the following questions.

1. What is the most common nosocomial infection?
   a. Bacteremias
   b. Genitourinary infections
   c. Respiratory infections
   d. Surgical site infections

2. When providing routine patient care, which type of handwashing is most appropriate?
   a. Handwash with soap or detergent to remove soil and transient microorganisms
   b. No specific handwash is necessary
   c. Perform a surgical hand scrub
   d. Use antimicrobial soap or detergent to perform asepsis

3. The minimum time to scrub hands, wrists, and lower forearms during handwashing is:
   a. 5 seconds.
   b. 10 to 15 seconds.
   c. 30 seconds.
   d. 45 to 60 seconds.

4. Healthcare workers can develop latex allergies due to:
   a. improper handwashing.
   b. previous allergies.
   c. the powder in latex gloves.
   d. wearing masks.

5. Soaps work as antimicrobial agents by:
   a. altering microbial cellular proteins.
   b. disrupting microorganisms' enzyme functions.
   c. lowering surface tension of oil on the skin.
   d. melting microorganisms' inner cellular membrane.

CHAPTER 42

Infection Control

■ Terminology Review

Match the following definitions with the correct terms and acronyms.

1. _____ precautions used during care of all patients, regardless of diagnosis or infection status

2. _____ Hospital Infection Control Practices Advisory Committee

3. _____ personal protective equipment

4. _____ used when a patient must be protected from the outside environment

5. _____ precaution used for diseases transmitted through direct or indirect contact between a susceptible host's body surface and an infected or colonized person

6. _____ Centers for Disease Control and Prevention

7. _____ used with patients who have a weakened immune system

8. _____ precautions designed for patients with specific infections or diagnoses

9. _____ blood-borne pathogens

10. _____ occurs when a microorganism is present in a patient but the patient shows no clinical signs or symptoms of infection

11. _____ tuberculosis

12. _____ type of precaution used for diseases that are transmitted from evaporated droplets suspended in the air or are carried on dust particles

13. _____ precaution used for microorganisms that at propelled as droplets through the air from an infected person and deposited on the host's eyes, nose, or mouth

14. _____ methods using standard precautions and transmission-based precautions to prevent disease transmission

a. airborne precautions
b. BBP
c. CDC
d. colonization
e. contact precautions
f. droplet precautions
g. HICPAC
h. isolation
i. neutropenic isolation
j. PPE
k. protective isolation
l. Standard Precautions
m. TB
n. transmission-based precautions

■ Short Answers

1. Indicate the appropriate PPE you would use for the following patients. Provide rationale for each. Use the following abbreviations: Gl for gloves, M for mask on nurse, MC for mask on patient, H for handwashing, E for eyewear, G for gown, and N for nothing.

   a. Patient on airborne precautions and you need to look at a bedside monitor.

   b. Examining a patient's mouth, teeth, and gums.

c. Assisting with an operative procedure with high possibility of blood splashing.

d. Talking with a patient who is not on transmission-based precautions.

e. Transporting a patient who is on droplet precautions.

f. Changing bed linen on a patient with diarrhea who is on contact precautions.

g. Irrigating a wound on a patient who is on contact precautions for a wound infection.

h. Adjusting intravenous (IV) rate on a patient who is on droplet precautions.

i. Inserting an IV on a patient.

j. Administering oral medications to a patient on contact isolation.

2. A patient is admitted to your nursing unit with tuberculosis. What type of transmission-based precautions would this patient need? How would you prepare the room?

3. Summarize why Standard Precautions are used.

4. A new patient with cancer is admitted to your nursing unit and is undergoing chemotherapy. The patient is on protective isolation. Describe the nursing measures you would take to ensure patient safety.

5. Describe the role of the infection control committee.

■ Multiple Choice

Circle the best answers in the following questions.

1. When adhering to Standard Precautions, the most appropriate nursing action after giving an injection is:
   a. discard without recapping
   b. leave the needle at the bedside for further use.
   c. recap the needle and discard.
   d. remove the needle and discard.

2. To which of the following patients would Standard Precautions apply?
   a. Patients on contact precautions
   b. Every patient the nurse encounters
   c. Only patients with infectious diseases
   d. Only patients on neutropenic isolation

3. A patient is admitted with suspected chickenpox. The nurse's first action would be:
   a. complete a physical examination.
   b. orient the patient to the unit.
   c. place in a private negative air flow room.
   d. take the patient's vital signs.

4. A patient on the nursing unit has pneumonia and is on droplet precautions. Which of the following would be most appropriate for the nurse to teach the patient to prevent the transmission of the disease?
   a. Cover mouth with tissue when coughing
   b. Good oral hygiene is essential
   c. Wash hands frequently
   d. Wear gloves when bathing

5. A patient is admitted to your unit and needs to be placed on contact precautions. There are no private rooms available. Which intervention would be appropriate?
   a. Discharge a different patient from the hospital to free up a room
   b. Encourage the patient to go to a different hospital
   c. Have the patient wait in the hall until a room is available
   d. Place in a room with patient infected with the same microorganism

6. When setting up a patient's room for isolation, where is the best location to store supplies?
   a. By the patient's bed in the bedside table
   b. Inside the room by the entrance door
   c. Outside the room by the entrance door
   d. Outside the room and across the hall

7. Which nursing intervention would be appropriate for a patient on isolation?
   a. Avoid communication with the patient
   b. Organize care to spend longer periods of time with the patient
   c. Remain in the patient's room as short of time as possible to prevent disease transmission
   d. Remind visitors to spend as little time in the room with the patient as possible

8. Which would be the best method to take vital signs for someone who is on isolation?
   a. Take vital signs only as often as absolutely necessary
   b. Teach the patient how to take his or her own vital signs
   c. Use disposable equipment to the take vital signs
   d. Wear gloves, gown, mask, and eyewear

CHAPTER 43

Emergency Care and First Aid

■ Terminology Review

Match the following definitions with the correct terms and acronyms.

1. _____ occurs in hot environments when people do not take in enough water and sodium to replace lost fluids and electrolytes, resulting in a serious blood flow disturbance similar to shock

2. _____ nosebleed

3. _____ the most common cause of death in infants

4. _____ method used to clear complete airway obstruction, also called Heimlich maneuver

5. _____ occurs anytime breathing and heartbeat stop abruptly or unexpectedly

6. _____ tie used on an extremity over a pressure point to stop hemorrhage

7. _____ oxygen is provided to a victim by rescuer inflating victims lungs

8. _____ communicable disease transmitted through animal bites

9. _____ any substance that threatens a person's health when it is absorbed or comes into contact with the body

10. _____ freezing of body tissues that results from exposure to extremely cold temperatures

11. _____ potentially life-threatening condition when the body's heat-regulating mechanisms fail and the core body temperature soars

12. _____ treatment that includes starting intravenous (IV) lines, administering fluids and medications, using defibrillation and cardiac monitoring, administering oxygen, and opening and maintaining the airway

13. _____ poisonous substances

14. _____ basic technique used to resuscitate victims and the maintain airway, breathing, and circulation

15. _____ open chest wound that allows air to enter the chest cavity and compress the lung

16. _____ drowning in which recovery has occurred after submersion

17. _____ results when the body loses its ability to circulate an adequate supply of oxygenated blood to all its components, particularly the brain

18. _____ occurs when air leaks out of the lung into the chest cavity and cannot escape

19. _____ substance that neutralizes poisons

20. _____ displacement of a bone from a joint

21. _____ includes rapid entry into EMS, performance of CPR, and use of techniques to clear an obstructed airway

22. _____ medications that dissolve clots and clear blocked blood vessels

23. _____ broken bone

24. _____ substances that are extremely irritating

25. _____ tension pneumothorax that remains uncorrected

26. _____ type I allergic life-threatening reaction to a substance

27. _____ service to contact in life-threatening situations

28. _____ high-pitched wheezing due to partially obstructed airway

29. _____ direct pressure applied to victim's sternum to compress the heart to simulate a heart contraction

30. _____ occurs when a person's breathing and heartbeat stop

31. _____ piece of material used to hold a dressing or splint in place, to give support, or to apply pressure

32. _____ causes vomiting

33. _____ inserting a tube into the trachea

34. _____ twisting of a joint with rupture of ligaments and other possible damage

35. _____ to cut away

36. _____ definitive initial treatment of victims in cardiac arrest

37. _____ twisting or stretching that damages a muscle or tendon

38. _____ occur after hard exertion and are frequently found in physically fit young people, who usually have been sweating profusely and drinking plain water

39. _____ major bleeding

40. _____ slang term for person who dies from airway obstruction when eating, often rushing from a restaurant to avoid embarrassment

41. _____ condition in which a person is exposed to extreme cold or is cold for long enough to lower his or her core body temperature to < 94° Fahrenheit

42. _____ permanent damage of brain cells due to lack of oxygen

43. _____ moving victim onto side, while moving the head, shoulders, and torso simultaneously after spontaneous breathing has occurred during rescue breathing

44. _____ wound or injury caused by an outside force

a. abdominal thrusts
b. advanced cardiac life support
c. anaphylaxis
d. antidote
e. automated external defibrillator
f. bandage
g. basic cardiac life support
h. biologic death
i. cafe coronary
j. cardiopulmonary resuscitation
k. caustic
l. clinical death
m. debride
n. dislocation
o. emergency medical service
p. emetic
q. epitasis
r. external chest compression
s. fracture
t. frostbite
u. heat cramps
v. heat exhaustion
w. heat stroke
x. hemorrhage
y. hypothermia
z. intubation
aa. mediastinal shift
bb. near drowning
cc. pneumothorax
dd. poison
ee. rabies
ff. recovery position
gg. rescue breathing
hh. shock
ii. sprain
jj. strain
kk. stridor
ll. sudden death
mm. sudden infant death syndrome
nn. tension pneumothorax
oo. thrombolytic
pp. tourniquet
qq. toxin
rr. trauma

■ Correct the False Statements

Circle the word True *or* False *that follows the statement. If the word* false *has been circled, change the underlined word/words to make the statement true. Place your answer in the space provided.*

1. When administering first aid, <u>it is not necessary to follow Standard Precautions</u>.

   True   False   _____

2. Look for all signs of shock. A <u>falling blood pressure</u> is a late sign of shock and is ominous.

   True   False   _____

3. The most common airway obstruction in an unconscious person is caused by <u>food stuck in the trachea</u>.

   True   False   _____

4. <u>Mask-to-mouth breathing</u> has replaced mouth-to-mouth breathing as the preferred method.

   True   False   _____

5. Use a one-way filtered breathing mask for cardiopulmonary resuscitation (CPR) whenever possible to <u>protect the rescuer</u>.

   True   False   _____

6. <u>Always</u> finger sweep a child's mouth. It is <u>unlikely</u> to cause complications.

   True   False   _____

7. The ABCs of Basic Life Support
   A = <u>Airway</u>
   B = <u>Breathing</u>
   C = <u>Circulation</u>

   True   False   _____

8. When working in a cold climate, you will likely see frostbite among <u>very few people.</u>

   True   False   _____

9. Hypothermia that accompanies frostbite is <u>an expected finding</u>.

   True   False   _____

10. Massaging cramped muscles <u>will not cure heat cramps</u>; in fact, it may increase pain.

    True   False   _____

11. Any person with <u>heat exhaustion</u> needs immediate medical attention.

    True   False   _____

12. The most frequent common denominator in heart attack is <u>pain radiating to the right arm</u>.

    True   False   _____

13. If a person with a <u>nosebleed has a fractured skull</u>, do not attempt to stop the bleeding.

    True   False   _____

14. <u>Anaphylaxis</u> is a true medical emergency. Time is crucial.

    True   False   _____

15. <u>Induce vomiting</u> for a person who has ingested a poison.

    True   False   _____

■ Short Answers

Complete the following questions by providing the most appropriate answer.

1. What should you do at an emergency scene before rushing in to provide assistance?

2. What is the purpose of a Medic Alert tag?

3. Describe the correct order for assessing a person in an emergency.

4. Review the differences for CPR for adults, children, and infants. After reviewing, complete the following table.

	Adults	Children Ages 1–8	Infants
Pulse position			
Hand position			
Used for compression			
Depth of compression			
Compression per minute			
Compression to ventilation ratio			

5. What findings indicate that resuscitation measure have been successful?

6. Why can some victims of near drowning respond to resuscitation without sustaining brain damage?

7. What does the acronym RICE stand for, and when would you use it?

8. When should a tourniquet be used?

9. Indicate which pressure point would be used to stop bleeding in each of the following examples.

   a. Amputated finger _____

   b. Lacerated side of the head above the ear
   _____

   c. Bleeding shoulder _____

   d. Slit wrist _____

   e. Crushed knee _____

   f. Cut lip _____

10. Describe measures to take with a victim who has been poisoned or taken an overdose.

11. Describe factors that would indicate that a person has suicidal tendencies or is a potential risk for harming self or others.

■ Multiple Choice

Circle the best answer for each of the following questions.

1. Most states have laws to protect emergency care rescuers from legal liability. These laws are called:

   a. EMT Protection Laws.

   b. Good Samaritan Laws.

   c. Rescuer Laws.

   d. Safe Care Laws.

2. Which of the following are early signs of shock?

   a. Anxiety, mental confusion, restlessness

   b. Cold and clammy skin, nausea, thirst

   c. Nausea, vomiting, falling blood pressure

   d. Shaking of limbs, unresponsiveness, feeling of impending doom

3. Which of the following interventions would be your priority when treating a victim suspected of being in shock?

   a. Establish, maintain, and monitor the airway

   b. Immobilize fractures

   c. Maintain body temperature

   d. Monitor level of consciousness

4. How long should you take to determining breathlessness in an unresponsive victim?

   a. None, start rescue breathing immediately

   b. 1 to 3 seconds

   c. 3 to 5 seconds

   d. 5 to 10 seconds

5. When starting rescue breathing on an infant, what action is appropriate if the initial ventilation is unsuccessful?

   a. Begin chest compressions

   b. Complete a mouth sweep

   c. Perform back thrusts

   d. Reposition baby's head and try again

6. Which action would need to be performed before transporting a victim with a suspected neck or back injury?

   a. Assess vital signs

   b. Drag the person to safety

   c. Estimate blood loss

   d. Immobilize the neck and back

7. Which action would be appropriate when caring for a victim with an object that has punctured the chest?

   a. Do not remove the object, but stabilize it

   b. Gently pull on the object and remove it if it is loose

   c. Remove any loose pieces of the object that are in the rescuers way

   d. Remove the object and cover with an occlusive dressing

8. A person is suspected of having frostbite to the hands and feet. Which action would be appropriate?

   a. Apply a mild ointment

   b. Gently rub extremities to warm them

   c. Place in tepid water

   d. Wrap in cool blankets to prevent rapid warming

9. During which condition would heat injuries most likely occur?

   a. High humidity, high temperatures, and no breeze

   b. High humidity, high temperatures, and strong breeze

   c. High humidity, moderate temperatures, and no breeze

   d. Low humidity, high temperatures, and no breeze

10. A victim has fallen from the second floor of a two-story building and complains of pain in the right leg. Which action is most appropriate?

    a. Ask the person to walk on the leg to see if it is broken

    b. Do not move the person

    c. Question the person as to why he or she fell

    d. Remove the victim's pants

11. Which maneuver would not be used on an adult with an obstructed airway?

    a. Abdominal thrusts

    b. Back blows

    c. Heimlich maneuver

    d. Mouth sweep

12. Which medication would be used for the treatment of anaphylaxis?

    a. Activated charcoal

    b. Allerdryl

    c. Benadryl

    d. Epinephrine

CHAPTER 44

Therapeutic Communication Skills

■ Terminology Review

Match the following definitions with the correct terms and acronyms.

1. _____ area around each person

2. _____ communication using action

3. _____ physician's order given over the telephone

4. _____ giving, receiving, and interpreting of information through any of the five senses by two or more interacting people

5. _____ using a name other than one's own name

6. _____ goal-directed conversation in which one person seeks information from the other

7. _____ physician's order given in person

8. _____ type of communication using words

9. _____ also known as

10. _____ elicits only brief and predictable responses in an interview

11. _____ helpful and healing for one or more of the communicating participants

12. _____ order that requires nursing judgment

13. _____ information about the patient cannot be given out without this form

14. _____ sharing information without using words or language

15. _____ inability to communicate verbally

16. _____ feeling of harmony

17. _____ encourages longer and more thorough answers during the interview

18. _____ looking directly into the eye of another person

a. alias
b. aphasia
c. body language
d. closed-ended question
e. communication
f. eye contact
g. interview
h. nonverbal communication
i. open-ended question
j. personal space
k. rapport
l. therapeutic communication
m. verbal communication
n. AKA
o. PRN
p. ROI
q. TO
r. VO

■ Correct the False Statements

Circle the word True *or* False *that follows the statement. If the word* false *has been circled, change the underlined word/words to make the statement true. Place your answer in the space provided.*

1. The <u>goal of therapeutic communication</u> is to help patients to talk about and resolve their feelings and problems related to health, illness, treatments, and nursing care.

   True   False   _____

2. During communication, <u>the sender and receiver participate individually</u>.

   True   False   _____

3. It is important for the nurse to note the <u>volume of a patient's speech</u>, which may relate to culture or a physical impairment.

   True   False   _____

4. The nurse should always communicate with a patient <u>with aphasia</u> as if the patient can hear.

   True   False   _____

5. A patient with a hearing impairment <u>might invade someone's personal space</u> to hear.

   True   False   _____

6. Patients may have <u>difficulty communicating</u> due to not bringing glasses or hearing aids to the facility.

   True   False   _____

7. Reflection may be used to echo the patient's words or <u>to allow the patient to collect his or her thoughts.</u>

   True   False   _____

8. <u>"Bien"</u> means bad in Spanish.

   True   False   _____

9. <u>"Por favor"</u> means please in Spanish.

   True   False   _____

10. Verbal orders <u>do not need to be signed</u> by a physician.

    True   False   _____

■ Short Answers

Complete each of the following questions with the most appropriate answer.

1. You are a student nurse caring for a patient. The patient's physician comes in, talks to the patient briefly, and then says to you, "Her output is down, I want you to give her another 30 milligrams of Lasix." How do you respond?

2. List the five components of effective communication.

3. Explain ways to establish rapport with patients and why it is important in nursing.

4. How would you interpret differences in personal space?

5. A patient has just returned from having surgery. The patient has not had any pain medication. His vital signs are elevated, which could indicate he is in pain. He has a calm facial expression. What would you do?

6. Indicate if the following questions are open-ended (O) or closed-ended (C) questions.

   a. _____ Tell me about your health history.

   b. _____ Are you nauseated?

   c. _____ What have you been doing for the skin rash?

   d. _____ What would you like to discuss?

   e. _____ Did you take any aspirin for your headache?

7. In the following examples, use paraphrasing to restate the patient's statements.

   a. "I haven't been sleeping well. I can't get to sleep at night until after midnight."

   b. "I don't believe all this stuff about smoking. I am healthy and have smoked for 20 years."

8. In the following examples, use reflection in your response to the patient.

   a. "My husband was supposed to be here an hour ago. What time is it?"

   b. "I don't feel like doing anything or even talking."

9. You need to obtain vital signs on each of the following patients. Describe how you would modify communication to explain this procedure the each patient.

   a. Young child

   b. Visually impaired

   c. Patient who is aggressive

   d. Patient who speaks a different language

10. What would you do to ensure accurate message taking from a telephone conversation?

■ Multiple Choice

Circle the best answer for each of the following questions.

1. When a nurse communicates with a patient and family, the nurse's gestures, appearance, and eye contact are forms of which type of communication?

   a. Ineffective communication
   b. Nonverbal communication
   c. Therapeutic communication
   d. Verbal communication

2. A patient begins to tell the nurse about the death of her husband. During the conversation, she stops talking and becomes teary eyed. The best response by the nurse would be to use which of the following therapeutic communication techniques?

   a. Clarifying
   b. Questioning
   c. Reflection
   d. Silence

3. As a student nurse, you can use effective communication techniques by:

   a. crossing your arms and legs during the interview.
   b. holding your hands on your hips to stress a point.
   c. leaning toward the patient to express acceptance.
   d. pointing finger at the patient during the interview.

4. Verbal communication includes:

   a. eye contact.
   b. gestures.
   c. personal space.
   d. writing.

5. Which of the following actions would be appropriate when caring for an unconscious patient?

   a. Assume the patient can hear you
   b. Discuss the patient when completing care
   c. Enter the room quietly without talking
   d. Perform all care without talking

6. A patient is scheduled for surgery. She tells the nurse, "I've never had surgery before. I'm worried about it." The nurse's most appropriate response would be:

   a. "Don't worry, everything will be okay."
   b. "Having surgery can be scary. Do you want to talk about it?"
   c. "The doctor says you need this surgery and knows what's best for you."
   d. "You shouldn't have gotten yourself into this mess."

CHAPTER 45

Admission, Transfer, and Discharge

■ Terminology Review

Match the following definitions with the correct terms and acronyms.

1. _____ performs formal admission interviews, nursing diagnoses, and admission charting

2. _____ when a patient is absent without leave

3. _____ measurements of body temperature, pulse, respiration, and blood pressure

4. _____ process of depriving a person of personality, spirit, and other human qualities

5. _____ Joint Commission on Accreditation of Healthcare Organizations

6. _____ intensive care unit

7. _____ intravenous

8. _____ abbreviation for temperature, pulse, and respiration

9. _____ sling-type apparatus that looks like a suspended hammock, used to weigh immobile patients

10. _____ blood pressure

11. _____ when a patient leaves a healthcare facility without a physician's permission

a. dehumanization
b. litter scale
c. vital signs
d. AMA
e. AWOL
f. BP
g. ICU
h. IV

i. JCAHO
j. RN
k. TRP

■ Short Answers

Complete the following questions by providing the best response.

1. Explain measures you can take during the following situations to prevent dehumanization.
   a. An 8-year-old child is admitted to the nursing unit

   b. A 52-year-old is being transferred to another unit due to a deterioration in status

   c. A 75-year-old is being discharge to home tomorrow

2. Indicate whether the following actions are part of admission (A), transfer (T), or discharge (D). Some items may have more than one answer.
   a. _____ determine how the patient will be moved

   b. _____ teach the patient the proper operation of equipment and care of tubes

   c. _____ provide information about public health and home nursing services

   d. _____ assemble all the patient's personal belongings, double-check for all clothes and other articles

e. _____ be sure the patient receives and wears and identification band

f. _____ treat the patient as a person

g. _____ teach patient how to use communication system

h. _____ review dietary restrictions

i. _____ provide for patient safety

j. _____ notify all departments of patient's location

3. List admission information that you should report to the registered nurse (RN) or team leader.

4. Identify three reasons a patient may be transferred to another unit.

5. Describe the procedure when a patient leaves a healthcare facility AMA.

■ Correct the False Statements

Circle the word True *or* False *that follows the statement. If the word* false *has been circled, change the underlined word/words to make the statement true. Place your answer in the space provided.*

1. <u>During admission</u>, patients sign documents giving consent and for accepting financial responsibility.

   True   False   _____

2. The healthcare facility <u>assumes liability</u> for articles left at the bedside.

   True   False   _____

3. On admission, patients should be weighed <u>in their street clothes</u> .

   True   False   _____

4. <u>Patients should supply</u> essential toilet articles as toothbrushes, toothpaste, combs, tissues, and soap.

   True   False   _____

5. Inform patients on admission that their equipment is <u>for their use alone</u>.

   True   False   _____

6. <u>Valuables, such as jewelry, credit cards, and cash</u> should not be brought to the facility.

   True   False   _____

7. The nurse should always think of each patient as a person whose need for <u>physical and emotional support is greater</u> than normal because of illness.

   True   False   _____

8. <u>After transferring a patient</u>, the nurse should give a verbal report and ensure the receiving unit is ready.

   True   False   _____

9. Discharge preparation should include explaining danger signs <u>the patient should be alert for</u>.

   True   False   _____

10. When undressing an immobile patient, if the patient cannot raise his or her hips, the nurse should <u>roll the patient side to side</u>.

   True   False   _____

■ Multiple Choice

Circle the best answer for each of the following questions.

1. Advance directives:

   a. allow the family to specify choices of healthcare treatment without patient input.

   b. are only to provide information about healthcare choices.

   c. are required by law to be discussed on admission to healthcare facilities.

   d. are verbal agreements allowing an individual to specify healthcare choices.

a. granulation tissue

b. guaiac

c. herniation

d. Homans' sign

e. hyperopia

f. hypoxemia

g. infection

h. inspection

i. kyphosis

j. lipoma

k. malaise

l. necrosis

m. nodule

n. observation

o. palpation

a. percussion

b. purulent

c. pustule

d. rhonchi

e. serosanguineous

f. sign

g. strabismus

h. striae

i. stridor

j. symptom

k. thrombophlebitis

l. turgor

m. ulcer

n. vesicle

o. wheal

Match the following definitions with the correct terms.

31. _____ crowing, whining sound, mainly heard on inspiration

32. _____ blood clot formation within the vein

33. _____ exudates that contain pus

34. _____ transient superficial elevated area of localized edema

35. _____ continuous dry rattling heard on auscultation

36. _____ skin resiliency and plumpness

37. _____ elevated superficial cavity filled with pus with a well-defined border

38. _____ subjective data of a disease

39. _____ stretch marks

40. _____ tapping the fingers against the body

41. _____ exudates containing clear and bloody fluid

42. _____ objective data of a disease that can be measured

43. _____ small, elevated, cavity filled with serous fluid with a well-defined border

44. _____ cross-eyed

45. _____ local unhealed area of epithelial tissue

■ Correct the False Statements

Circle the word True *or* False *that follows the statement. If the word* false *has been circled, change the underlined word/words to make the statement true. Place your answer in the space provided.*

1. The medical diagnosis focuses on the person and his or her needs in response to the disease, rather than on the disease itself.

   True   False   _____

2. The nurse assesses the patient in almost every nursing interaction.

   True   False   _____

3. Excess intake of fatty foods can increase the risk of developing cholecystitis.

   True   False   _____

4. A low intake of calcium can place a patient at risk for poor wound healing.

   True   False   _____

5. Signs of inflammation include heat, redness, or swelling.

   True   False   _____

6. The purpose of <u>UTox</u> is to determine if a patient is pregnant.

   True   False   _____

7. <u>Endoscopy</u> can be used to determine a patient's digestive or reparatory structure and function.

   True   False   _____

8. Before any procedure using dye, the healthcare worker should ask the patient if he or she is allergic to <u>strawberries or nuts</u>.

   True   False   _____

9. A urinalysis is obtained <u>to evaluate for blood in the urine</u>.

   True   False   _____

10. <u>A biopsy</u> is used to determine a patient's respiratory status.

    True   False   _____

■ Assessment Review

Indicate if the following assessment findings are normal (N) or abnormal (A).

1. _____ anorexia

2. _____ no cough

3. _____ bluish colored skin

4. _____ pitting edema

5. _____ no complaints of nausea

6. _____ pyrexia

7. _____ induration

8. _____ macule

9. _____ papule

10. _____ fissure

11. _____ white sclera

12. _____ 20/20 vision

13. _____ myopia

14. _____ low-pitched bubbling breath sounds

15. _____ wheezing

16. _____ symmetrical face

17. _____ orientated to person, place, and time

18. _____ dysphasia

19. _____ accommodation of eyes

20. _____ pain

21. _____ strong hand grasps bilaterally

22. _____ 40 degree hip abduction

23. _____ positive Homans' sign

24. _____ tender mass

25. _____ lordosis

26. _____ PMI at fifth intercostals space, left midclavicular line

27. _____ regular S_1 and S_2

28. _____ bilateral, equal popliteal pulses

29. _____ bowel sounds of 10 gurgles in one minute

30. _____ hemorrhoids

■ Multiple Choice

Circle the best answer for each of the following questions.

1. The primary purpose of nurses examining patients is to:
   a. determine the patient's physical condition.
   b. establish a professional relationship with the patient.
   c. identify sources of pain.
   d. make a diagnosis of the underlying pathology.

2. A patient has returned from having a cholecystogram and complains of feeling cold and having an itchy nose. Which action should the nurse take?
   a. Assess for return of gag reflex
   b. Continue to monitor the patient's status
   c. Notify the registered nurse/medical doctor

d. Reassure the patient these are normal feelings

3. Which of the following is the most important tool when examining a patient?

   a. Thermometer

   b. Tongue blade

   c. Stethoscope

   d. Use of examiner's senses

4. Which assessment technique would provide the most information about a patient's ability to move air into and out of the lungs?

   a. Auscultation

   b. Inspection

   c. Palpation

d. Percussion

5. Which format of examination provides a complete picture of the patient?

   a. Focused physical assessment

   b. Functional assessment

   c. Head-to-toe assessment

   d. Structural assessment

CHAPTER 48

Body Mechanics and Positioning

■ Terminology Review

Match the following definitions with the correct terms and acronyms.

1. _____ imaginary vertical line through the top of your head, center of gravity, and base of support

2. _____ style of walking

3. _____ use of the safest and most efficient methods of moving and lifting

4. _____ inability to move the body or body parts because of damage to the brain or spinal cord

5. _____ hard plastic device used to help move patients

6. _____ located in the pelvic area with half the body weight distributed above and below the area

7. _____ paralysis on one side of the body

8. _____ protective device such as a restraint

9. _____ muscle-setting exercises

10. _____ feet provide this and prevent us from tipping over

11. _____ another name for line of gravity

12. _____ paralyzed from the waist down

13. _____ sturdy webbed belt with a buckle that easily secures around the waist

14. _____ shortening the length of the muscles to move the bones of a joint

a. base of support
b. body mechanics
c. center of gravity
d. contracture
e. gait

f. gravital plane
g. hemiplegia
h. isometric
i. line of gravity
j. paralysis
k. paraplegic
l. transfer belt
m. transfer board
n. safety device

Match the following definitions with the correct terms.

15. _____ method of turning the patient that keeps the body in straight alignment

16. _____ position used for pelvic examinations

17. _____ another name for a wheeled stretcher

18. _____ lying on the back with legs straight of flexed

19. _____ patient lies on abdomen

20. _____ allowing to hang unsupported

21. _____ left side lying with the right knee flexed against the abdomen and left knee slightly flexed

22. _____ four-wheeled bedlike cart with a moisture-proof mattress

23. _____ head of bed elevated and knees flexed

a. dangling
b. dorsal lithotomy
c. Fowler's
d. gurney
e. litter
f. logroll turn
g. prone
h. recumbent
i. Sims'

Match the following definitions with the correct movement terms.

24. _____ moving backward or back into anatomic position

25. _____ turning the hand so the palm faces downward and backward

26. _____ decreasing the angle between two bones

27. _____ every body joint has a opening and closing motion

28. _____ turning the foot so the sole faces away from the other foot

29. _____ moving a bone on a longitudinal axis

30. _____ if a patient is unable to move, the nurse assists with range of motion (ROM)

31. _____ increasing the angle between two bones

32. _____ moving a body part away from the midline of the body

33. _____ moving forward or anteriorly

34. _____ inversion, turning the foot so its sole faces the other foot

35. _____ patient doing his or her own exercise

36. _____ moving an extremity in circles

37. _____ mechanical device that provides continuous motion to a specific joint

38. _____ turning a part so that it faces medically or inside

39. _____ moving a body part toward the midline of the body

40. _____ opposite side

a. abduction

b. active range of motion (AROM)

c. adduction

d. circumduction

e. continuous passive motion (CPM)

f. contralateral

g. eversion

h. extension

i. flexion

j. inversion

k. passive range of motion (PROM)

l. pronation

m. protraction

n. range of motion (ROM)

o. retraction

p. rotation

q. supination

■ Sequencing

Number the following actions in the correct order for dangling a patient. The first action should be number 1. Continue to number the items.

_____ roll a pillow and tuck it firmly behind the patient's back

_____ place one arm around the patient's shoulders and your other arm under his or her knees

_____ measure the record the patient's pulse and blood pressure for baseline

_____ after some time, help the patient lie down again by supporting his or her shoulders and knees and turning him or her back around

_____ recheck pulse and blood pressure, wash hands, and document the procedure

_____ dangle the patient's legs for as long as ordered, if tolerated

_____ elevate the head of the bed as high as it will go

_____ turn the patient toward you so his or her feet touch the floor

_____ place bed in low position, explain procedure, and position bed covers

Number the following actions in the correct order for moving a patient from the bed to stretcher. The first action should be number 1. Continue to number the items.

_____ place stretcher next to bed with rails down and wheels locked

_____ on signal, all nurses move patient to edge of bed and then onto the stretcher

_____ place draw sheet under patient and bath blanket on top of patient

_____ all nurses grasp the edge of draw sheet, close to patient's body

_____ assess for body alignment, cover patient, and position safety devices

_____ lock the bed wheels and raise the bed to same height as stretcher

_____ position two nurses next to stretcher and 1 to 2 nurses next to the bed

Number the following actions in the correct order for helping a patient into a wheelchair from the bed. The first action should be number 1. Continue to number the items.

_____ assist patient to sit at side of bed.

_____ wash your hands.

_____ put on patient's robe and slippers on patient; obtain help if needed

_____ reposition footrests, secure patient, cover patient, and provide nurse call button

_____ bed, lock wheels, and remove footrests

_____ pivot patient into position in front of wheelchair and lower patient into chair

_____ raise the head of the bed

_____ apply transfer belt, spread patient's feet, and brace your knees against the patient; place your arms around the patient's waist

_____ wash hands and explain procedure to the patient

_____ use the rocking motion of the legs to assist the patient to stand.

■ Appropriate Actions

Indicate if the following actions would be appropriate (A) or inappropriate (I).

1. _____ when logroll turning the patient, keep the body in a straight alignment

2. _____ place a patient in a protective prone position with head turned sideways for long periods to prevent aspiration and minimize headache

3. _____ use pillows to support the head, neck, arms, and hands when a patient is lying on his or her back

4. _____ in a modified Sims' position (alternate side-lying) you ask the patient to keep knees straight

5. _____ when moving an immobile patient to the side of the bed, bend at the back and pull with your arms

6. _____ use a transfer board or bridge for patients who are unable to stand

7. _____ use a broad base of support when transferring patients

8. _____ instruct the patient to move the nonsupportive leg with the unaffected leg when using crutches using the three-point gait

9. _____ use a hydraulic lift to move a heavy patient

10. _____ maintain the stability of the neck when using the logroll turn on a patient with a spinal cord injury

11. _____ medicate a patient in pain 1 hour before assisting with ambulation

■ Multiple Choice

Circle the best answer for each of the following questions.

1. When a patient is in bed, the straps of safety devices should be tied to the:
   a. bedside stand.
   b. chair at the bedside.
   c. moveable part of the bed frame.
   d. immovable bed frame.

2. Which instruction would the nurse teach a patient learning to use a walker?
   a. Pick up the walker and move it 12 to 18 inches at a time
   b. Position the walker to the side of the patient
   c. When one side is weak, move the strong leg first
   d. When both sides are weak, move the right leg first

3. When completing AROM exercises on a patient's elbow, which of the following is a correct motion?
   a. Abduction
   b. Adduction
   c. Flexion
   d. Pronation

4. Which of the following reflects a basic principle of body mechanics?
   a. More energy is needed to keep an object moving than to stop it
   b. Pushing or pulling is easier than lifting
   c. Rocking to use you body weight is not recommend
   d. Using the back muscles is recommended

5. Which position is used for most of the physical examination and can be uncomfortable for a patient with a back problem?
   a. Horizontal recumbent
   b. Knee-chest
   c. Prone
   d. Sims'

6. Which type of crutch-walking gait is the safest and easiest to use?
   a. Swing-through
   b. Two-point
   c. Three-point
   d. Four-point

7. A swing-through gait is most often used with which type of patient?
   a. Patient with one leg amputated
   b. Patient with bilateral leg fractures
   c. Patient with both legs of equal strength
   d. Patient with one leg disabled on one leg strong

8. Patient safety devices can be used when:
   a. a patient is verbally abusive.
   b. a physician orders them.
   c. anytime a nurse chooses to use them.
   d. only with a court order.

9. Which finding best indicates that a patient is able to correctly use a cane?
   a. Patient holds cane on the weak side
   b. Patient keeps arm extended in a straight position
   c. Patient moves at a pace to maintain balance
   d. Patient moves stronger leg with the cane

CHAPTER 49

Beds and Bedmaking

■ Terminology Review

Match the following definitions with the correct terms and acronyms.

1. _____ assistive devices on the bed that prevent patients from falling out of bed

2. _____ foam rubber mattress shaped like and egg carton

3. _____ bed that is prepared so a patient may easily be transferred from a stretcher or wheelchair into a newly made bed

4. _____ system used to provide tension or pull on a body part

5. _____ device attached to the foot of the bed to prevent footdrop

6. _____ any bed that is empty at the time it is made

7. _____ type of fold on a sheet that provides a neat appearance and keeps the sheet secure

8. _____ changing bed linens when the patient is still in the bed

9. _____ horizontal bar attached to a large overhead frame, which itself attaches to the bed

10. _____ linens are turned down, making it easier for the patient to get into bed

11. _____ frame used to prevent the bedclothes from touching all or part of the patient's body

12. _____ type of mattress that is used for patients on prolonged bed rest or with poor skin integrity

a. bed cradle
b. closed bed
c. egg crate mattress
d. flotation mattress
e. footboard
f. mitered corner
g. occupied bed
h. open bed
i. postoperative bed
j. side rails
k. traction
l. trapeze

■ Sequencing

Number the following actions in the correct order for making a closed or unoccupied bed. The first action should be number 1. Continue to number the items.

_____ put on clean pillowcase and place pillow at top of the bed

_____ slide mattress to the head of bed and put on mattress pad

_____ refold the spread or any item that is to be reused

_____ move to the other side of the bed and tuck in linens

_____ fanfold the top linens, position call signal, and overbed table

_____ wear gloves if the linens are soiled; remove, roll up and place soiled linens in hamper

_____ remove soiled pillowcases and place in linen hamper

_____ place draw sheet on the bed

_____ place bottom sheet on the bed

_____ gather supplies, wash hands, and adjust bed to correct height

_____ place the top sheet on the bed, centering it in the same manner as the bottom sheet

_____ make a toe pleat at the foot of the bed

_____ tuck the sheet securely under the head of the mattress using a mitered corner

_____ discard linens and wash your hands

_____ tuck the sheet under the entire bed

_____ cover the top sheet with a blanket and/or bedspread

Number the following actions in the correct order for making an occupied bed. The first action should be number 1. Continue to number the items.

_____ loosen bottom bed linens from the side of the bed and wedge them close to the patient

_____ adjust the bed to a comfortable height, remove call bell, lower side rail on the near side

_____ make a toe pleat or loosen top linens over the patient's feet

_____ grasp clean linens and gently pull them out from under the patient; spread them over the bed's unmade side

_____ gather supplies, explain procedure, wash hands, and put on gloves

_____ place the top sheet over the bath blanket, remove bath blanket, and replace spread

_____ discard linens, remove gloves, and wash hands.

_____ loosen top bed lines, remove the spread, and place a bath blanket on patient

_____ assist the patient back to the center of the bed

_____ raise the side rail, lower the bed and replace call bell

_____ raise the side rail, move to the other side of the bed, and help patient roll over the folded linen

_____ assist the patient to turn toward the other side of the bed, and adjust the pillow

_____ remove the soiled bottom linens.

_____ place the clean bottom sheet on the bed folded lengthwise with the centerfold as close to the patient's back as possible.

▪ Correct the False Statements

Circle the word True *or* False *that follows the statement. If the word* false *has been circled, change the underlined word/words to make the statement true. Place your answer in the space provided.*

1. The nurse should prepare a <u>closed bed</u> for a patient returning from the operating room.

   True   False   _____

2. The top linens should be <u>fanfolded to the bottom of the bed</u> when making a closed bed.

   True   False   _____

3. Stained sheets should be changed <u>as soon as the nurse has time</u>.

   True   False   _____

4. The nurse should <u>make an occupied bed</u> when the patient has generalized weakness.

   True   False   _____

5. <u>A footboard</u> is used to prevent a deformity called footdrop.

   True   False   _____

6. The purpose of bedmaking in the healthcare facility is to <u>make the patients comfortable</u>.

   True   False   _____

7. Bed cradles are used for patients with <u>intravenous lines</u>.

   True   False   _____

8. Side rails should <u>be down</u> when changing an occupied bed.

   True   False   _____

9. The purpose of having a detachable headboard is so that it <u>may be placed under a patient in the event that CPR is needed for that patient.</u>

   True   False   _____

10. A Stryker frame keeps the patient immobile when rotating the patient from <u>head to toe.</u>

   True   False   _____

■ Completion

Complete the following sentences by filling in the blanks.

1. Side rails _____ patients from falling out of bed and are _____ devices for changing position when patients are in bed.

2. _____ and _____ are two patient conditions that might require the use of a bed cradle.

3. A bed board may be placed under the mattress to _____ the body in _____ _____ .

4. Therapeutic beds are used to treat patients with severe joint _____, prolonged _____, or skin _____ such as burns or pressure ulcers.

5. Therapeutic beds reduce or relieve the effects of _____ against the skin through various mechanisms.

6. A _____ _____ is used to move a patient from prone to supine position while keeping the body in straight, flat alignment.

7. _____ _____ are more comfortable for patients with severe contractures.

CHAPTER 50

Personal Hygiene and Skin Care

■ Terminology Review

Match the following definitions with the correct terms and acronyms.

1. _____ brownish deposits on the tongue and the mouth's mucus membranes

2. _____ breath odor caused by food particles between the teeth

3. _____ eggs of lice

4. _____ intravenous

5. _____ inflammation of the tooth sockets

6. _____ lice

7. _____ ear wax

8. _____ bathing the genitalia and surrounding area

a. cerumen

b. halitosis

c. nits

d. pediculosis

e. perineal care

f. pyorrhea

g. sordes

h. IV

■ Nursing Actions

Indicate if the following actions would be appropriate (A) or inappropriate (I).

1. _____ offer the patient the opportunity to brush his or her teeth before and after each meal and in the morning and evening

2. _____ when providing mouth care, wear gloves and assist the patient to an upright position with an emesis basin in hand

3. _____ keep dentures dry in a clean cloth when the patient leaves the dentures out of the mouth

4. _____ encourage the patient to wear the dentures at all times to prevent gum-line changes

5. _____ when providing mouth care, open the patient's mouth and insert a padded tongue blade to keep the mouth open

6. _____ when giving routine eye care, soak cotton balls or gauze squares in peroxide or alcohol

7. _____ special eye care for the patient who cannot blink includes keeping the eye and surrounding area dry to prevent cross-infection

8. _____ wipe the patient's eyelid from the inner canthus to the outer canthus to prevent infection

9. _____ remove ear wax with a moist Q-tip and warm saline

10. _____ use scissors to cut the patient's nails if the nails are torn or jagged

▪ Sequencing

Number the following actions in the correct order for giving a bed bath. The first action should be number 1. Continue to number the items.

_____ put the towel over the patient's chest and fold the bath blanket back, wash, rinse, and dry the patient's chest

_____ raise the bed to a comfortable height for you

_____ fill the basin about two-thirds full with warm water and place it on the bedside table

_____ close the curtain or the door

_____ uncover the patient's far leg; wash, rinse, and dry it

_____ lower the side rails and assist the patient to turn away from you onto the side; uncover the back and buttocks; wash, rinse, and dry this area

_____ provide the patient an opportunity to use a bedpan

_____ give a back rub at this time; tie or snap the patient's gown at the back of the neck

_____ keeping the towel over the patient's chest, lower the bath blanket just above the pubic area and wash, rinse and dry the abdomen

_____ moisten the mitt with plain water and wash the patient's eye

_____ place the basin on a folded bath towel and immerse the patient's foot in water; wash, rinse, and dry each foot (immerse on at a time)

_____ change the bath water at this point

Number the following actions in the correct order for giving a back rub. The first action should be number 1. Continue to number the items.

_____ stand with one foot slightly forward and knees bent; rock on your feet as you rub

_____ wash hands and document

_____ provide privacy and place patient in comfortable position

_____ rub in the hollow at the back of the neck with a circular motion

_____ apply warmed lotion all over the patient's back

_____ rub the neck under the hairline with a circular motion

_____ rub the shoulders with a circular motion

_____ rub the length of the neck with a circular motion

_____ wash hands and apply gloves if needed

_____ repeat the massaging steps three times

_____ rub hands up and down the spine from the coccyx to the hairline

_____ use circular motion down each side of the spine to the coccyx

Number the following actions in the correct order for providing denture care. The first action should be number 1. Continue to number the items.

_____ soak dentures in commercially prepared solution and rinse with tap water

_____ apply denture adhesive

_____ position patient, wash hands, apply gloves, and remove dentures

_____ assist patient to rinse mouth

_____ remove and discard gloves, wash hands, and document

_____ place washcloth in sink or basin and fill with water

_____ inspect dentures and oral mucosa

_____ replace in patient's mouth or store dentures

_____ rinse the dentures with tap water

_____ scrub dentures one at a time

■ Multiple Choice

Circle the best answer for each of the following questions.

1. At which degree angle should the nurse instruct a patient to hold a toothbrush against the gum line?
   a. 15
   b. 30
   c. 45
   d. 90

2. Which of the following actions should the nurse take if a patient constantly removes his or her dentures?
   a. Ask family members to take dentures home
   b. Inform the physician
   c. Inspect the mouth for irritated areas
   d. Place the dentures in water in a denture cup.

3. A patient is using a toothpick to remove cerumen from his ear. Which of the following instructions is appropriate?
   a. Inform the patient that ear wax should not be removed and protects the ear canal
   b. Instruct patient to stop using a toothpick in the ear to prevent injury
   c. Teach patient to use alcohol on a washcloth to remove the wax
   d. Warn patient to use a Q-tip instead of a sharp toothpick.

4. For which of the following patients could the nurse safely cut his or her toenails?
   a. A newborn
   b. Patient with hemophilia
   c. Patient with diabetes
   d. Healthy adult

5. Which technique can be used to prevent pulling of the hair when brushing?
   a. Comb through hair with your fingers before brushing
   b. Hold lock firmly and leave slack between hand and head
   c. Use only a pick
   d. Use slow gently strokes with a comb

6. The nurse knows that foot soaks should:
   a. be completed after the bedbath.
   b. be completed daily for patients with diabetes.
   c. use hot water for very short periods of time.
   d. use warm water and last 10 to 20 minutes.

7. Which of the following indicates that the patient needs further instruction about the purpose of bathing?
   a. "Baths remove sweat."
   b. "Baths refresh me."
   c. "I must shower daily to be healthy."
   d. "Taking a bath increases circulation."

8. Which of the following would be an appropriate bath for a patient who is comatose?
   a. Complete bed bath
   b. Partial bed bath
   c. Shower using a shower chair
   d. Towel bath

9. Which of the following correctly describes the method for cutting toenails?
   a. Cut straight across
   b. Cut straight across and round the corners
   c. Cut straight with a "V" in the center
   d. Cut toenails in a rounded shape

CHAPTER 51

Elimination

■ Terminology Review

Match the following definitions with the correct terms.

1. _____ stones
2. _____ desire or sensation of needing to void immediately
3. _____ amount of urine is less than 100 mL/day
4. _____ passing urine from the body
5. _____ latex or vinyl tube whose purpose is to remove urine
6. _____ involuntary voiding in bed
7. _____ inflammation of the bladder
8. _____ painful urination
9. _____ inability to empty the bladder of urine
10. _____ voiding more often that usual without an increase in volume
11. _____ penetrating pain in the lower back
12. _____ increase amount of urine voided over a period of time
13. _____ voiding during the night
14. _____ decrease in the expected amount of urine a person excretes
15. _____ gentle pressure applied to the bladder to assist in bladder emptying

a. anuria
b. calculi
c. Crede's maneuver
d. cystitis
e. dysuria
f. enuresis
g. frequency
h. micturition
i. nocturia
j. oliguria
k. polyuria
l. renal colic
m. retention
n. urgency
o. urinary catheter

Match the following definitions with the correct terms.

16. _____ excretion of feces
17. _____ stomach contents
18. _____ intestinal gas
19. _____ digested blood in the stools
20. _____ expulsion of loose, watery, unformed stools
21. _____ body's solid waste product
22. _____ involuntary action that expels stomach contents
23. _____ straight-back chair with an open seat and a receptacle beneath
24. _____ involuntary loss of urine from the bladder
25. _____ introduction of a solution into the rectum and colon to stimulate peristalsis that empties the bowel of stool
26. _____ hard dry stools resulting from the rectum not being emptied for some time and excess liquid has been absorbed
27. _____ stool that is so hard and dry or putty-like that it cannot be expelled by the patient
28. _____ emesis expelled with great force

a. commode
b. constipation
c. defecation
d. diarrhea
e. emesis
f. enema
g. fecal impaction
h. feces
i. flatus
j. incontinence
k. melena
l. projectile
m. vomitus

■ Acronym Review

Match the following definitions with the acronyms.

1. _____ inserted into the bladder by way of surgical incision through the abdominal wall to the bladder to remove urine

2. _____ as needed

3. _____ measurement of fluids that enter and leave the body

4. _____ most common type of cleansing enema

5. _____ bowel movement

6. _____ noise produced from peristaltic movement

7. _____ infection in the urinary tract system

8. _____ bathroom privileges

9. _____ type of cleansing enema that uses a soap solution

a. BM
b. BRP
c. BS
d. I & O
e. PRN
f. SP
g. SSE
h. TWE
i. UTI

■ Assessment Review

Indicate if the following assessment findings are normal (N) or abnormal (A) findings.

1. _____ output > input
2. _____ colorless urine
3. _____ transparent urine
4. _____ aromatic urine
5. _____ void of 250 mL
6. _____ dysuria
7. _____ incontinence
8. _____ urgency
9. _____ yellowish brown feces
10. _____ gray-colored stool
11. _____ melena
12. _____ stools that float
13. _____ bowel sounds q 10 seconds
14. _____ hard abdomen
15. _____ bowel sounds in all quadrants
16. _____ projectile vomiting
17. _____ pus in stool
18. _____ urinary catheter
19. _____ afebrile
20. _____ soft formed stool

■ Sequencing

Number the following actions in the correct order for administering an enema. The first action should be number 1. Continue to number the items.

_____ wash hands and document procedure

_____ apply the clamp and remove the rectal tube when the enema is completed; ask patient to retain solution

_____ place a waterproof pad under the patient's buttocks

_____ separate the patient's buttocks and gently insert the rectal tube 3 to 4 inches toward the umbilicus

_____ assist the patient into the bathroom or onto the bedpan with the head of bed elevated

_____ place the enema bag on the IV pole or raise the container 18 inches above the patient's anus

_____ return the patient to a comfortable position

_____ assist patient onto the left side with right knee flexed

_____ prepare the enema, wash hands, and apply gloves

_____ hold the tube in place with one hand while opening the clamp with the other hand, allowing the solution to flow into the rectum

_____ close the curtain or door to the room

Number the following actions in the correct order for removing impacted feces. The first action should be number 1. Continue to number the items.

_____ assist patient to bathroom, commode, or bedpan; leave signal cord in reach

_____ drape patient, place waterproof pad under buttocks, and instruct patient

_____ before removing your finger, gently stimulate the anal sphincter with a rotating motion

_____ document procedure and results

_____ wash hands, apply gloves, explain procedure, and position patient on left side.

_____ dispose of gloves and wash hands

_____ lubricate fingers, insert into rectum, and rotate finger to break up stool

Number the following actions in the correct order for giving and removing a bedpan. The first action should be number 1. Continue to number the items.

_____ assist patient onto the bedpan

_____ place call light and toilet tissue within patient's reach and leave patient alone

_____ explain procedure, wash hands, put on gloves, and provide privacy

_____ cleanse area with soap and water if necessary

_____ wash hands, put on gloves, and wipe patient from front to back; remove the bedpan

_____ remove gloves, wash hands, and document

_____ replace line over patient, elevate head of bed

_____ raise bed to comfortable height, fold linen away from patient to expose as little of patient as possible.

■ Case Study

Maria Ortez, a 79-year-old female, was admitted to your long-term care facility one month ago. She was continent of urine and stool when she was admitted. Since admission, she been incontinent of urine and the staff has been using incontinent pads continuously. Mrs. Ortez is sitting in her room with you and tells you that she doesn't know what has happened to make her incontinent. All laboratory results are normal, as well as her vital signs.

1. What additional information would you like to have regarding this patient?

2. As the nurse talks with Mrs. Ortez, she finds out that the patient is experiencing urgency. She has stated that staff do not usually assist her quick enough to get to the bathroom on time, so she has just given up trying. Outline a plan of care as well as teaching for Mrs. Ortez and staff.

■ Multiple Choice

Circle the best answer for each of the following questions.

1. A patient is complaining of nausea. In which position should the nurse place the patient?
   a. Prone
   b. Right side
   c. Sim's
   d. Supine

2. When preparing a cleansing enema, how much solution should the nurse use for an adult patient?

   a. 100 to 300 mL

   b. 400 to 600 mL

   c. 750 to 1,000 mL

   d. 1,500 mL

3. A patient with a urinary catheter is complaining of lower abdominal cramping. The nurses first action should be:

   a. check the tubing for kinks and placement.

   b. encourage the patient to ambulate.

   c. medicate with an analgesic.

   d. notify the physician or team leader.

4. When auscultating the bowel sounds, which technique is correct?

   a. Listen for audible bowel sounds

   b. Use either the bell or diaphragm of the stethoscope

   c. Use the bell of the stethoscope

   d. Use the diaphragm of the stethoscope

5. A patient is admitted with renal calculi. It is most important for the nurse to put which item in the patient's room?

   a. Bedpan

   b. Catheter

   c. Extra pillows

   d. Urine strainer

6. Your patient had the following data for your shift: broth—200 cc; Jello—120 cc; water—50 cc and 150 cc; voided—200 cc, 150 cc, and 100 cc; emesis—100 cc. You would record the I & O as:

   a. Intake 620 mL and output 450 mL.

   b. Intake 520 mL and output 450 mL.

   c. Intake 520 mL and output 550 mL.

   d. Intake 620 mL and output 550 mL.

7. Which of the following enemas should be retained by the patient?

   a. Medicated enema

   b. Normal saline enema

   c. Soap suds enema

   d. Tap water enema

8. You have just administered an enema to your patient. The patient complains of not being able to expel the enema. What action would you take?

   a. Allow more time for the patient to expel the enema

   b. Encourage the patient to breathe deeply and relax

   c. Instruct the patient to wipe rectum to stimulate removal of enema

   d. Withdrawn the solution with the rectal tube

CHAPTER 52

Specimen Collection

■ Terminology Review

Match the following definitions with the correct terms.

1. _____ method used to collect a sputum specimen

2. _____ hidden blood

3. _____ measurement to determine the concentration of urine

4. _____ test used to detect the presence of occult blood in the stool

5. _____ using a needle to withdraw blood from a vein

6. _____ laboratory test that determines the specific components of urine

7. _____ another name for a hydrometer

8. _____ a person's fluid intake and fluid output for a 24-hour period

9. _____ tests referred to as guaiac tests

10. _____ device that measures urine specific gravity

a. expectorate
b. guaiac
c. Hemoccult and Hematest
d. hydrometer
e. intake and output
f. occult
g. specific gravity
h. urinalysis
i. urinometer
j. venipuncture

Match the following definitions with the correct acronyms.

11. _____ nasogastric

12. _____ as needed

13. _____ intake and output

14. _____ number that indicates whether a substance is acidic or alkaline

15. _____ gastrointestinal

16. _____ identifies the disease-causing organism and what medications will kill or arrest the growth of the organism

17. _____ milliliters

18. _____ urine volume and specific gravity

19. _____ ova and parasites

20. _____ cubic centimeters

21. _____ intravenous

22. _____ nonsteroidal anti-inflammatory drug

a. cc
b. C & S
c. GI
d. I & O
e. IV
f. mL
g. NG
h. NSAID
i. O & P
j. pH
k. PRN
l. V & S

■ Sequencing

Number the following actions in the correct order for collecting a urine specimen from a retention catheter. The first action should be number 1. Continue to number the items.

_____ Unclamp the catheter and prepare container for transport to laboratory.

_____ Cleanse the aspiration port with alcohol prep or a povidone-iodine (Betadine) swab.

_____ Gather supplies, explain procedure, wash hands, and put on gloves.

_____ Dispose of used equipment.

_____ Clamp drainage tube for 15 minutes or less.

_____ Send specimen to the laboratory immediately and document appropriately.

_____ Insert needle into aspiration port and withdraw urine into the syringe.

Number the following actions in the correct order for collecting a stool specimen. The first action should be number 1. Continue to number the items.

_____ Give bedpan when client is ready.

_____ Take container immediately to the laboratory.

_____ Remove the bedpan, use a tongue blade to transfer stool from three different areas into the container.

_____ Maintain body substance precautions, explain procedure, and label container.

_____ Cover container, remove and discard gloves, and wash hands.

■ Multiple Choice

Circle the best answer.

1. Which measure, if used by the nurse, would be most effective in preventing the transmission of disease when obtaining specimens?
   a. Attach laboratory cards to each specimen.
   b. Instruct client to take specimen to the laboratory.
   c. Label each specimen container.
   d. Place all specimens in leak-proof containers.

2. When teaching a client to prepare for a guaiac stool specimen, it is most important to tell the client to:
   a. avoid smoking before the test.
   b. bring a family member to drive you home from the test.
   c. do not take aspirin for 3 days before the test.
   d. drink plenty of fluids for 3 days before the test.

3. When measuring urine output, which method should the nurse use to measure urine output correctly?
   a. Fill beaker with urine and measure meniscus at eye level.
   b. Insert a Foley catheter before each void.
   c. Record amount of urine in the toilet hat.
   d. Teach the client how to measure urine in the toilet hat.

4. At the end of the 24-hour urine collection, the nurse should:
   a. instruct client to void and discard this urine.
   b. instruct client to void and include this in the specimen.
   c. take the specimen to the laboratory at the end of the shift.
   d. take the last specimen to the laboratory in a biohazard bag.

5. To obtain a clean-catch urine specimen, the male client should be instructed to:
   a. cleanse the penis using a circular motion outward from the urethral meatus.
   b. cleanse the penis using downward strokes starting at the urethra meatus.
   c. void the last stream of the urine into the sterile cup.
   d. wear gloves when collecting the specimen.

6. A client had a 240-mL cup of ice chips, 120 mL of coffee, and a 4-ounce cup of juice. The client voided 250 mL at noon and vomited 120 mL in the emesis basin a 2 pm. Calculate the intake and output for this client.
   a. Intake: 364 mL; output: 370 mL
   b. Intake: 360 mL; output: 250 mL
   c. Intake: 360 mL; output: 370 mL
   d. Intake: 480 mL; output: 120 mL

7. Which of the following would be recorded as intake for a client?

    a. Emesis of 200 mL

    b. Intravenous fluid of 1,000 mL

    c. Nasogastric fluid of 25 mL

    d. Urine of 500 mL

8. Which of the following urine specific gravity measurements indicates the most dilute urine?

    a. 1.010

    b. 1.019

    c. 1.020

    d. 1.025

9. When is the best time to collect a sputum specimen?

    a. In the morning soon after the client awakens

    b. In the early afternoon

    c. Before the evening meal

    d. Before hours of sleep

CHAPTER 53

Bandages and Binders

■ Terminology Review

Match the following definitions with the correct terms and acronyms.

1. _____ abbreviation for antiembolism stockings

2. _____ most commonly used bandage

3. _____ binder used to hold perineal or rectal dressings in place

4. _____ gauze dressing used to hold dressings in place

5. _____ all-cotton elastic bandage

6. _____ skin softening and breakdown due to moisture accumulation and lack of circulation

7. _____ assessment of color, motion, and sensitivity

8. _____ stockings used postoperatively to ensure adequate return circulation and to prevent blood clots

9. _____ used with frequent dressing changes

a. ACE bandage
b. antiembolism stockings
c. Kerlix
d. maceration
e. Montgomery straps
f. T-binder
g. ACE
h. CMS
i. TED

■ Sequencing

Number the following actions in the correct order for applying Montgomery straps. The first action should be number 1. Continue to number the items.

_____ Document procedure and condition of the wound.

_____ Secure the ends of the straps with ties across the dressing.

_____ Wash hands, apply gloves, and use Standard Precautions.

_____ Cut holes into the ends of the straps if the adhesive-backed strip does not contain them.

_____ Cover the incision with the dressing.

_____ Use premade products or make straps with tape for both sides of the dressing.

_____ Untie straps for dressing changes. Leave in place until soiled, need to be changed, or discontinued.

Number the following actions in the correct order for applying antiembolism stockings. The first action should be number 1. Continue to number the items.

_____ Instruct the client to report any extreme discomfort.

_____ Grasp the stocking's heel and turn it inside out.

_____ Apply a small amount of talcum powder to the client's feet and legs if not contraindicated.

_____ Explain procedure, determine stocking size for client, and gather supplies.

_____ Support the client' ankle and ease the stocking smoothly over the calf and remainder of the leg.

_____ Slip the client's foot, toes, and heel into the stocking. Center heel and slide over the foot.

_____ Pull forward slightly on the stocking's toe section.

_____ Remove gloves and wash hands. Document procedure.

_____ Wash hands, wear gloves if needed, and assist client to supine position.

■ Correct the False Statements

Circle the word True or False that follows the statement. If the word false has been circled, change the underlined word/words to make the statement true. Place your answer in the space provided.

1. The purpose of a bandage is <u>to give support or to hold dressings in place</u>.

   True   False   _____

2. A <u>bandage</u> must be checked to make sure it is not too tight or too loose.

   True   False   _____

3. Gentle pressure of a bandage against tissues <u>promotes healing</u>.

   True   False   _____

4. When ACE bandages are in place, CMS checks should be <u>completed every 4 hours.</u>

   True   False   _____

5. A <u>binder</u> is a wide, flat piece of fabric that is applied to support a specific body part or to hold a dressing in place.

   True   False   _____

6. T-binders are used to <u>support the arm</u>.

   True   False   _____

7. A abdominal binder may be used <u>after abdominal surgery or childbirth</u>.

   True   False   _____

8. Tape <u>should never be used</u> to give support to sprained ankles.

   True   False   _____

9. <u>Ace bandages</u> help prevent skin irritation by maintaining skin integrity with frequent dressing changes.

   True   False   _____

10. When completing CMS checks on an extremity, it is normal for the skin <u>to remain lighter when touched</u>.

    True   False   _____

■ Multiple Choice

Circle the best answer.

1. When using acetone to remove tape adhesive, which precaution should the nurse take?
   a. Avoid pulling the hair with removal of tape.
   b. Avoid slow movements; pull tape off quickly.
   c. Never use acetone on an open wound.
   d. Never use acetone on the client's skin.

2. Which roller bandage width would be appropriate for an average adult client's extremity?
   a. 1/2 inch
   b. 2 inch
   c. 5 inch
   d. 8 inch

3. When applying a roller bandage to an upper extremity, which technique should the nurse use?
   a. Wrap from the fingers to the shoulder.
   b. Wrap from the hip to the toes.
   c. Wrap from the shoulder to the fingers.
   d. Wrap from the toes to the hip.

4. A roller bandage should be released every 4 hours (unless contraindicated) to:

   a. ensure that the proper size of bandage is used.

   b. examine for color, motion, and sensitivity.

   c. prevent the area from becoming macerated.

   d. prevent deformities and discomfort.

5. A client has a bandage on the arm. When the nurse presses a client's hand, an imprint remains. Which action is most appropriate?

   a. Apply ice to the arm.

   b. Notify RN or MD.

   c. Restrict fluid intake.

   d. Take the client's temperature.

CHAPTER 54

Heat and Cold Application

Terminology Review

Match the following definitions with the correct terms and acronyms.

1. _____ while awake
2. _____ method of applying deep, penetrating heat to muscles and tissues
3. _____ penetrating type of dry heat rays
4. _____ its purpose is to apply heat to the pelvic area
5. _____ ultrasound
6. _____ ultraviolet rays
7. _____ type of dry heat by flowing temperature-controlled distilled water through a waterproof pad
8. _____ flat, oval, rubber bag with a leak-proof, screw-in top
9. _____ type of rays that are not as penetrating dry heat as infrared rays
10. _____ a plastic mattress pad through which very cold water flows continuously
11. _____ infrared rays
12. _____ type of bath used to reduce a client's elevated temperature

a. aquathermia pad
b. hypothermia blanket
c. icecap
d. infrared rays
e. sitz bath
f. tepid sponge
g. ultrasound
h. ultraviolet rays
i. IR
j. US
k. UV
l. WA

Application of Heat and Cold Therapy

Indicate whether the following rules or guidelines for application are for heat (H) or cold (C) therapy.

1. _____ Used to slow or stop bleeding.
2. _____ Prolonged exposure to extreme levels may cause frostbite.
3. _____ Promotes drainage (draws infected materials out of wounds).
4. _____ Relieves local pain or aching, particularly of muscles or joints.
5. _____ Often applied to a sprain, strain, or fracture to help remove blood and lymph congestion.
6. _____ Used to control pain and fluid loss in the initial treatment of burns.
7. _____ Raises the body's temperature.
8. _____ Used to relive pain in an engorged breast.
9. _____ Assists in wound healing.
10. _____ Can be used to loosen scabs and crusts from encrusted wounds.

Fill-in-the-Blank

Complete the following statements by filling in the blanks.

1. Cold application prevents escape of heat from the body by _____ circulation, which also relieves _____ and often relieves muscle pain.

2. When using cold, moist compresses, wring the compress thoroughly and _____ compresses frequently.

3. Fill an icecap about _____ full using small pieces of ice to help the bag fit close to the body.

4. When applying a warm compress to the eye, wash your hands and wear _____ to prevent infecting the eye.

5. Apply _____ _____ to the client's skin before applying a warm, moist compress.

6. A warm compress or pack is covered with a dry, moisture-proof cover to insulate against _____ _____ and _____ .

7. Cold humidity is often ordered for clients who have _____ difficulties.

8. When giving a tepid sponge bath, place moist cool, cloths in the client's _____ and on the _____ because blood vessels lie close to the skin in these areas.

9. After providing a whirlpool bath, the tub should be _____ to prevent the spread of disease.

10. A heat lamp should be used by a person trained to use the lamp and only with a _____ _____ .

Nursing Actions

Indicate whether the following actions are appropriate (A) or inappropriate (I).

1. _____ When giving a tepid sponge bath, use alcohol to bring down an elevated temperature quickly.

2. _____ Give clients who are receiving radiation therapy or chemotherapy warm compresses or hot packs for a longer period of time because these clients need extra warmth for comfort.

3. _____ Before applying an electric heating pad, connect it to an electric outlet and turn the heating switch to high to see whether the pad heats promptly.

4. _____ Inspect the skin of a client receiving heat therapy frequently to prevent burning.

5. _____ Apply a cold pack to an ankle that was sprained 24 hours ago to reduce the swelling that is present.

6. _____ Set the temperature no higher than 105°F when giving a tub soak.

7. _____ Change cold compresses every hour.

8. _____ Provide a tepid sponge bath for a client with cardiovascular disease.

9. _____ Discontinue a sponge bath when the client begins to shiver.

10. _____ Assess a client's skin at least every 30 minutes when receiving a warm, moist compress.

11. _____ Remove cold therapy if a client's skin looks white or spotty.

CHAPTER 55

Client Comfort and Pain Management

■ Terminology Review

Match the following definitions with the correct terms.

1. _____ normal pain transmission, which has four phases

2. _____ lowest intensity of a stimulus that causes the subject to recognize pain

3. _____ process through which a client receives a suggestion that helps control pain

4. _____ another name for acute pain

5. _____ another name for chronic pain

6. _____ chronic pain that resists therapeutic interventions

7. _____ sensation that results abruptly and lasts for 6 months or less

8. _____ feelings that one experiences by listening to his/her body rhythm

9. _____ denotes the point at which a person can no longer tolerate pain

10. _____ pain that continues for a period of 6 months or longer and interferes with a person's normal functioning

11. _____ medications that relieve pain

12. _____ substances produced by the central nervous system that help control pain perception

a. acute pain
b. analgesics
c. chronic pain
d. cue
e. endorphins
f. guided imagery
g. intractable
h. neuropathic pain

i. nociception
j. nociceptive pain
k. pain threshold
l. pain tolerance

Match the following definitions with the correct terms.

13. _____ method that allows clients to administer their own analgesics

14. _____ nonsteroidal anti-inflammatory drugs

15. _____ agency that states a client's self-report of pain is the single best indicator of pain

16. _____ transcutaneous electrical nerve stimulation

17. _____ organization that requires healthcare facilities to use a pain scale to help clients determine their level of pain

a. AHCPR
b. JCAHO
c. NSAIDs
d. PCA
e. TENS

■ Nursing Actions

Indicate whether the following actions by a nurse would be appropriate (A) or inappropriate (I).

1. _____ Encourage a client with chronic pain to withdraw from social activities because the stimulation might cause increased discomfort.

2. _____ Explain to clients that acute pain is short term and disappears once the underlying cause is identified and treated.

3. _____ Help a client with chronic pain set goals and target dates to gain control over one part of his or her life at a time to reduce the sense of loss of control that aggravates pain.

4. _____ Encourage the client with chronic pain to join a support group and bond with family when pain is intense.

5. _____ Give pain medication when pain is most intense so that endorphins are present to help the analgesics work more effectively.

6. _____ Tell the client at 2 weeks after surgery that there should be no pain at this time so what the client is experiencing is probably a memory of previous real pain.

7. _____ Provide a back rub to help relax the client.

■ Correct the False Statements

Circle the word True or False that follows the statement. If the word false has been circled, change the underlined word/words to make the statement true. Place your answer in the space provided.

1. Transmission involves the brain recognizing, defining, and responding to pain.

   True   False   _____

2. Physical causes of pain include trauma, injury, surgical incision, and tumor growth.

   True   False   _____

3. Muscle spasms can cause pain because of engorgement of tissues.

   True   False   _____

4. Acute pain results from the nervous system's normal processing of trauma to the skin, muscles, and visceral organs.

   True   False   _____

5. Clients with nociceptive pain report burning, tingling sensations and shooting pain.

   True   False   _____

6. Anticonvulsants and antidepressants can help improve a client's mood, thus assisting with muscle relaxation and pain control.

   True   False   _____

7. Pain medication should be given prior to painful procedures.

   True   False   _____

8. Nurses can help provide client comfort by positioning the client comfortably and ensuring proper nutrition.

   True   False   _____

9. Vigorous massage may relieve congestion and promote circulation and oxygenation and thus help relieve pain.

   True   False   _____

10. Applying heat and cold is a nonpharmocologic technique proven to help relieve pain.

   True   False   _____

11. Client and family teaching should focus on relieving pain when it becomes severe.

   True   False   _____

■ Multiple Choice

Circle the best answer.

1. Which of the following symptoms experienced by a client with chronic pain would require a referral?
   a. Lack of interest in surroundings
   b. Periods of pain
   c. Sleeps 8 hours every night
   d. Stable weight

2. Which of the following may decrease endorphin production?
   a. Exercise and laughter
   b. Fruits and vegetables
   c. Nicotine and alcohol
   d. Social activities

3. Which of the following statements by the client would indicate that further instruction is needed?

   a. "I should administer medications as prescribed."

   b. "I should change my position frequently when lying in bed."

   c. "I should practice guided imagery to help control my pain."

   d. "I should request pain medication when my pain becomes unbearable."

4. Which of the following is an example of passive relaxation?

   a. Deep breathing

   b. Exercise

   c. Sewing

   d. Traveling

5. Which assessment data relates most directly to pain?

   a. Blood pressure 120/80 mmHg

   b. Dilated pupils

   c. Pulse 80 beats/min

   d. Respirations 14/min

CHAPTER 56

Preoperative and Postoperative Care

■ Terminology Review

Match the following definitions with the correct terms.

1. _____ opening or separation of the surgical incision

2. _____ complete or partial loss of sensation

3. _____ occurs when a piece of clot or thrombus breaks off and enters the person's circulatory system

4. _____ phase of surgical nursing when the client is in the operating room and postanesthesia care unit

5. _____ collapse of a portion of the lung caused by mucous plugs that close the bronchi

6. _____ inadequate oxygen

7. _____ type of surgery that is optional for the client to have done

8. _____ lowered body temperature after surgery

9. _____ type of process by which an incision is made into the body or part is removed

10. _____ edges of the surgical wound separate and the abdominal organs protrude

a. anesthesia
b. atelectasis
c. dehiscence
d. elective surgery
e. emboli
f. evisceration
g. hypothermia (postoperative)
h. hypoxia
i. intraoperative
j. invasive

Match the following definitions with the correct terms.

11. _____ supporting the operative area with a pillow, folded bath towel, or blanket during coughing

12. _____ material used to close a surgical wound

13. _____ after surgery

14. _____ formation of a blood clot in a vein

15. _____ time before surgery

16. _____ heparin or saline lock

17. _____ urinalysis

18. _____ time span that includes preparation for, process of, and recovery from surgery

19. _____ consists of temperature, pulse, and respirations

20. _____ inflammation of the lungs

21. _____ measurements of the client's basic body functioning

a. perioperative
b. pneumonia
c. postoperative
d. preoperative
e. splinting
f. suture
g. thrombophlebitis
h. venous access lock
i. TPR
j. UA
k. VS

Match the following definitions with the correct terms.

22. _____ electrocardiogram

23. _____ postanesthesia care unit

24. _____ complete blood count

25. _____ intake and output

26. _____ operating room

27. _____ diet as tolerated

28. _____ intravenous

29. _____ turn, cough, and deep breathe

30. _____ postanesthesia recovery

31. _____ recovery room

32. _____ oxygen saturation

33. _____ blood pressure

34. _____ nothing by mouth

a. BP

b. CBC

c. DAT

d. ECG

e. I & O

f. IV

g. NPO

h. O$_2$ sat.

i. OR

j. PACU

k. PAR

l. RR

m. TCDB

■ Nursing Actions

Indicate whether the following actions by a nurse would be appropriate (A) or inappropriate (I) when receiving the preoperative client in the nursing unit.

1. _____ Ensure that the surgical consent is signed before surgery.

2. _____ Arrange for preoperative client to speak with spiritual advisor.

3. _____ Instruct client on preoperative procedures before surgery and wait to teach about the postoperative after surgery.

4. _____ Obtain CXR, CBC, UA, and ECG results before surgery.

5. _____ Instruct the client to cleanse the skin using an antibacterial soap.

6. _____ Instruct the client to remain NPO for 24 hours before surgery.

7. _____ Encourage ambulation after administration of preoperative medications.

8. _____ Note on the front of the chart any drug allergies or if client is taking cortisone, insulin, an anticonvulsant, or an anticoagulant.

9. _____ On receiving a client from the PACU after surgery, keep the client flat, often in Sims' position, until he or she awakens.

10. _____ Clamp all tubes and drains before the PACU nurse leaves your unit.

11. _____ Carry out any orders for immediate drug or oxygen administration.

12. _____ If vomiting occurs, turn the client's head to the side.

13. _____ If the client is receiving IV fluids from the PACU, discontinue infusions and give the client clear liquids to maintain hydration.

■ Correct the False Statements

Circle the word True or False that follows the statement. If the word false has been circled, change the underlined word/words to make the statement true. Place your answer in the space provided.

1. An example of a <u>nonelective surgery</u> is a hernia repair.

   True   False   _____

2. An <u>urgent surgery</u> must be performed immediately to save the client's life.

   True   False   _____

3. <u>Halothane (Fluothane)</u> is commonly used as an inhalation anesthetic.

   True   False   _____

4. During the first stage of analgesia, the heart rate and blood pressure <u>rise rapidly</u>.

   True   False   _____

5. During the forth stage of anesthesia, <u>no flexes are present and pupils are widely dilated</u>.

   True   False   _____

6. A common concern for many preoperative clients is <u>fear of pain</u>.

   True   False   _____

7. An electrocardiogram is usually obtained for <u>all clients older than 20 years of age</u> before surgery.

   True   False   _____

8. Three types of medication used preoperatively are <u>sedatives, narcotics, and drying agents</u>.

   True   False   _____

9. Immediate postoperative complications include <u>paralytic ileus and infection</u>.

   True   False   _____

10. <u>Early postoperative ambulation</u> helps prevent lung congestion and improves respiration and circulation.

    True   False   _____

■ Case Study

You are arriving at work at 1400 on the surgical unit. You have just received the following information about your clients:

   Mr. J has just returned from OR 2 hours ago. His vital signs are TPR-97, 96, 8 and BP 112/60. His VS are scheduled to be taken in 15 minutes.

   Mr. M had abdominal surgery 2 days ago and is complaining of abdominal gas pains.

   Mrs. P returned from surgery at 1000 today for repair of hip fracture. The CNA reports that the sequential machine is not working properly.

   Mrs. H had surgery yesterday and wants her Foley catheter removed.

How would you prioritize you care? Provide rationale for your actions.

■ Multiple Choice

Circle the best answer.

1. A client has just returned from surgery. After assessing the client, the nurse determines that the client has active reflexes, increased heart rate, irregular breathing, increased BP, pupils widely dilated and divergent. The nurse recognizes that the client is in which stage of general anesthesia?

   a. Stage of analgesia/amnesia

   b. Stage of dreams and excitement

   c. Stage of surgical anesthesia

   d. Stage of toxic or extreme depression

2. A 79-year-old man is scheduled for surgery. He has a history of smoking for the past 60 years, weighs 50 lb more than desired weight, and has a large family who will be at the hospital. Which factors place the client at risk for surgery?

   a. Age, weight, and use of chemicals

   b. Large family places the client at risk for excessive stimulation postoperatively.

   c. Psychological status places client at risk for excessive fear and dementia.

   d. Weight only

3. During the preoperative period, the nurse would explain which of the following?

   a. Directly before the operation, the nurse will see that all blood samples have been collected and sent to the laboratory.

   b. On admission, the client is asked to void, and this information is documented on the front of the chart.

   c. Directly before the operation, the client will need to remove dentures and glasses.

   d. Showering before surgery will not need to be done if the client has bathed in the past 24 hours.

4. Which of the following represents an immediate postoperative complication and the appropriate nursing action to address it?

   a. Constipation, which should be treated with a stool softener such as docusate (Surfak)

   b. Hypoxia, which is treated by administering oxygen by nasal cannula or mask if necessary

   c. Nausea, which would be treated with sips of cool fluid and an antiemetic such as Compazine

   d. Urinary retention, which should be monitored and the client catheterized if not resolved

5. Which of the following medications when used as an anesthetic agent during conscious sedation helps produce an amnesic effect after surgery?

   a. etomidate (Amidate)

   b. fentanyl citrate with droperidol (Innovar)

   c. midazolam HCl (Versed)

   d. propofol (Diprivan)

6. Which of the following would a nurse expect to complete before surgery for a client undergoing abdominal surgery?

   a. Enema

   b. Heart monitor

   c. NG tube with irrigation

   d. Urinary catheterization

7. A drying agent is given preoperatively to:

   a. decrease mucus production.

   b. relax the client.

   c. sedate the client.

   d. stabilize blood pressure.

8. Which team member assists the surgeon with sterile instruments during surgery?

   a. Anesthesiologist

   b. Circulating assistant

   c. Circulating nurse

   d. Scrub nurse

9. A client has an indwelling urinary catheter post-operatively. The nurse notices that the urine out-put has been 100 mL over the past hour. The nurse should:

   a. continue to monitor urinary output.

   b. determine whether the catheter is patent.

   c. notify the physician immediately.

   d. remove the catheter.

10. Which of the following assessment findings in a postoperative client are signs of shock?

    a. Brisk capillary refill

    b. Normal oxygen saturation

    c. No signs of cyanosis

    d. Rapid pulse

CHAPTER 57

Surgical Asepsis

■ Terminology Review

Match the following definitions with the correct terms and acronyms.

1. _____ is used to obtain one urine sample only and then is removed

2. _____ technique used to maintain sterility

3. _____ item that is free of all microorganisms and spores

4. _____ central sterile supply

5. _____ process of exposing articles to heat or to chemical disinfectants long enough to kill all microorganisms or spores

6. _____ many or most harmful microorganisms have been removed

7. _____ an example is a Foley

8. _____ object that was clean or sterile before it touched a dirty object

9. _____ central supply room

10. _____ synonymous with sterile technique

11. _____ pressure steam sterilizer

12. _____ any object or person that has not been cleaned or sterilized for removal of microorganisms

13. _____ destruction of most pathogens, but not spores

14. _____ remains inside the bladder

a. autoclave
b. clean
c. contaminated
d. dirty
e. disinfection
f. indwelling catheter
g. retention catheter
h. sterile
i. sterile technique
j. sterilization
k. straight catheter
l. surgical asepsis
m. CSR
n. CSS

■ Correct the False Statements

Circle the word True or False that follows the statement. If the word false has been circled, change the underlined word/words to make the statement true. Place your answer in the space provided.

1. Medical asepsis is used when changing dressings, administering parenteral medications, and performing surgical procedures.

   True   False   _____

2. Boiling for 10 minutes destroys most but not all organisms.

   True   False   _____

3. Chemical disinfectants powerful enough to destroy germs can be used on plastic.

   True   False   _____

4. Radiation and gas sterilization <u>do not</u> destroy spores.

   True   False   _____

5. When applying a sterile gown, touch only <u>the inside of the gown</u>.

   True   False   _____

6. Below the waist level and <u>above the neck</u> are considered contaminated when wearing a sterile gown.

   True   False   _____

7. Generally, no more than <u>1,500 to 2,000 mL</u> of urine should be removed from the bladder at any one time.

   True   False   _____

8. Sterile to <u>sterile</u> remains sterile.

   True   False   _____

9. The first step in opening a sterile package is to <u>open the flap toward you</u>.

   True   False   _____

10. Touching contaminated items with sterile gloves makes the gloves <u>contaminated</u>.

   True   False   _____

■ Sequencing

Number the following actions in the correct order for putting on sterile gloves. The first action should be number 1. Continue to number the items.

_____ Use your nondominant hand to grasp the inside upper surface of the glove's cuff for your dominant hand.

_____ Slip the fingers of your sterile gloved hand under (inside) the cuff of the remaining glove while keeping your thumb pointed outward.

_____ Open the outer glove package on a clean, dry, flat surface at waist level or higher.

_____ Insert you nondominant hand into the glove.

_____ Insert your dominant hand into the glove, placing your thumb and fingers in the proper openings.

Number the following actions in the correct order for catheterizing a female client with an indwelling catheter. The first action should be number 1. Continue to number the items.

_____ Ensure adequate lighting.

_____ Open lubricant and apply to catheter's tip for 1 to 2 inches.

_____ Dry the client's perineal area, remove gloves, reposition client and bed. Dispose of equipment.

_____ With your dominant hand use the forceps and cleanse the labial folds front to back.

_____ Provide privacy and adjust bed height.

_____ Advance the catheter another 1 to 2 inches.

_____ Wash hands and document type of catheter and client's response.

_____ Set up equipment on the tray, opening antiseptic and pouring it over the cotton balls.

_____ Spread the labia using your nondominant hand to expose the urinary meatus.

_____ Explain the procedure, check physician's order, and wash hands.

_____ Put on clean gloves, wash and rinse the woman's perineal area with soap. Wash hands again.

_____ Attach prefilled syringe and check balloon.

_____ Secure catheter and position bag below bladder level.

_____ Move catheterization tray with equipment onto the sterile drape between the client's thighs.

_____ Open the sterile catheterization tray on the bedside table. Apply sterile gloves and position sterile drape under edge of buttocks.

_____ Have client breathe deeply, and advance the catheter until urine begins to drain.

CHAPTER 58

Wound Care

■ Terminology Review

Match the following definitions with the correct terms.

1. _____ drainage

2. _____ sterile moist dressing that is left in place until dry and then removed, causing débridement of the wound

3. _____ torn, ragged edges

4. _____ also called pressure ulcers

5. _____ the end result of constant skin pressure; also called bed sores or decubitus

6. _____ lack of blood supply

7. _____ wound with clean, intentional edges

8. _____ removal of infected tissues or tissue debris

9. _____ abnormal opening in the skin

10. _____ eschar that separates from living tissue

11. _____ stitches

12. _____ stab wound

13. _____ rubbing off of the skin's surface

14. _____ leathery black crust of dead tissue that develops in the fourth stage of wound healing

a. abrasion
b. débridement
c. decubitus ulcer
d. eschar
e. exudate
f. incision (surgical)
g. ischemia
h. laceration
i. pressure ulcer
j. puncture
k. sloughing
l. sutures
m. wet-to-dry dressing
n. wound

■ Nursing Actions

Indicate whether the following actions are appropriate (A) or inappropriate (I).

1. _____ Position the client to irrigate a wound so that the solution will run from the lower end of the wound toward the upper end.

2. _____ Use clean gloves to remove a soiled dressing from an open wound.

3. _____ Before putting on sterile gloves when changing a sterile dressing, open sterile dressings and uncap sterile saline.

4. _____ When irrigating a wound, hold the syringe just inside the wound edges to prevent splashing.

5. _____ Teach the client to observe for excess drainage and report severe pain.

6. _____ Limit elevation of head of bed to 30 degrees.

7. _____ Turn clients who are bedridden every 4 hours.

8. _____ Use barrier ointment on client who is incontinent.

9. _____ Irrigate sinus tracts of wounds to remove dead tissue.

10. _____ Use a cotton-tipped applicator to assess depth of wounds.

■ Sequencing

Number the following actions in the correct order for changing a sterile dressing. The first action should be number 1. Continue to number the items.

_____ Provide privacy; position and prepare client.

_____ Put on sterile gloves. Moisten sterile dressings and cleanse the wound.

_____ Remove and dispose of gloves. Apply tape or tie Montgomery straps.

_____ Explain procedure to the client. Gather supplies and check physician's order. Wash hands.

_____ Remove gloves and place in the plastic bag. Wash hands.

_____ Open sterile dressings on the bedside table. Uncap the sterile saline.

_____ Wash your hands. Document wound care and assessments.

_____ Apply a layer of dry sterile dressing over the incision and wound area. Pad with additional dressings if needed.

_____ Put on clean gloves and remove soiled dressing.

_____ Prepare a plastic bag as a receptacle for soiled dressings.

_____ Reposition and cover the client. Dispose of supplies.

_____ Assess the drainage, wound, and surrounding tissue.

Number the following actions in the correct order for irrigating a sterile wound. The first action should be number 1. Continue to number the items.

_____ Wash hands, check physicians order, and gather supplies.

_____ Open irrigation tray using sterile technique. Pour solution into irrigation tray.

_____ Position client so that solution will run from the upper end of the wound downward.

_____ Assess drainage, wound, and surrounding tissue.

_____ Provide privacy and explain procedure to client.

_____ Apply sterile dressings as ordered.

_____ Put on clean gloves and an eye shield or face guard.

_____ Open sterile dressing tray, put on sterile gloves, and prepare inside irrigation and dressing trays.

_____ Draw up solution into syringe. Irrigate slowly and continuously.

_____ Pat dry wound's edges with sterile 4 X 4's.

_____ Remove old dressing and discard. Discard gloves and wash hands.

_____ Make client comfortable. Discard materials, wash hands, and document procedure.

■ Multiple Choice

Circle the best answer.

1. A client has an area of redness over the sacrum. The area does not blanche when pressed with a finger. What nursing intervention would be most appropriate?
   a. Apply ice to the area.
   b. Keep the client off the area.
   c. Massage the area.
   d. Place a heating pad on the area.

2. The nurse knows that a large decubitus ulcer must heal through granulation. This healing process is best described as:
   a. débridement.
   b. primary intention.
   c. second intention.
   d. third intention.

3. Which of the following vitamins promote wound healing?
   a. Vitamin B_1
   b. Vitamin B_{12}
   c. Vitamin C
   d. Vitamin K

4. The nurse ensures that deep open wounds heal from the inside outward to:

a. minimize scarring.

b. prevent abscess formation.

c. promote circulation.

d. provide easy access for dressing changes.

5. Which of the following indicates a healthy healing process for a wound?

a. Pink granulation tissue

b. Purulent drainage

c. Strong odor in wound

d. Very painful tissues surrounding wound

CHAPTER 59

Care of the Dying Person

■ Terminology Review

Match the following definitions with the correct terms.

1. _____ fast, labored, and deep respirations usually occurring if a person experiences acidosis

2. _____ rapid breathing

3. _____ periods of apnea and hyperpnea

4. _____ examination of the body after death

5. _____ absence of breathing

6. _____ a document in which clients state the types of treatment they will accept if a terminal situation arises

7. _____ irreversible cessation of total brain function

8. _____ designates a person of the client's choice to make healthcare decisions should the client become incompetent in the future

9. _____ another name for autopsy

a. apnea
b. autopsy
c. brain death
d. Cheyne-Stokes respiration
e. durable power of attorney
f. hyperpnea
g. Kussmaul's breathing
h. living will
i. postmortem examination

Match the following definitions with the correct terms.

10. _____ do not hospitalize

11. _____ electroencephalogram

12. _____ law passed by Congress that increases autonomy of dying persons

13. _____ total parenteral nutrition

14. _____ do not intubate

15. _____ cardiopulmonary resuscitation

16. _____ intravenous

17. _____ expressions of the wishes of clients about the kinds of treatment and care they want to receive at the point of death

18. _____ activities of daily living

19. _____ do not resuscitate

a. AD
b. ADL
c. CPR
d. DNH
e. DNI
f. DNR
g. EEG
h. IV
i. PSDA
j. TPN

■ Short Answer

Complete the following questions.

1. List two nursing interventions that might be performed during the process of dying related to each of the following:

   a. Care of the mouth, nose, and eyes

   b. Breathing difficulties

   c. Incontinence

   d. Nutrition

   e. Odor control

2. List two signs of approaching death.

3. Discuss how a body should be cared for after death.

4. Discuss what should be done with a dead person's belongings.

5. Describe methods to increase self-esteem and personal dignity in dying clients.

6. Your client is a 79-year-old woman whose condition has steadily deteriorated. Her son tells you that the dying person wants to plan her own funeral. The son is upset and says he does not want to think about planning his mother's funeral yet. How would you respond?

■ Correct the False Statements

Circle the word True or False that follows the statement. If the word false has been circled, change the underlined word/words to make the statement true. Place your answer in the space provided.

1. Nurses should examine their own feelings about death before helping dying individuals and families.

   True   False   _____

2. Clients who have a living will should keep a copy readily available to take to the acute care facility in an emergency.

   True   False   _____

3. It is not the nurse's responsibility to know which clients are DNR or full code.

   True   False   _____

4. Clients should be positioned on their stomachs to prevent choking on secretions.

   True   False   _____

5. The physician should be notified if a dying client has not voided for 2 hours.

   True   False   _____

6. It is important to <u>keep the room darkened</u> in the dying client's hospital room.

   True   False   _____

7. The dying process proceeds from <u>distal portions of the body inward</u>.

   True   False   _____

8. <u>Diminished circulation and diaphoresis</u> are signs of approaching death.

   True   False   _____

9. The nurse <u>should</u> continue to speak to the client until the final moment of death.

   True   False   _____

10. Family members should understand that crying or being sad in front of the dying client is <u>unacceptable</u>.

    True   False   _____

CHAPTER 60

Review of Mathematics

■ Terminology Review

Match the following definitions with the correct terms and acronyms.

1. _____ first and last numbers of a proportion

2. _____ two equal rations

3. _____ 1,000 grams

4. _____ top number of a common fraction

5. _____ study of chemicals and their effects on the body

6. _____ numbers that have practical meaning

7. _____ apothecary measurement approximately equal to one drop

8. _____ metric base measurement unit of weight

9. _____ the relationship of one quantity to another

10. _____ 1/1,000 of a gram

11. _____ second and third number of a proportion

12. _____ metric base measurement unit of length

13. _____ 1/100 of a meter

14. _____ type of fraction in which the denominator is always 10

15. _____ decimal system based on the number 10

16. _____ bottom number of a common fraction

17. _____ oldest system of measurement

18. _____ metric base measurement unit of liquid

a. apothecary

b. centimeter

c. decimal

d. denominator

e. extreme

f. gram

g. kilogram

h. liter

i. mean

j. meter

k. metric

l. milligram

m. minim

n. numerator

o. pharmacology

p. proportion

q. ratio

r. significant figure

■ Matching

Match the prefix with the appropriate meaning.

1. _____ Deci

2. _____ Kilo

3. _____ Deca

4. _____ Micro

5. _____ Centi

a. Multiply by 10; × 10

b. Multiply by 100; × 100

c. Divide by 100; 1/100

d. Multiply by 1,000; × 1,000

e. Divide by 10; 1/10

f. Divide by 1,000,000; 1/1,000,000

■ Short Answer

Complete the following with the best answer.

1. If you need grams of a medication and you have the medication in milligrams, how would you convert the amount?

2. List the steps involved in dividing fractions.

3. In a fraction, the larger denominator denotes _____ pieces. Therefore, 1/100 is _____ as much as 1/50.

4. What can nurse do if unsure about the dosage she or he has calculated?

5. Why is it essential that the nurse have a basic understanding of mathematics?

6. Describe three rules that apply when using ratio and proportions.

7. Describe how to convert from a percentage to a fraction.

■ Matching

Match the unit of measurement with the system of measurement. The system of measurements may be used more than once.

1. _____ Teaspoon
2. _____ Milligram
3. _____ Minim
4. _____ Drop
5. _____ Pint
6. _____ Liter
7. _____ Kilogram
8. _____ Tablespoon
9. _____ Ounce
10. _____ Cubic centimeter
11. _____ Dram
12. _____ Milliliter
13. _____ Quart

a. Metric
b. Household
c. Apothecary

■ Multiple Choice

Circle the best answer.

1. Which of the following measurements would be used to administer a liquid medication?
   a. Grams
   b. Kilograms
   c. Meter
   d. Milliliter

2. Which system of measurement is the least accurate?
   a. Apothecary
   b. Household
   c. Metric

3. The doctor ordered aspirin gr 1/100. The medication is available in aspirin gr 1/200 tablets. How many tablets would you administer with each dose?

    a. One-half
    b. One
    c. One and one-half
    d. Two

4. The doctor orders 3,000 mL of IV fluid for a client. The first hour, the client is to receive 30% of the fluid. How much should you administer over the first hour?

    a. 30 mL
    b. 90 mL
    c. 300 mL
    d. 900 mL

5. The doctor order 60 mg Tylenol (acetaminophen). The mediation available is Tylenol 120 mg/5 mL. How much medication should be given with each dose?

    a. 0.25 mL
    b. 2.5 mL
    c. 5 mL
    d. 10 mL

6. You must administer 2 teaspoons of syrup of ipecac. You have available a 20-mL syringe and the syrup. How much medication will you administer in the syringe?

    a. 0.1 mL
    b. 1.0 mL
    c. 10 mL
    d. 20 mL

7. You must infuse a 250-mL bag of medication at 50 mL/hr. How long will it take you to administer the full amount?

    a. 5 hours
    b. 2.5 hours
    c. 0.5 hours
    d. 0.25 hours

CHAPTER 61

Introduction to Pharmacology

■ Terminology Review

Match the following definitions with the correct terms.

1. _____ medications taken into the GI tract by the mouth

2. _____ parenteral route of medication administration

3. _____ actions of drugs

4. _____ new form of solid medication that dissolves instantly when placed on the tongue

5. _____ medication that enhances the effects of another medication

6. _____ route of medication that is absorbed into the skin

7. _____ same as a synergistic medication

8. _____ route of medication administration

9. _____ compressed, spherical form of a medication

10. _____ science that deals with the origin, nature, chemistry, effects, and uses of medications

11. _____ another name for brand name

12. _____ name identified in the USP

13. _____ medicinal agent that modifies body functions

14. _____ medication that does not dissolve until the tablet reaches the intestine because the medication can irritate that stomach mucosa

15. _____ medication that produces a desired response

16. _____ contains the dose and scheduled time

17. _____ medication in powdered or pellet form enclosed in soluble, cylindrical, gelatin-like material

18. _____ describes medication's chemical composition

19. _____ medication that has an opposing effect or acts against another medication

20. _____ copyrighted name assigned by the company making the medication

21. _____ type of medication that is breathed into the lungs or nose

22. _____ name assigned by the medication's first manufacturer

23. _____ tablet in the shape of a capsule

a. agonist
b. antagonist
c. brand name
d. caplet
e. capsule
f. chemical name
g. dosage
h. enteric-coated
i. generic name
j. inhalant
k. injectable
l. medication
m. official name
n. oral
o. pharmacokinetics
p. pharmacology
q. potentiating
r. synergistic
s. tablet
t. topical
u. trade name
v. transdermal
w. zydis

■ Acronym Review

Match the following definitions with the acronyms.

1. _____ personal identification number

2. _____ publications that define standards for medication approval

3. _____ verbal order

4. _____ *Physician's Desk Reference*

5. _____ healthcare professional who is licensed to prepare and dispense medications on the order of licensed practitioner of medicine

6. _____ telephone order

7. _____ medications purchased without a prescription

8. _____ ensures that medications and therapeutic agents are safe and effective for public use

9. _____ lists the official and unofficial names of medications

10. _____ Department of Health and Human Services

11. _____ National Formulary

a. DEA
b. FDA
c. NF
d. OTC
e. PDR
f. PIN
g. RPh
h. TO
i. USD
j. USP
k. VO

■ Abbreviation Review

Write the definition of the following abbreviations used in medication administration. Refer to Tables 37-4 and 37-5 if you need help.

1. BID _____

2. IM _____

3. ou _____

4. q _____

5. qd _____

6. QID _____

7. QOD _____

8. stat _____

9. subq _____

10. susp _____

■ Short Answers

Complete the following questions with the best answer.

1. List three things the nurse should know about the medication being administered.

2. List the four parenteral administration routes.

3. List four factors healthcare professionals must consider when prescribing medication.

4. Name persons who are able to write prescriptions; include the acronym for each.

5. Describe the procedure to verify the scheduled drug count.

6. Identify and briefly explain the five types of doses.

■ Multiple Choice

Circle the best answer.

1. Which category of controlled substances has no accepted medical use and a high potential for abuse?
   a. I
   b. II
   c. III
   d. IV

2. The physician orders Mylanta 30 mL po AC and HS. When is this medication to be administered?
   a. Before and after meals
   b. Bedtime and after meals
   c. Before meals and at bedtime
   d. When the client requests the mediation

3. When handling controlled substances, which of the following is an appropriate action for the nurse?
   a. Keep narcotic key in possession at all times.
   b. Only document medications that are wasted.
   c. Share your PIN with other staff members.
   d. Share the key with trustworthy colleagues.

4. The nurse is preparing to administer an enteric-coated medication. What instructions should be given to the client?
   a. Allow the medication to dissolve slowly under the tongue.
   b. Crush the tablet and mix with food.
   c. Do not chew this medication.
   d. Do not take with any liquids.

5. How will the pain medication dose need to be adjusted for a client with a relatively high threshold for pain?
   a. Administer a higher dose of medication.
   b. Administer a lower dose of medication.
   c. Do not administer to this type of client.
   d. No adjustment is needed

CHAPTER 62

Classification of Medications

■ Terminology Review

Match the following definitions with the correct terms.

1. _____ toxic effect caused by damage to the eighth cranial nerve that results in dizziness, tinnitus, and gradual hearing loss

2. _____ neurotransmitters that play an important part in the body's response to stress

3. _____ medications that constrict the blood vessel

4. _____ antibiotics that are effective against only a few microorganisms

5. _____ generalized infection throughout the body

6. _____ able to kill bacteria

7. _____ pain-relieving medications derived from opium or having opium-like actions

8. _____ retards the growth of bacteria

9. _____ speed up certain mental and physical processes

10. _____ antibiotics that are effective against many organisms

11. _____ medications used to relieve constipation

12. _____ toxic effect manifested by blood and protein in the urine

13. _____ slow down certain mental and physical processes

14. _____ side effect in which the person is sensitive to light

a. bactericidal
b. bacteriostatic
c. broad spectrum
d. catecholamine
e. cathartic
f. depressant
g. narrow spectrum
h. nephrotoxicity
i. opiate
j. ototoxicity
k. photosensitivity
l. septicemia
m. stimulant
n. vasoconstrictor

■ Acronym Review

Match the following definitions with the correct acronyms.

1. _____ hypertension

2. _____ medication that inhibits the growth of susceptible bacteria

3. _____ antimetabolite

4. _____ potassium-wasting diuretic

5. _____ given to reduce symptoms caused by hormonal deficiencies

6. _____ vaccine used to prevent diphtheria, pertussis, and tetanus

7. _____ lab value that is monitored when a client is on anticoagulant therapy

8. _____ nonsteroidal ant-inflammatory drugs

9. _____ vaccine to protect against measles, mumps, and rubella

10. _____ nonnarcotic analgesic derived from salicylic acid

11. _____ morphine sulfate

12. _____ potent vasodilator used to treat acute angina pectoris

13. _____ dangerous organism that can cause life-threatening illness because it is resistant to antibiotics

14. _____ angiotensin-converting enzyme, which is used to treat resistant hypertension

15. _____ gastroesophageal reflux disease

16. _____ used as a cathartic

a. ACE
b. ASA
c. DPT
d. GERD
e. HCTZ
f. HRT
g. HTN
h. MMR
i. MOM
j. MRSA
k. MS
l. NSAID
m. NTG
n. PCN
o. PT
p. 5-FU

■ Medication Table

Complete the following table, filling in the action/use, side effects, and nursing considerations for each of the medications listed.

Classification/Medication	Action/Use	Side Effects	Nursing Considerations
Penicillins (amoxicillin/[Amoxil])			
Hypnotics (phenobarbital/[Luminal])			
Nonsteroidal anti-inflammatory drugs (NSAIDs)			
Adrenergic medications (epinephrine/[Adrenaline])			
Steroids (prednisone/[Delt-Cortef])			

Continues

Medication Table (Continued)

Classification/Medication	Action/Use	Side Effects	Nursing Considerations
Narcotic analgesic (morphine)			
Anticoagulants (heparin)			

▪ Matching

Match the following commonly prescribed medications with the classification.

1. _____ tetracycline

2. _____ lanolin

3. _____ diazepam (Valium)

4. _____ morphine (morphine sulfate)

5. _____ dexamethasone (Decadron)

6. _____ captopril (Capoten)

7. _____ lidocaine (Xylocaine)

8. _____ aminophylline (Aminophyllin)

9. _____ pseudoephedrine (Sudafed)

10. _____ dimenhydrinate (Dramamine)

11. _____ tamoxifen (Nolvadex)

12. _____ omperazole (Prilosec)

13. _____ digitalis (Lanoxin)

14. _____ furosemide (Lasix)

a. Antiarrhythmic

b. Antiemetic

c. Antibiotic/anti-infective

d. Bronchodilator

e. Adrenal gland medication

f. Decongestant

g. Sedative/hypnotic

h. Dermatologic

i. Narcotic

j. Antihypertensive

k. Cardiotonic

l. Loop diuretic

m. Proton pump inhibitor

n. Antineoplastic hormone

▪ Multiple Choice

Circle the best answer.

1. Before surgery, the client should be instructed to discontinue which medication 7 to 10 days before the surgery?

   a. Aspirin

   b. Digoxin

   c. Furosemide

   d. Theophylline

2. Which medications are used for inflammation, for analgesia, and as an antipyretic?

   a. Nonsalicylate analgesics and opiates

   b. Narcotic analgesics and NSAIDs

   c. Opiates and salicylates

   d. Salicylates and NSAIDs

3. When evaluating the effectiveness of phenytoin (Dilantin), the nurse would assess for:

   a. absence of fever.

   b. absence of seizure activity.

   c. presence of thin secretions.

   d. presence of stable vital signs.

4. The nurse would administer a miotic ophthalmic preparation to:

   a. constrict the pupils.

   b. control inflammation.

   c. decrease absorption of aqueous humor.

   d. dilate the pupils.

5. Which insulin may be given safely intravenously?

   a. NPH

   b. Regular

   c. Lente

   d. Semilente

6. A client is allergic to penicillin. Which antibiotic would be administered cautiously to this client?

   a. Aminoglycosides

   b. Cephalosporins

   c. Erythromycins

   d. Tetracylines

7. Which data would be most important for the nurse to assess in a client taking steroids?

   a. Changes in appetite

   b. Moodiness

   c. Signs of infection

   d. Stable heart rate

8. A client has been taking digitalis (Digoxin) for the past 6 months. He complains of nausea, blurred vision, and constipation. The cardiac monitor shows atrial fibrillation. The nurse recognizes that:

   a. atrial fibrillation is a sign of digitalis toxicity.

   b. blurred vision is a sign that the client needs more medication.

   c. constipation is a sign that the client needs a digitalizing dose.

   d. nausea is a sign of digitalis toxicity.

9. The nurse administers morphine to a client after surgery. Later the client is drowsy, pupils are constricted, pulse rate is 65 beats/min, and respiration rate is 6 breaths/min. The nurse realizes that the:

   a. constriction of the pupils is an unexpected effect of the morphine.

   b. drowsiness is a sign that the morphine is having a negative effect.

   c. pulse rate indicates that the client needs a higher dose of morphine.

   d. respiratory rate indicates a dangerous side effect of morphine.

10. Common side effects of thyroid replacement hormones include:

   a. bradycardia.

   b. coughing.

   c. palpitations.

   d. urinary retention.

CHAPTER 63

Administration of Medications

■ Terminology Review

Match the following definitions with the correct terms and acronyms.

1. _____ semisolid medication designed to melt at body temperature

2. _____ undesired harmful effect that results from an increased blood level of medication beyond the therapeutic level

3. _____ method of injecting that helps prevent the medication from leaking back onto the skin

4. _____ medication causes the client to experience severe, life-threatening allergic reaction

5. _____ large quantities of solution given IV

6. _____ glass container equipped with a self-sealing rubber stopper

7. _____ computer-generated sheet used to document the administration of medications

8. _____ absence of ability to generate a sensitivity reaction

9. _____ powders are mixed with this before using as an injectable medication

10. _____ the same as a side effect

11. _____ desired effect of a medication

12. _____ effect is limited to the area of application

13. _____ blood or blood products administered IV

14. _____ response from an administered medication that is not intended or desired

15. _____ glass container that holds a premeasured, single medication dose

16. _____ for eye administration

17. _____ IV intermittent access site

18. _____ drugs that the body absorbs into the general circulation

19. _____ IV fluids enter into surrounding tissues

20. _____ medications applied to the skin that release a constant dosage

a. adverse effect
b. ampule
c. anaphylactic effect
d. anergic
e. diluent
f. Hep-Lock
g. infiltration
h. infusion
i. local
j. medication administration record (MAR)
k. ophthalmic
l. side effect
m. suppository
n. systemic
o. therapeutic effect
p. toxicity
q. transdermal
r. transfusion
s. vial
t. z-track

■ Acronym Review

Match the following definitions with the acronyms.

1. _____ medication given IV at scheduled intervals using additional IV tubing connected to an existing infusion

2. _____ should be applied to clean, dry, hairless skin

3. _____ dextrose in half-normal saline

4. _____ right eye

5. _____ gastrostomy tube

6. _____ normal saline

7. _____ Purified Protein Derivative

8. _____ hours of sleep

9. _____ diameter of a needle

10. _____ left eye

11. _____ given per vagina

12. _____ medication to be given immediately

13. _____ jejunosotomy tube

14. _____ total parenteral nutrition or alimentation

15. _____ both eyes

16. _____ metered dose inhaler

17. _____ IV inserted in the antecubital site and threaded to a large central vein

18. _____ nasogastric

19. _____ stop an infusion

20. _____ dextrose in sterile water

21. _____ number of drops per milliliter

22. _____ sodium chloride

23. _____ dextrose in normal saline

a. D-5-W 5%

b. D-51/2-NS 5%

c. D-5-NS 5%

d. D/C

e. DRF

f. G

g. G-tube

h. HS

i. IVPB

j. JT

k. MDI

l. NaCl

m. NG

n. NS

o. OD

p. OS

q. OU

r. PICC

s. PPD

t. STAT

u. TD

v. TPA/TPN

w. V

■ Sequencing

Number the following actions in the correct order for administering oral medications. The first action should be number 1. Continue to number the items.

_____ Prepare medication as needed.

_____ Complete necessary assessments before giving medication.

_____ Check client within 30 minutes after giving medications.

_____ Select medication and compare label of medication to the MAR (first check). Complete calculations. Dish up medication.

_____ Remain with the client until the medication is taken.

_____ When you have prepared all medications, compare each medication to the MAR (third check).

_____ Wash your hands and record medication administration.

_____ Identify the client before giving the medication.

_____ Administer the medication.

_____ Wash your hands, gather equipment, and unlock medication cart or drawer.

_____ Recheck each medication with the MAR (second check).

_____ Assist the client to a comfortable position.

Number the following actions in the correct order for drawing up a medication from a vial. The first action should be number 1. Continue to number the items.

_____ Use your dominant hand to pull back on the syringe's plunger. Withdraw an accurate dose into the syringe.

_____ Hold the needle and recheck the syringe's content for presence of air. Tap the barrel of the syringe to move air bubbles upward before expelling them.

_____ Invert the vial; brace your little finger against the plunger.

_____ Insert the needle through the center of the rubber stopper and inject air into the vial, keeping the needle above the solution.

_____ Wash hands, remove the needle cap, and add the amount of air to the syringe equal to the amount of medication that you will withdraw from the vial; change the needle if necessary, recap the needle or pull the safety sheath over it.

Number the following actions in the correct order for giving a subcutaneous injection. The first action should be number 1. Continue to number the items.

_____ Hold the syringe in your dominant hand like a pencil or dart.

_____ Release the skin and move your nondominant hand to steady the syringe's lower end.

_____ Aspirate for blood return by pulling back on the plunger with your dominant hand.

_____ Wash hands; record the medication administration indicating that you used the subcutaneous site.

_____ Remove the needle cap; use your nondominant hand to bunch or spread tissue gently at the injection site.

_____ Massage the site gently with the alcohol swab unless contraindicated for specific medication.

_____ Assist the client to a comfortable position. Select the appropriate site using anatomic landmarks.

_____ Insert the needle quickly at the correct angle (45° to 90°).

_____ Inject the medication at a slow and steady rate. Safely dispose of the needle.

_____ Put on gloves and close the door or pull the bed curtains.

Number the following actions in the correct order for administering medications through a gastric tube. The first action should be number 1. Continue to number the items.

_____ Check placement of G-tube. Clamp tubing and remove the syringe.

_____ Wash hands; gather supplies, set up medication following "five rights."

_____ Assist client to comfortable position, wash hands, and document.

_____ Release the clamp and pour the medication into the syringe.

_____ Explain procedure and don gloves.

_____ After administering medications, flush tube, clamp tube, and remove syringe.

_____ Remove the plunger from the syringe and reconnect the syringe to the tube.

■ Matching

Match the definition in Part A with the route in Part B and the administration method in Part C. Each definition should have two letters; Part C letters may be used more than once.

PART A

1. _____ Medications are placed under the tongue where they are dissolved and absorbed.

2. _____ Medications are shallow and given just beneath the epidermis.

3. _____ Medication is administered into adipose tissues located below the dermis.

4. _____ Medication is placed between the client's cheek and gum.

5. _____ Medication is introduced directly into the bloodstream; medication is absorbed rapidly.

6. _____ Medications are given in muscles below the dermal and subcutaneous skin layers.

7. _____ Medications given into the anal canal.

PART B

a. Buccal

b. Sublingual (SL)

c. Intravenous (IV)

d. Intradermal (ID)

e. Subcutaneous (SubQ)

f. Intramuscular (IM)

g. Rectal (R, PR)

PART C

h. Enteral

i. Parenteral

■ Case Study

Your client is 71 years old with hypertension, headache, anxiety, and a productive cough. The client sometimes has difficulty taking all the medications. The client is to receive all the following medications at 0800 hr:

Capoten tablet for hypertension
Robitussin cough syrup
Tylenol for headache
Valium for anxiety

How would you handle this situation and what actions would you take?

■ Multiple Choice

Circle the best answer.

1. When teaching a parent to instill ear drops in a child, it is most important for the nurse to teach the parents to:

   a. avoid shaking the medication.

   b. chill the drops before administration.

   c. pull the ear down and back to instill the medication.

   d. pull the ear up and back to instill the medication.

2. Which of the following medications cannot be administered by a transdermal patch?

   a. Antibiotics

   b. Hormones

   c. Nicotine

   d. Nitroglycerin

3. The nurse should apply ophthalmic medications to the:

   a. cornea.

   b. conjunctival surface.

   c. iris.

   d. pupil.

4. How far should a vaginal applicator be inserted when administering a vaginal medication?

   a. 1/2 to 1 inch

   b. 2 to 4 inches

   c. 5 to 7 inches

   d. 8 to 10 inches

5. Which syringe would be most appropriate for the nurse to use to give an intramuscular injection to an average-sized man?

   a. $\frac{1}{2}$ inch, 21 gauge

   b. $\frac{2}{8}$ inch, 25 gauge

   c. $1\frac{1}{2}$ inch, 22 gauge

   d. 2 inch, 17 gauge

6. A medication is scheduled to be administered at 1000 hours. In which time frame may the medication be given?

   a. Only exactly at 1000

   b. Between 0800 and 1000

   c. Between 1000 and 1100

   d. Between 0930 and 1030

7. Which information assures the nurse that an intradermal medication was administered in the correct area?

   a. Client complains that the injection stung.

   b. Formation of a wheal.

   c. Mild bleeding at the site.

   d. No bleeding during aspiration.

8. After administration of ear drops, the nurse:
   a. asks client to lie on the side of the unaffected ear.
   b. asks client to lie on the side of the affected ear.
   c. asks client to sit at bedside with head erect.
   d. asks client to sit with head tilted forward.

9. After administration of eye drops, the nurse should place gentle pressure on the inner canthus to:
   a. minimize risk for systemic effects.
   b. minimize swelling of the eye.
   c. prevent medication from stinging.
   d. prevent the client from blinking.

10. Which of the following anatomic landmarks are used in correctly identifying the ventrogluteal injection site?
    a. Acromium process
    b. Anterior superior iliac spine
    c. Lateral aspect of thigh
    d. Posterior superior iliac spine

11. The physician has ordered an IV of 1,000 mL of solution to be administered over 8 hours. The DRF (drops per milliliter) is 15. How many drops per minute will you infuse?
    a. 15
    b. 26
    c. 31
    d. 500

CHAPTER 64

Normal Pregnancy

■ Terminology Review

Match the following definitions with the correct terms.

1. _____ a morula or decidua once it is fully implanted

2. _____ a definite pigmentation of the abdomen often appears as a dark line extending from the umbilicus to the pubis

3. _____ the developing organism after the eighth week in the 40-week system

4. _____ a fluid-filled sac in which the fetus floats

5. _____ a vascular and glandular organ that supplies the developing organism with food and oxygen, carries waste away to the woman, and produces hormones that help maintain pregnancy

6. _____ a hollow ball of developing cells with an inner and outer layer of cells

7. _____ means that the fetus is mature enough to survive outside the uterus; usually 20 weeks

8. _____ fertilized ovum

9. _____ total time from the moment of fertilization of the egg until birth of the newborn

10. _____ a suntanned, bronzed masking across the face of dark-haired pregnant women

11. _____ pregnancy

12. _____ three 3-month periods

13. _____ parting of mother and baby

14. _____ egg of female fertilized with sperm

15. _____ pregnant woman

a. embryo
b. fetus
c. placenta
d. amnion
e. viability
f. chorion
g. gestation
h. melasma
i. linea nigra
j. conception
k. trimester
l. gravida
m. para
n. antepartum
o. zygote

Match the following definitions with the correct terms.

16. _____ opening between the right and left atria

17. _____ breastfeeding

18. _____ area where the umbilical cord enters the fetus

19. _____ soft jelly-like substance that protects the umbilical cord

20. _____ inward curve of the lower back

21. _____ first fetal movements that a pregnant female feels

22. _____ pattern of normal fetal growth and development

23. _____ measurement of the size of the uterus

24. _____ nausea or vomiting lasting beyond the fourth month

25. _____ connection between the pulmonary artery and aorta that allows shunting of blood around the fetal lungs

26. _____ twins or more

27. _____ born with

28. _____ clear or slightly milky fluid that breasts begin to produce by the 14th week of pregnancy

29. _____ education about expected changes

30. _____ short duct found only in the fetus where oxygenated blood enters

31. _____ increase in salivation

a. congenital
b. cephalocaudal
c. Wharton's jelly
d. umbilicus
e. ductus venosus
f. ductus arteriosus
g. foramen ovale
h. hyperemesis gravidarum
i. quickening
j. colostrum
k. lactation
l. lordosis
m. participatory guidance
n. multifetal
o. fundal height
p. ptyalism

■ Acronym Review

Match the following definitions with the acronyms.

1. _____ previous menstrual period

2. _____ sexually transmitted infections

3. _____ estimated delivery date

4. _____ last normal menstrual period

5. _____ test completed at 15 to 19 weeks of gestation to screen for neural tube defects

6. _____ recommended weight gain for each woman based on her height and what she weighed before she got pregnant

7. _____ pregnancy test to check for the presence of human chorionic gonadotropin

8. _____ nurse specialists working with pregnant women during their pregnancies, helping them maintain wellness, and attending vaginal births

9. _____ estimated date of confinement

a. BMI
b. CNM
c. EDC
d. EDD
e. hCG
f. LMP/LNMP
g. MS-AFP
h. PMP
i. STI

■ Assessment Review

Indicate whether the following signs of pregnancy are presumptive, probable, or positive signs of pregnancy.

1. _____ softening of the cervix

2. _____ quickening

3. _____ basal body temperature elevation

4. _____ amenorrhea

5. _____ visualization of the fetus

6. _____ nausea

7. _____ positive urine pregnancy test

8. _____ bluish or purple color of the cervix

9. _____ fetal heartbeat

10. _____ pigmentation changes

11. _____ frequent urination

12. _____ softening of the lower uterine segment

13. _____ fatigue

14. _____ enlarged breasts

15. _____ ballottement

■ Completion

Complete the following statements by filling in the blanks.

1. The pregnant woman needs an increase in caloric intake by approximately _____ calories.

2. If a woman experience constipation, she may take a stool _____ or increase _____ to prevent constipation; however, _____ and enemas should be avoided.

3. A woman should bathe as usual and use minimal or little _____ on her nipples.

4. Sexual intercourse during pregnancy is _____ as long as it is not unduly uncomfortable or consists of risky sexual practices.

5. Most teratogenic effects occur in the _____ trimester of pregnancy.

6. _____ _____ is the most common discomfort of early pregnancy that may be relieved with _____ _____ meals and _____ carbohydrate foods.

7. _____ _____ are held for the expectant mother and significant other, spouse, or friend.

8. A woman's feelings about her pregnancy are likely to be influenced by her personal _____ and the _____ and _____ support she receives from family members and others close to her.

9. Human chorionic gonadotropin hormone can be detected in small amounts in the woman's urine or blood by about the _____ to _____ days of pregnancy.

10. An examiner can hear fetal heart tone with a _____ as early as the 10th week and with a _____ at about the 18th to 20th week.

11. During the first trimester, the pregnant woman should have a prenatal visit every _____.

12. If a woman is _____, she should receive RhoGAM at the 28th week and following any episode of bleeding or invasive procedure.

13. Weight loss is _____ _____ during pregnancy.

14. _____ is the most well-known model for childbirth preparation.

15. During the first trimester, fathers often fear losing their _____ and _____.

■ Case Study

Your client presents at the clinic and suspects that she is pregnant. She complains of amenorrhea, nausea, and breast tenderness.

1. What other assessment data would you obtain?

2. What instructions would you provide to this client?

3. It is determined that the client is pregnant. What development tasks will this client need to adapt? What assessment findings will you anticipate seeing in this client?

■ Multiple Choice

Circle the best answer.

1. Which of the following is a danger sign during the first trimester of pregnancy?

   a. Epigastric pain

   b. No longer feeling pregnant

   c. Preterm rupture of the membranes

   d. Visual changes

2. Using Naegle's Rule, calculate the estimated date of delivery if the woman's LNMP was October 1.

   a. June 23

   b. July 8

   c. December 23

   d. January 8

3. Which of the following would be appropriate to teach the pregnant woman regarding exercise?

   a. Avoid any physical activity during the second trimester.

   b. Contact sports are allowed during the first trimester.

   c. Extremely active women should reduce the level of exertion.

   d. Relaxation and stretching exercises should be discontinued.

4. The functions of amniotic fluid is to:

   a. exchange nutrients from mother to fetus.

   b. immobilize the fetus.

   c. protect the woman's uterus.

   d. regulate temperature.

5. Which category drugs may be safely administered during pregnancy?

   a. Category A

   b. Category B

   c. Category C

   d. Category D

6. During the last months of pregnancy, the nurse should instruct the client to:

   a. rest on her left side for at least 1 hour in the morning and afternoon.

   b. sleep on her back during the night and during naps.

   c. start nipple exercises and stimulation twice a day.

   d. start to cut back on water intake, especially at night.

7. When teaching a pregnant woman about traveling during the pregnancy, it is most important to focus on which of the following?

   a. If traveling by car, stop every 2 hours for 10 minutes.

   b. Get plenty of rest before long trips made in automobiles.

   c. Travel in any type of aircraft is acceptable.

   d. Travel can be completed anytime throughout the pregnancy.

8. Which of the following is recommended for all women of childbearing age?

   a. Additional B vitamins

   b. Additional vitamin A

   c. Folic acid supplement

   d. Vitamin C supplement

9. Between 24 and 28 weeks, all pregnant women should be screened for:

   a. anemia.

   b. bladder infections.

   c. diabetes.

   d. neural tube defects.

10. Which of these measures would be helpful for the pregnant client complaining of sleeplessness?

    a. Eat evening meal close to bedtime.

    b. Sit in a sitz bath before bedtime.

    c. Try to remain in one position when sleeping.

    d. Use pillows to help find a comfortable position.

11. The first 8 weeks of pregnancy are known as the critical period of human development because:

    a. by the time this period ends, the embryo is completely safe from any damage.

    b. many embryos die during this time period.

    c. the infant's sex is determined at the end of the eighth week.

    d. the major structures of the embryo are forming, and damage can result in major birth defects.

12. Which of these statements is most accurate about the placenta?

    a. The blood of the baby mixes with the mother's blood to permit exchange of nutrients and oxygen.

    b. The blood of the baby and the mother do not mix; exchange occurs across blood vessels and the walls of the villi.

    c. The placenta lets the blood from the fetus cross to the mother, but not the mother's blood cross to the fetus.

    d. The placenta serves as a complete barrier between the baby and mother so that any drugs the mother takes do not cross to the baby.

13. Which of the following is the best recommendation about taking medicines during pregnancy?

    a. All over-the-counter (OTC) drugs are safe during pregnancy.

    b. All herbal preparations are safe during pregnancy.

    c. Don't take anything during pregnancy without asking your health care provider.

    d. Take an OTC diuretic if you have swelling during pregnancy.

14. A feeling of ambivalence about pregnancy is:

    a. a sign of an unwanted pregnancy.

    b. normal in early pregnancy.

    c. rare at any stage of pregnancy.

    d. typical in late pregnancy.

CHAPTER 65

Normal Labor, Delivery, and Postpartum Care

■ Terminology Review

Match the following definitions with the correct terms.

1. _____ opening of the softened cervix

2. _____ response of the breasts to the presence of an increased volume of milk and a sudden change in hormones

3. _____ incision in the perineum

4. _____ mouth of the uterus

5. _____ purpose of this device is to record the rate and quality of the fetal heartbeat during contraction and relaxation

6. _____ thinning out of the cervix

7. _____ procedure of artificially rupturing the membranes

8. _____ painful uterine cramps for a few days after delivery

9. _____ freestanding setting for labor and birth

10. _____ thin, yellowish secretion that provides vitamins and immune substances that protect the newborn against infection

11. _____ room where both labor and delivery occur

12. _____ painless, short, and irregular contractions, also called false labor

13. _____ during the second stage of labor when the rectum dilates, the perineum bulges, and the top of the fetal head appears

14. _____ special hook used to perform amniotomy

15. _____ upper curve of the uterus

a. after-pains
b. amnihook
c. amniotomy
d. birthing center
e. birthing room
f. Braxton Hicks contractions
g. cervical os
h. colostrum
i. crowning
j. dilation
k. effacement
l. engorgement
m. episiotomy
n. fetal monitor
o. fundus

Match the following definitions with the correct terms.

16. _____ period from the start of one contraction to the start of the next one

17. _____ occurs during the fourth stage of labor when the woman's reproductive organs begin to return to their normal prepregnant size

18. _____ staining the sticky mucous plug a pinkish color

19. _____ discharge after delivery

20. _____ cause the uterus to open and move the fetus downward into the birth canal, delivering the baby and expelling the placenta

21. _____ newborn

22. _____ contractions that occur more often than every 2 minutes, or if each lasts more than 90 seconds

23. _____ after delivery

24. _____ consists of four stages

25. _____ production of milk caused by release of prolactin and oxytocin

26. _____ pressure-sensitive device used to monitor the frequency of contractions

27. _____ time period during which labor and delivery take place

28. _____ loops of umbilical cord wrapped around the infant's neck

29. _____ settling of the fetus into the pelvis; "baby has dropped"

a. intrapartum
b. involution
c. labor
d. labor contractions
e. interval
f. lactation
g. lightening
h. lochia
i. neonate
j. nuchal cord
k. postpartum
l. "show"
m. tetanic/tonic contraction
n. tocodynamometer

■ Stages of Labor Review

Match the following occurrence or definition with the correct stage of labor. Answers may be used more than once.

1. _____ placenta is delivered

2. _____ cervix dilates

3. _____ crowning occurs

4. _____ show is noted

5. _____ lochia flow is bright red and moderate

6. _____ baby is delivered

7. _____ placenta moves into the vagina

8. _____ woman complains of feeling chilled and shakes uncontrollably

9. _____ generally lasts 1 to 2 hours in a primigravida

10. _____ uterus becomes smaller in size with contractions

a. First stage of labor
b. Second stage of labor
c. Third stage of labor
d. Fourth stage of labor

■ Assessment Review

Indicate whether the following assessment findings are normal (N) or abnormal (A).

1. _____ ability to press fingers into fundus with mild contraction

2. _____ cloudy amniotic fluid

3. _____ amniotic fluid with a pH of 7.0

4. _____ cervix fully effaced and dilated at end of stage one of labor

5. _____ second stage of labor lasting more than 2 hours

6. _____ uterus is boggy feeling after expulsion of the placenta

7. _____ 500 mL of blood loss with delivery

8. _____ parents bonding with newborn

9. _____ no bright-red bleeding during onset of labor

10. _____ numbness in the legs in women receiving anesthesia

11. _____ hypotension

12. _____ FHR of 150 beats/min

13. _____ FHR decelerates early and mirrors contraction pattern

14. _____ late deceleration

15. _____ FHR of 100 beats/min

16. _____ woman is exhausted after delivery

17. _____ uterus feels firm and is situated midline after delivery

18. _____ bright red lochia on fourth day after delivery

19. _____ no edema at episiostomy

20. _____ engorgement of breast on third day after delivery

21. _____ negative Homans' sign

■ Short Answer

Complete the following short answers.

1. What is the normal position of the fetus?

2. In which position can the fetus not be delivered?

3. List the danger signs of labor.

4. List three differences between true labor and false labor.

5. Outline topics that the nurse should instruct the postpartum client in before discharge.

6. Explain why urinary catherizaiton may be needed during labor.

■ Case Study

Your client is a 25-year-old primagravida who has just delivered a healthy baby girl. During your initial assessment, you assess the fundus and it is not firm.

1. What action will you take? Describe in detail how you will complete the nursing procedure.

2. You taught the client how to assess her fundus. She demonstrates the correct technique. What additional information would you provide for the client?

■ Multiple Choice

Circle the best answer.

1. Which assessment relates most directly to ruptured membranes and release of amniotic fluid?
   a. Bloody show
   b. Woman complains of urge to push.
   c. Fluid with a pH of 5.0 with nitrazine test
   d. Fluid with a pH of 7.0 to 7.5 with nitrazine test

2. When the placenta is delivered with the dull side out (Duncan presentation), the woman is at risk for:
   a. excessive bleeding.
   b. hemorrhoids.
   c. increased lacerations of the perineum.
   d. sterility.

3. To assess the uterine contraction, the nurse:
   a. asks the woman if she is having a contraction.
   b. palpates above the symphysis pubis.
   c. palpates just below the xyphoid process of the sternum.
   d. performs a sterile vaginal examination.

4. The nurse knows that a postpartum client's susceptibility to hemorrhage is most likely related to a:

   a. boggy uterus.

   b. firm fundus.

   c. long labor.

   d. negative Homans' sign.

5. Which of the following indicates that the new mother understands how to handle breast milk safely?

   a. "I can store fresh breast milk in the refrigerator for only 24 hours."

   b. "I can store frozen breast milk for up to 1 month."

   c. "I need to express my breast milk into a clear glass."

   d. "I should never store my breast milk in a frozen-food locker."

6. To prevent infection of the perineal area after delivery, the nurse should instruct the client to:

   a. begin sitz baths at the first sign of infection.

   b. pull panties straight down.

   c. use hot water to cleanse the area after bowel movements.

   d. wipe with sweeping motion, from front to back.

7. Analgesics given too late in labor can result in which of the following?

   a. Elevated blood pressure

   b. Increased bleeding

   c. Lethargy in the newborn

   d. Stopping of the labor process

8. During the labor process, which of the following would require immediate action by the nurse?

   a. Contractions that increase in intensity

   b. Early deceleration

   c. FHR dropping to 100 beat/min

   d. Pain during contractions

9. In evaluating the effects of oxytocin (Pitocin) after delivery, the nurse should monitor for:

   a. effective breastfeeding.

   b. engorged breasts.

   c. relief of pain.

   d. the uterus remaining firm.

10. During active labor, the mother usually exhibits which of the following behaviors?

    a. Difficulty following directions

    b. Excited and talkative

    c. Frustration and irritability

    d. Serious expression and apprehension

11. When providing postpartum teaching about self-care, one of the danger signs that a lactating woman should know to report to the birth attendant is:

    a. breast fullness just before feeding.

    b. breast engorgement to a degree that the baby can't latch on.

    c. nipple soreness after feedings.

    d. nipple dryness before feedings.

12. "Show" is usually present in:

    a. Braxton Hicks contractions.

    b. false labor.

    c. true labor.

    d. second stage of labor only.

CHAPTER 66

Care of the Normal Newborn

■ Terminology Review

Match the following definitions with the correct terms.

1. _____ accumulation of blood between the bones of the skull and the periosteum

2. _____ peel

3. _____ white, thick, cheesy material that may cover newborn's skin

4. _____ small amount of bloody mucus expelled from the vagina of the female newborn

5. _____ chemical that stabilizes the walls of the alveoli

6. _____ newborn extremities appear cyanotic because of slow peripheral circulation

7. _____ inherited disorder in which the newborn cannot digest glucose

8. _____ inherited disorder caused by the body's inability to digest protein normally

9. _____ newborns during the first 28 days of life

10. _____ mark on the newborn's eyelid or forehead

11. _____ the foreskin covers the glans penis or extends beyond it with an opening that is very small

12. _____ soft spots in the newborn's skull

a. acrocyanosis
b. cephalohematoma
c. desquamate
d. fontanels
e. galactosemia
f. neonate
g. phenylketonuria
h. phimosis

i. pseudomenstruation
j. surfactant
k. stork bites
l. vernix caseosa

Match the following definitions with the correct terms.

13. _____ urinary meatus located on the upper side of the penis

14. _____ red, hive-appearing, raised lesions on some sensitive newborns' skin

15. _____ fine, downy hair on face, shoulders, and back of the newborn

16. _____ set amount stored fat in infants

17. _____ mother and baby align their heads as they look at each other

18. _____ urinary meatus located on the underside of the penis

19. _____ quick and accurate way to assess the newborn's physical condition at the time of birth

20. _____ part or all of the foreskin is removed

21. _____ accumulation of fluid within the newborn's scalp

22. _____ lung sacs

23. _____ corners of the eye

24. _____ process by encouraging parent to see, touch, and hold their newborn baby

a. alveoli
b. Apgar score
c. brown fat
d. bonding
e. canthus, inner and outer
f. caput succedaneum

g. circumcision

h. *en face* position

i. epispadias

j. erythema toxicum

k. hypospadias

l. lanugo

Match the following definitions with the correct terms.

25. _____ phenylketonuria

26. _____ elongation of neonate's head

27. _____ breast infection caused by bacteria from the baby's mouth

28. _____ placing the newborn on its back or side while sleeping helps reduce the risk for this disorder

29. _____ pinhead-sized white spots on the neonate's nose and cheeks

30. _____ neonate blindness caused by infective organisms

31. _____ excess secretions and dead skin cells

32. _____ purple-red permanent birthmark

33. _____ greenish-black, tarry first stool that the newborn passes

34. _____ foreskin

35. _____ appear on the buttocks, lower back, or upper legs of nonwhite babies

36. _____ acronym for breastfeeding

a. mastitis

b. meconium

c. milia

d. molding

e. Mongolian spots

f. opthalmia neonatorum

g. port-wine stain

h. prepuce

i. smegma

j. LATCH

k. PKU

l. SIDS

■ Assessment Review

Indicate whether the following assessment data for a newborn indicate a normal finding (N) or an abnormal finding (A).

1. _____ Apgar score at 5 minutes = 10

2. _____ Apgar score at 1 minute = 6

3. _____ birth weight of 4.5 lb

4. _____ length of 20 inches

5. _____ head circumference of 13.5 inches

6. _____ molding

7. _____ presence of anterior fontanel

8. _____ gray or blue eyes

9. _____ swollen genitals

10. _____ foreskin that cannot be retracted

11. _____ hypospadias

12. _____ acrocyanosis at 48 hours

13. _____ small white spots on the cheeks

14. _____ downy hair over the shoulders and back

15. _____ difficulty awaking

16. _____ newborn respiratory rate of 50 breaths/min

17. _____ newborn heart rate of 170 beats/min

18. _____ grunting noises when breathing

19. _____ first stool is greenish black and tarry looking

20. _____ no voiding for more than 24 hours

21. _____ hemoglobin of 16 g/100 mL

22. _____ blood glucose of 45 mg/100 mL

23. _____ turns head toward stimulus when cheek is stroked

24. _____ does not grasp finger when placed into newborn's hand

25. _____ fans toes when sole of foot is scraped from heel to toe

■ Sequencing

Number the following actions in the correct order for weighing the newborn. The first action should be number 1. Continue to number the items.

_____ Keep your hand close above the newborn at all times and do not leave newborn unattended.

_____ Wash hands and record the weight in grams; convert to pounds for the mother.

_____ Wash hands, clean scale, pad scale, and deduct weight of towel.

_____ Remove the newborn's clothes, paper the scale, and weigh newborn.

_____ Dress the newborn and place back in the crib.

Number the following actions in the correct order for bathing the newborn. The first action should be number 1. Continue to number the items.

_____ Keep newborn warm and secure. Support the newborn and assess as you bathe the newborn.

_____ Moisten, wash, and dry the hair.

_____ Place baby on back to sleep.

_____ Begin the bath by wiping each eye with a cotton ball dampened with clear water only.

_____ Cleanse genital area. If baby boy is circumcised, provide circumcision care.

_____ Wash hands; gather equipment.

_____ Dress newborn, folding diaper below the cord stump, and wrap in a blanket.

_____ Wash hands and document all observations.

_____ Check baby's vital signs; undress and weigh if needed.

_____ Wipe all surfaces with prescribed antiseptic and discard trash.

■ Short Answer

Complete the following questions.

1. List the three purposes of the newborn taking his or her first few breaths.

2. List the components of the Apgar score.

3. List methods of proper identification of newborns. Explain the rationale for using these methods.

4. Describe measures to promote bonding between infant and parents.

5. Describe methods to conserve heat in the newborn.

6. Describe what instructions you would teach a new mother regarding cord care.

7. Discuss advantages of breastfeeding.

8. Explain the process of bubbling (burping) the newborn. How often should it be done?

■ Multiple Choice

Circle the best answer.

1. Apgar score assessments are completed at:
   a. birth and 10 minutes.
   b. 1 and 5 minutes.
   c. 5 minutes and upon arrival to the nursery.
   d. the time of birth.

2. A newborn of 4 hours displays grunting respirations and a respiratory rate of 70 breaths/min. The priority nursing intervention would be to:
   a. begin resuscitative measures and call for help.
   b. continue to monitor respiratory status; variations are normal.
   c. obtain vital signs every 15 minutes.
   d. transfer the newborn to the mother's room for feeding.

3. Which measure would be used to prevent heat loss in the newborn?
   a. Immediately give the baby a bath.
   b. Offer the baby warm glucose water.
   c. Place the baby on the mother's bare stomach.
   d. Wrap the baby in room-temperature blankets.

4. Which measure would be most effective in preventing the transfer of gonorrhea or chlamydia to the infant's eyes from the mother?
   a. Administering vitamin K
   b. Applying erythromycin ointment
   c. Bathing the newborn
   d. Instructing the father to bathe the baby

5. A newborn will respond to sudden noises or jarring movement by throwing out the arms and drawing up the legs. This is called a:
   a. Babinski reflex.
   b. Moro reflex.
   c. Stepping reflex.
   d. Tonic neck reflex.

6. The nurse is caring for a newborn at 12 hours of life. The newborn has just voided. The most appropriate response by the nurse would be:
   a. continue to monitor voiding patterns.
   b. immediately check vital signs.
   c. notify the physician.
   d. obtain an order for a straight catheterization.

7. Which position should newborns be placed when sleeping?
   a. Back
   b. Head of bed elevated
   c. Prone
   d. Side lying with pillow

8. Most babies should be fed:
   a. every 1 to 2 hours
   b. every 2 to 4 hours
   c. every 4 to 6 hours
   d. on demand

9. When evaluating the effectiveness of instruction regarding breastfeeding, which of the following responses by the mother indicate that she understands the teaching?
   a. "I need to rub my nipples to toughen them up."
   b. "I should apply lotion to my nipples to prevent cracking."
   c. "I should nurse at least 10 minutes on one breast before offering the next breast."
   d. "I should use soap and water to gently cleanse my breasts daily."

10. Which of the following would the nurse recommend to the breastfeeding mother to limit in her diet?
    a. cheese
    b. fruit
    c. strongly flavored foods
    d. vegetables

11. The fontanels are soft spots formed by the:
    a. blood accumulated between the bone and periosteum.
    b. edema of the scalp from birth pressure.
    c. junction of individual skull bones.
    d. pressure of a vacuum extractor.

12. Signs of respiratory distress include:
    a. grunting with expiration.
    b. respiratory rate of 50 breaths/min.

c. synchronized movements of the baby's chest and abdomen.

d. the baby's chest expands as a whole.

13. The most efficient way for a baby to regulate temperature is to:

a. burn body fat.

b. move arms and legs.

c. shiver.

d. use brown fat.

CHAPTER 67

High-Risk Pregnancy and Childbirth

■ Terminology Review

Match the following definitions with the correct terms.

1. _____ most severe complication of pregnancy that results in tonic-clonic seizures, very rapid pulse, and very high blood pressure

2. _____ surgical procedure used to deliver the baby through an incision in the abdomen and the uterus

3. _____ nonabsorbable suture or ring placed on cervix to keep it closed during pregnancy

4. _____ lack of uterine muscle tone that prevents contracting and closing of the venous sinuses

5. _____ pregnancy that implants outside the uterus

6. _____ inflammation of the bladder

7. _____ premature separation of the normally implanted placenta from the uterine wall

8. _____ double-bladed curved instruments used to assist delivery of the fetus

9. _____ newborn born with disorder that is a result of the Rh-negative mother who has produced antibodies to a Rh-positive fetus

10. _____ type of delivery that results in higher fetal mortality

11. _____ condition in which the HCG remains high after delivery of a hydatidiform mole

12. _____ insertion of a needle through the maternal abdominal wall into the amniotic sac and withdrawing amniotic fluid

13. _____ occurs when the mother and fetus have different blood types

14. _____ prolonged, painful labor that does not result in effective cervical dilation or effacement

a. ABO incompatibility
b. abruption placentae
c. amniocentesis
d. atony
e. breech
f. cerclage
g. cesarean delivery
h. choriocarcinoma
i. cystitis
j. dystocia
k. eclampsia
l. ectopic
m. erythroblastosis fetalis
n. forceps delivery

Match the following definitions with the correct terms.

15. _____ placenta implants in the lower segment of the uterus, rather than the upper wall

16. _____ excessive amount of amniotic fluid; more than 2 liters

17. _____ stimulating labor to begin using a medication

18. _____ retained placenta after delivery

19. _____ oversized fetus

20. _____ embryo dies in utero and the chorionic villi degenerate, forming grapelike clusters of vesicles

21. _____ diabetes that occurs during the time of pregnancy

22. _____ pregnancy in which physiologic or psychological factors could significantly increase the chances of mortality or morbidity of woman or fetus

23. _____ umbilical cord becomes wrapped around the neck of the fetus

24. _____ another name for polyhydramnios

a. gestational diabetes

b. high-risk pregnancy

c. hydatidiform mole

d. hydramnios

e. induction

f. macrosomia

g. nuccal cord

h. placenta accrete

i. placenta previa

j. polyhydramnios

Match the following definitions with the correct terms.

25. _____ test used to evaluate response of the fetal heart to contractions

26. _____ round, soft plastic cup is placed on the fetal head to aid in delivery of the fetus

27. _____ occurs in a woman with a previously normal progressing pregnancy who then develops PIH with either edema, proteinuria, or both

28. _____ fetus lies across the woman's abdomen in the uterus

29. _____ placenta and fetus

30. _____ normal fetal presentation

31. _____ level of descent of the fetal presenting part in the birth canal

32. _____ manual rotation of the fetus

33. _____ complication occurring after delivery

34. _____ habitual and spontaneous abortions during the second or early third trimester of pregnancy

35. _____ bleeding into the subcutaneous tissue in the perineal area

a. postpartum hematoma

b. preeclampsia

c. premature cervical dilation

d. products of conception

e. puerperal

f. station

g. stress test

h. transverse lie

i. vacuum extraction

j. version

k. vertex

■ Acronym Review

Match the following definitions with the correct terms and acronyms.

1. _____ preferred method of intrauterine transfusion for Rh-sensitized fetuses

2. _____ test used to diagnose fetal defects early in pregnancy

3. _____ screening tool used to detect fetal neural tube defects and open abdominal wall defects early in pregnancy

4. _____ combines an NST with ultrasonic fetal assessment to evaluate fetal breathing, fetal movement, fetal tone, amniotic fluid volume, and placental grade

5. _____ characterized by hypertension, edema, and proteinuria

6. _____ direct occiput posterior position

7. _____ provides information on the fetal heart rate in response to fetal activity

8. _____ disseminated intravascular coagulation

9. _____ emergency delivery outside of healthcare facility

10. _____ natural or artificial termination of a pregnancy before the fetus is viable

11. _____ right occiput posterior position

12. _____ lecithin-sphingomyelin ratio

13. _____ provides information on how well the placenta is supplying oxygen to the fetus

14. _____ left occiput posterior position

15. _____ surgical procedure used to remove products of incomplete abortion

16. _____ magnesium sulfate

17. _____ premature rupture of membranes

18. _____ presenting part, usually the fetal head, is too large to pass through the woman's pelvis

a. AB

b. BOA

c. CPD

d. CVS

e. D & C

f. DIC

g. FBP

h. LOP

i. LS Ratio

j. $MgSO_4$

k. MSAFP

l. NST

m. OCT

n. OP

o. PIH

p. PROM

q. PUBS

r. ROP

■ Assessment Review

Indicate whether the following assessment findings are normal (N) or abnormal (A) findings for the pregnant female of fetus/infant.

1. _____ painless vaginal bleeding

2. _____ excessive weight loss

3. _____ end of morning sickness at 12th week of pregnancy

4. _____ protein in urine

5. _____ edema in lower extremities

6. _____ blood pressure of 190/110

7. _____ sudden rise in fundus

8. _____ less than 2,000 mL of amniotic fluid

9. _____ placenta expelled within 20 minutes of delivery

10. _____ labor occurring after the end of 37th week of gestation

11. _____ labor lasting less than 3 hours

12. _____ sharp, tearing pain followed by sudden cessation of pain

13. _____ vertex position

14. _____ laceration

15. _____ blood loss of 300 mL during delivery

16. _____ negative Homans' sign

17. _____ pain in lower extremity

18. _____ temperature of 101°Ft

19. _____ headache

20. _____ hyperreflexia

■ Correct the False Statements

Circle the word True or False that follows the statement. If the word false has been circled, change the underlined word/words to make the statement true. Place your answer in the space provided.

1. Down syndrome can be diagnosed <u>from an amniocentesis</u>.

   True   False   _____

2. The nurse should prepare a woman for an <u>oxytocin challenge test</u> by having the woman drink large amounts of water.

   True   False   _____

3. <u>Ritodrine</u> in used to stimulate contractions during an OCT.

   True   False   _____

4. A nonstress test is considered reactive when at least <u>two episodes of fetal heart rate accelerations of 15 beats/min last at least 15 seconds within a continuous 10-minute period</u>.

   True   False   _____

5. <u>Maternal alcohol use and cigarette smoking</u> can contribute to spontaneous abortions.

   True   False   _____

6. <u>Hemorrhage and infection</u> are major risk factors when criminal or illegal abortions are performed.

   True   False   _____

7. <u>Severe eclampsia</u> is treated with rest and limiting sodium intake.

   True   False   _____

8. <u>Cardiac problems</u> in the mother often result in higher birth weight in the infant.

   True   False   _____

9. ABO incompatibility is usually treated with <u>blood transfusions</u>.

   True   False   _____

10. Pregnancy continuing <u>beyond 42 weeks</u> is known as a prolonged pregnancy.

    True   False   _____

11. Pregnancy in a girl younger than 16 years often results in infants being <u>preterm and small for their gestational age.</u>

    True   False   _____

12. Intrauterine infection is a complication of <u>SROM.</u>

    True   False   _____

13. A complete breech presentation is when <u>the buttocks present with the legs extended straight up.</u>

    True   False   _____

14. <u>A fourth-degree laceration</u> extends to the anal canal.

    True   False   _____

15. <u>Forceps delivery</u> is indicated when the mother is exhausted, has heart disease, or has prolonged labor.

    True   False   _____

16. After a caesarean section, the mother should be encouraged to <u>rest in bed.</u>

    True   False   _____

17. Severe pain during a bowel movement could indicate <u>uterine atony</u>.

    True   False   _____

18. Assessment of Homans' sign is done to screen for the presence of <u>thrombophlebitis</u>.

    True   False   _____

19. <u>Postpartum blues</u> are most likely due to gonadal hormone imbalances.

    True   False   _____

20. <u>Postpartum psychosis</u> rarely occurs in women with no previous psychiatric history.

    True   False   _____

■ Multiple Choice

Circle the best answer.

1. Which assessment most closely relates to a diagnosis of ectopic pregnancy?
   a. brownish red, tapioca-like vesicles.
   b. elevated temperature.
   c. spotting or bleeding 2 to 3 weeks after a missed menstrual period.
   d. sudden absence of fetal movement.

2. The drug of choice to treat pregnancy-induced hypertension is:
   a. iron and vitamins.
   b. magnesium sulfate.
   c. diazepam (Valium)
   d. furosemide (Lasix)

3. Which nursing intervention would be appropriate for a client who has a diastolic blood pressure of more than 20 mmHg on the "roll-over test"?
   a. Increase intake of oral fluids.
   b. Rest on left side as much as possible.
   c. Schedule follow-up care every 2 weeks.
   d. Use the stairs to increase activity level.

4. A mother receiving medications for pregnancy-induced hypertension should have her diastolic blood pressure maintained in the range of 90 to 100 mmHg to:
   a. avoid causing fetal anoxia.
   b. ensure progression of labor.
   c. prevent premature contractions.
   d. present sudden elevations in pulse.

5. Which of the following would be a priority intervention for a client with a prolapsed cord?
   a. Cover the cord with a dry sterile towel.
   b. Monitor mother's vital signs.
   c. Place woman in the Trendelenburg position.
   d. Start medications as ordered.

CHAPTER 68

The High-Risk Newborn

■ Terminology Review

Match the following definitions with the correct terms.

1. _____ vertical opening in the upper lip

2. _____ newborn with a complication

3. _____ upper end of the newborn's esophagus ends in a blind pouch

4. _____ genetic defect that renders the newborn incapable of metabolizing certain amino acids

5. _____ disorder or abnormality that exists at birth

6. _____ newborn's nostrils are closed at the entrance to the throat so that air cannot pass through to the lungs

7. _____ excess of CSF in the ventricles and subarachnoid spaces of the brain

8. _____ caused by abnormal development

9. _____ children born with all or part of their brain missing

10. _____ baby's rectum ends in a blind pouch, causing obstruction to the normal passage of feces

11. _____ elevated bilirubin levels

12. _____ split in the palate

13. _____ belongs to the herpes virus and can be transmitted to the fetus

a. anencephaly

b. choanal atresia

c. cleft lip

d. cleft palate

e. congenital

f. cytomegalovirus

g. esophageal atresia

h. exstrophy

i. galactosemia

j. high-risk newborn

k. hydrocephalus

l. hyperbilirubinemia

m. imperforate anus

Match the following definitions with the correct terms.

14. _____ protozoa found in cat feces that can cause possible fetal effects if the mother is exposed to the organism

15. _____ fusing together of two or more digits

16. _____ one or both feet turn out of the normal position

17. _____ congenital anomaly in which an increase in size of the musculature at the junction of the stomach and small intestine occurs

18. _____ use of fluorescent lights to alleviate jaundice

19. _____ congenital neural tube defect in which the vertebral spaces fail to close, allowing herniation or bulging of the spinal contents into the sac

20. _____ presence of an extra finger or toe

21. _____ fetus who remains in the uterus beyond 42 weeks

22. _____ yeast infection

23. _____ born before the end of the 37th week

24. _____ children with abnormally small heads

25. _____ results from the newborn's immature liver to handle bilirubin

a. microcephaly
b. phototherapy
c. physiologic jaundice
d. polydactylism
e. postterm
f. preterm
g. pyloric stenosis
h. spina bifida
i. syndactylism
j. talipes
k. thrush
l. toxoplasmosis

a. AGA
b. ASD
c. CMV
d. CSF
e. FAS
f. LBW
g. LGA
h. NEC
i. PKU
j. RDS
k. ROP
l. SGA
m. TORCH
n. VLBW
o. VSD

■ Acronym Review

Match the following definitions with the acronyms.

1. _____ cytomegalovirus

2. _____ leading cause of death, especially in the preterm newborn

3. _____ weighs less than 5.5 pounds

4. _____ serious disorder causing varying amounts of bowel wall to necrose

5. _____ birth weight is below the 10th percentile expected for that gestational age

6. _____ excess of this fluid in the ventricles and subarachnoid spaces causes hydrocephalus

7. _____ weighs between 1 and 3.5 pounds

8. _____ abnormal opening between the ventricles

9. _____ growth is within normal limits

10. _____ all newborns are tested for this before discharge from the hospital and at 6 weeks

11. _____ abnormal opening between the atria

12. _____ birth weight is higher than that of 90% of the babies born at that gestational age

13. _____ effects of this syndrome include growth deficiency, microcephaly, facial abnormalities, cardiac anomalies, and mental retardation

14. _____ complication of high concentration of oxygen

■ Assessment Review

Indicate whether the following assessment findings are normal (N) or abnormal (A).

1. _____ loose, dry skin

2. _____ vernix caseosa

3. _____ long fingernails

4. _____ transparent skin

5. _____ pink skin

6. _____ spitting up after feeding

7. _____ cyanosis

8. _____ high-pitched cry

9. _____ asymmetric Moro reflex

10. _____ folds of thigh are asymmetric

11. _____ protruding tongue

12. _____ cracks around anus

13. _____ pulse 150 beats/min

14. _____ diarrhea

15. _____ frequent sneezing

■ Nursing Actions

Indicate whether the following actions by a nurse would be appropriate (A) or inappropriate (I).

1. _____ Keeping environmental stimuli to a minimum when caring for a chemically dependent newborn

2. _____ Monitoring for symptoms including lethargy, poor feeding, and jitteriness as signs that a newborn is experiencing withdrawal from cocaine or crack

3. _____ Recognizing that microcephaly, being small for gestational age, and mental retardation are possible effects of cytomegalovirus on the newborn

4. _____ Informing a mother that her baby, whose birth weight is below the 10th percentile expected for that gestation age, is appropriate for gestation age (AGA) but very low birth weight

5. _____ Bathing a preterm newborn immediately after birth to remove skin organisms and prevent infection

6. _____ Providing the premature newborn with 2-hour feedings until the newborn tolerates 15 mL at each feeding

7. _____ Weigh only diapers of newborns that are at risk for dehydration or feeding difficulties

8. _____ Assessing the respiratory status of an infant who aspirated meconium

9. _____ Giving intravenous fluids, along with humidified oxygen, to dehydrated newborn

10. _____ Administer RhoGAM to Rh-negative mother at 28 weeks' gestation and after delivery to prevent Rh sensitization

11. _____ Perform range-of-motion exercises on the newborn with brachial plexus injury

12. _____ Instruct expectant mothers to increase vitamin E to prevent spina bifida

13. _____ Use special nipples to feed the infant with cleft palate

14. _____ Assess the newborn of a chemically dependent mother for signs of withdrawal

15. _____ Inform parents that no treatment is available for arterial septal defect

■ Multiple Choice

Circle the best answer.

1. Which of the following drugs can be given to the mother before a preterm birth to help reduce the severity of respiratory distress syndrome?
   a. betamethasone
   b. diazepam
   c. phenobarbital
   d. RhoGAM

2. Which intervention is the priority immediately after the delivery of a newborn who does not breathe?
   a. Clear air passages of obstructive substances.
   b. Keep the mother calm.
   c. Place bulb suction at head of the bed.
   d. Rub the baby's back

3. In which position should the newborn be placed who has intracranial hemorrhage?
   a. prone
   b. side-lying
   c. slightly elevated HOB
   d. supine

4. Prophylactic installation of antibiotic ointment in to the eyes of newborns prevents blindness when the mother is infected with:
   a. herpes simplex.
   b. HIV.
   c. gonorrhea.
   d. syphilis.

5. Which method, if used by the nurse, would be most effective in preventing the transmission of thrush?
   a. Assess the baby's mouth with every feeding.
   b. Use clean equipment and perform good handwashing.
   c. Teach family members to assess infant's mouth.
   d. Wipe newborn's mouth with gauze after feeding.

6. Which of the following is an important goal for a preterm infant with a nursing diagnosis stem of *Altered Nutrition, Less than Body Requirements*? Newborn will:

   a. demonstrate normal respirations.

   b. demonstrate heart rate within normal ranges.

   c. gain 20 to 30 g/d.

   d. learn to suck adequately on bottle.

CHAPTER 69

Sexuality, Fertility, and Sexually Transmitted Diseases

■ Terminology Review

Match the following definitions with the correct terms.

1. _____ birth control

2. _____ caused by herpes simplex virus type 2

3. _____ men who are sexually attracted to other men

4. _____ individuals who are not particularly attracted to either sex

5. _____ soft sore caused by *Haemophilus decreyi*

6. _____ individuals who are attracted to the opposite sex

7. _____ latex, plastic, or animal tissue sheaths applied to the penis to prevent conception and spread of STDs

8. _____ primary lesion of syphilis

9. _____ painful intercourse

10. _____ modern technology that is used to enhance fertility if the man's sperm count is too low of if the woman's body interferes with sperm motility

11. _____ also known as thrush

12. _____ individuals who are attracted to both sexes

13. _____ leading cause of preventable infertility in women

14. _____ birth control by the man withdrawing the penis before climax

15. _____ nonspecific vaginitis

a. artificial insemination
b. asexual
c. bacterial vaginosis
d. bisexual
e. candidiasis
f. *Chlamydia*
g. chancre
h. chancroid
i. coitus interruptus
j. condom
k. contraception
l. dyspareunia
m. gay
n. genital herpes
o. heterosexual

Match the following definitions with the correct terms.

16. _____ inability to enjoy or to engage in sexual activity

17. _____ absolute inability to procreate

18. _____ continued erection accompanied by pain

19. _____ most common and effective procedure for permanent sterilization in women

20. _____ women who are sexually attracted to women

21. _____ inability to conceive or to produce live babies after adequate sexual exposure

22. _____ culmination of sexual excitement

23. _____ individuals who are attracted to person of the same sex

24. _____ vas deferens are ligated

25. _____ involuntary contraction of vaginal outlet muscles that prevents penile penetration

26. _____ violent crime in which an individual has been sexually assaulted without his or her consent

27. _____ way in which individuals physically, mentally, emotionally, and socially experience and express themselves as sexual beings

28. _____ second most common vaginitis that has a foul-smelling greenish yellow or gray, frothy or bubbly discharge

29. _____ inability to achieve or to sustain erection

30. _____ tiny parasites that attach themselves to pubic hair

a. homosexual
b. impotence
c. infertility
d. lesbian
e. orgasm
f. pediculosis pubis
g. priapism
h. rape
i. sexual dysfunction
j. sexuality
k. sterility
l. trichomoniasis
m. tubal ligation
n. vaginismus
o. vasectomy

Match the following definitions with the acronym.

31. _____ human papillomavirus

32. _____ prevents implantation of a fertilized egg by interfering with the hormone balance

33. _____ rapid plasma reagin

34. _____ fertilization of the woman's or donor's egg outside the woman's body

35. _____ more commonly associated with common canker sores

36. _____ can lead to scar tissue and female infertility

37. _____ sexually transmitted disease

38. _____ impotence

39. _____ Venereal Disease Research Laboratory

40. _____ oral contraceptives

41. _____ device in the woman's uterus that prevent the fertilized ovum from implanting in the uterus

42. _____ posttraumatic stress disorder

43. _____ genital herpes

44. _____ fertility awareness methods

45. _____ potassium hydroxide

a. BCP
b. EC
c. ED
d. FAM
e. HPV
f. HSV-1
g. HSV-2
h. IUD
i. IVF
j. KOH
k. PID
l. PTSD
m. RPR
n. STD
o. VDRL

■ Short Answer

Complete the following questions.

1. Describe the most common type of sexual dysfunction in males. Identify causes of this problem.

2. Identify medical causes of female sexual dysfunction.

3. Discuss two tests used for diagnosing causes of female infertility.

4. Describe when emergency contraception can be used.

5. Discuss teaching that the nurse would include for the client wishing to use chemical barriers as a birth control method.

6. Discuss risk factors for developing STDs.

7. Why women are more easily infected with HIV during unprotected sex?

8. Discuss treatment methods for each of the following:

   a. HIV

   b. *Chlamydia*

   c. gonorrhea

   d. syphilis

   e. HSV-2

■ Multiple Choice

Circle the best answer.

1. Careful documentation and following hospital procedures are essential when caring for the rape victim to:
   a. ensure that appropriate information is available for legal purposes.
   b. help other victims come forward who have been assaulted.
   c. prevent posttraumatic stress disorder.
   d. provide emotional support for the victim.

2. In evaluating the effectiveness of yohimbine (Viagra), the nurse assess for:
   a. cardiac arrhythmias.
   b. erection.
   c. hypotension.
   d. priapism.

3. Which of the following procedures is used when a woman does not produce viable ova?
   a. artificial insemination
   b. fertility awareness method
   c. in vitro fertilization
   d. vasectomy

4. Which of the following contraceptive methods also offers protection against STDs?
   a. abstinence
   b. coitus interruptus
   c. fertility awareness methods
   d. oral contraceptives

5. The nurse knows that a client's choosing to continue to smoke and take oral contraceptives increases the risk for developing:
   a. asthma.
   b. cysts.
   c. gastritis.
   d. myocardial infarction.

6. In teaching the postoperative client who has just had a vasectomy, it is most important to focus on:

   a. asking how his partner feels about the surgery.

   b. alternate methods of expressing sexual needs and desires.

   c. discussing that a vasectomy does not make client less of a man.

   d. using birth control until sperm counts are zero for 6 weeks.

7. After a tubal ligation, it is not uncommon for the woman to complain of:

   a. breast tenderness.

   b. hemorrhoids.

   c. leg pain.

   d. shoulder pain.

8. Which assessment finding most closely relates to a diagnosis of *Chlamydia*?

   a. dry cough

   b. night sweats

   c. no symptoms

   d. memory loss

CHAPTER 70

Fundamentals of Pediatric Nursing

■ Terminology Review

Match the following definitions with the correct terms.

1. _____ along with health maintenance has proved to be the most effective method of promoting the growth and development of healthy children

2. _____ provides people with temporary or permanent protection against certain diseases

3. _____ primary emphasis in today's pediatric healthcare

4. _____ physician who provides care for children and adolescents

5. _____ area of care that deals with children and adolescents

6. _____ darkening of the skin color around the mouth due to poor oxygenation

7. _____ tool used to identify developmental delays in infants, toddlers, and preschoolers

a. circumoral cyanosis
b. Denver Developmental Screening Test
c. health maintenance
d. health supervision
e. immunization
f. pediatrician
g. pediatrics

Match the following definitions with the correct terms.

8. _____ type of central venous line used for long-term cancer chemotherapy or other IV medications

9. _____ upper respiratory infection

10. _____ immunization consisting of measles, mumps, and rubella

11. _____ American Academy of Family Physicians

12. _____ occipital-frontal circumference

13. _____ intermittent positive-pressure breathing

14. _____ total parenteral nutrition

15. _____ Advisory Committee on Immunization Practices

16. _____ immunization for *Haemophilus influenzae*

17. _____ nothing by mouth

18. _____ American Academy of Pediatricians

19. _____ Denver Developmental Screening Test

a. AAFP
b. AAP
c. ACIP
d. DDST
e. H flu
f. IPPB
g. NPO
h. OFC
i. MMR
j. PICC
k. TPN
l. URI

■ Fill-in-the-Blanks

Complete the following by filling in the blanks.

1. _____ is children's work and their means of communication.

2. Pediatrics requires knowledge of developmental _____; this knowledge helps you determine developmental _____.

3. Very _____ children are especially susceptible to communicable diseases.

4. Children may need _____ to remind them not to pull on tubes or pick at suture lines; these should be removed and reapplied every _____ to _____ hours and the child's skin and circulation checked _____ hour.

5. _____ substitute the safety device for good observation.

6. Early immunization is important to _____ small children.

7. Identify the appropriate age range in which the following immunizations should be administered:

   a. Hep B-1 _____

   b. Polio _____

   c. Varicella _____

   d. Measles, mumps, rubella _____

   e. Diphtheria, tetanus, pertussis _____

8. List four signs of respiratory distress in a child.

9. Do not use the _____ _____ for a child with respiratory distress to prevent closing of the airway.

10. Fevers above _____ degrees Fahrenheit must be immediately brought under control in children who have neurologic problems, history of febrile illness, or cardiac or respiratory problems.

11. Evaluation of _____, _____, and _____ is critical in the preschool years.

12. When examining the adolescent, the nurse should ensure _____.

13. The three stages of separation anxiety are _____, _____, and _____.

14. Infants should be weighed at the _____.

15. A bolus tube feeding is usually administered over _____ minutes.

■ Sequencing

Number the following actions in the correct order for using an Oxy-Hood. The first action should be number 1. Continue to number the items.

_____ Set up equipment. Attach flow regulator to the oxygen.

_____ Wash your hands.

_____ Document the time you started the oxygen, rate of flow, and assessments of the child.

_____ Connect the tubing to the hood's port and to the flow regulator.

_____ Turn the flow meter to the ordered rate to flush the hood.

_____ Check the physician's order, wash you hands, and collect equipment.

_____ Place the hood over the child's head and neck.

_____ Explain to caregivers what you are going to do and why.

_____ Monitor the child's respiratory status frequently. Report and document any significant changes or signs of respiratory distress.

■ Multiple Choice

Circle the best answer.

1. Which of the following instructions to a child would be most appropriate before a painful procedure?

   a. Do not tell the child anything, just do the procedure.

   b. "This is going to hurt."

   c. "This won't hurt at all."

   d. "Would you like to help me?"

2. Which of the following accurately describes how to collect a urine specimen for a urine culture in a 3-year-old girl?

   a. Apply a urine collector to the perineum sealing from the bottom up to the pubis.

   b. Cover the bag with a tight-fitting diaper or underpants to hold it in place.

   c. Clean the child's perineal area, adding powder to the thighs and labia to protect them from urine.

   d. Have the child lie on her stomach with a bedpan under her perineum.

3. The nurse assesses a 1-year-old and notes nasal flaring, tachypnea, and retractions. The most appropriate response is to:

   a. determine that this is unusual behavior and ask parents to sit with child.

   b. offer child a special treat to calm down.

   c. notify the physician and prepare to give oxygen by mist tent or oxyhood.

   d. recognize the child needs comfort and pick the child up and hold closely.

4. Which method would be helpful when administering liquid medication to a preschool-aged child?

   a. Ask the child if he or she would like to take the medication from a cup or spoon.

   b. Give the child a drop or two of liquid over an hour to prevent spitting it out.

   c. Tell the child the medicine is sweet candy syrup that he or she will like.

   d. Tell the child firmly to take the medicine.

5. Which of the following is particularly dangerous for small children because of potential fluid and electrolyte imbalances?

   a. Administer medication based on child's weight.

   b. Intramuscular injections

   c. Liquids administered through feeding tube

   d. Tap water enema

6. A child's temperature is 104.2°F. Which is the most appropriate nursing action?

   a. Administer aspirin.

   b. Apply alcohol to the skin to cool the child.

   c. Monitor the child's temperature every 2 hours.

   d. Sponge the child with lukewarm water.

7. When obtaining vital signs, which of the following is appropriate?

   a. Oral temperature in children younger than 6 years.

   b. Radial pulse in children older than 2 years.

   c. Rectal temperature in child with hematology disorder.

   d. Tympanic temperature in child with ventilating tubes.

8. When discharging a child from the hospital, it is most important for the nurse to document:

   a. that child's belongings were sent with caregivers.

   b. reaction of child to staff members.

   c. teaching follow-up care to family caregivers.

   d. weight of the child on discharge.

CHAPTER 71

Care of the Infant, Toddler, or Preschooler

■ Terminology Review

Match the following definitions with the correct terms.

1. _____ nosebleed

2. _____ multisystem chronic and incurable condition, is a major dysfunction of the exocrine glands

3. _____ severe atopic dermatitis

4. _____ incontinence of feces without physical cause

5. _____ deformities resulting from the failure of the upper lip and palate to close completely during the second and third gestational months

6. _____ defect in the bile ducts that prevents bile from escaping from the liver

7. _____ caused by protozoan that is ingested after water is contaminated by careless disposal of human excrement

8. _____ involuntary passage of urine

9. _____ brain inflammation

10. _____ viral respiratory infection resulting in inflammation of the bronchioles

11. _____ lazy eye

12. _____ undescended testicle

13. _____ most common malabsorption syndrome

14. _____ urinary meatus is located on the top of the penis

15. _____ paroxysmal abdominal pain, most common in the first 3 months of an infant's life

a. amblyopia
b. biliary atresia
c. bronchiolitis
d. celiac disease
e. cleft lip/palate
f. colic
g. cryptorchidism
h. cystic fibrosis
i. eczema
j. encephalitis
k. encorpresis
l. enuresis
m. epispadias
n. epistaxis
o. giardiasis

Match the following definitions with the correct terms.

16. _____ malignant lymphoma

17. _____ inherited disorder characterized by an inability to metabolize milk products

18. _____ changes in basement membrane of the glomeruli resulting in the kidneys excreting massive amounts of protein

19. _____ type of worm that enters host through bare feet

20. _____ shingles

21. _____ urinary meatus is located on the bottom of the penis

22. _____ small portion of the ileum ends in a blind pouch just before its junction with the colon

23. _____ general failure-to-thrive condition

24. _____ also known as Hirschsprung's disease

25. _____ sex-linked hereditary bleeding disorder

26. _____ most common form of nephritis in young children between the ages 5 and 10 years

27. _____ group of associated disorders characterized by malignancies in the bone marrow and lymphatic system

28. _____ telescoping of one bowel part into another

29. _____ most serious form of spina bifida in which the meninges and part of the spinal cord protrude through an opening

30. _____ child's colon lacks parasympathetic nerve supply

a. glomerulonephritis
b. hemophilia
c. Herpes zoster
d. Hirschsprung's disease
e. Hodgkin's disease
f. hookworm
g. hypospadia
h. intussusception
i. lactose intolerance
j. leukemia
k. marasmus
l. Meckel's diverticulum
m. megacolon
n. meningomyelocele
o. necrotic syndrome

Match the following definitions with the correct terms.

31. _____ lice infestation

32. _____ acute and potentially fatal childhood disease that usually occurs after a viral illness

33. _____ type of worm that is most common in warm climates with unclean living conditions

34. _____ vitamin C deficiency

35. _____ hereditary disease characterized by RBCs abnormally shaped like a sickle

36. _____ benign disease of infancy in which the infant has a high fever lasting a few days that is followed by a rash

37. _____ clubfoot

38. _____ malformation in which part of the vertebral or spinal column is open or missing

39. _____ "crossed eyes"

40. _____ also known as scarlatina

41. _____ potentially fatal condition when medications do not relieve an acute episode of asthma

42. _____ whooping cough

43. _____ infection of the upper urinary tract and kidneys

44. _____ child's pyloric sphincter thickens

45. _____ complication of rheumatic fever in which valvular lesions impair valve efficiency

a. pediculosis
b. pertussis
c. pyelonephritis
d. pyloric stenosis
e. Reye's syndrome
f. rheumatic carditis
g. roseola
h. roundworm
i. scarlet fever
j. scurvey
k. sickle cell anemia
l. spina bifida
m. status asthmaticus
n. strabismus
o. talipes

■ Assessment Review

Indicate whether the following assessment findings are normal (N) or abnormal (A).

1. _____ Sore throat and fever

2. _____ Swelling of the parotid gland

3. _____ Acne in teenager

4. _____ Bowel movement every day

5. _____ Anorexia

6. _____ Puncture wound

7. _____ Malaise

8. _____ Intact skin

9. _____ Apnea in infants for 5 seconds

10. _____ Unexplained bruises

11. _____ Rectal lesions

12. _____ Mongolian spots

13. _____ Buttock on infant has extra crease

14. _____ Strabismus

15. _____ Pulling on ears

■ Nursing Actions

Indicate whether the following actions are appropriate (A) or inappropriate (I).

1. _____ Provide a child with celiac disease a diet with carbohydrates supplied by wheat and barley.

2. _____ Administer acetaminophen and tepid sponge baths to a child experiencing febrile seizures.

3. _____ Place elbow restraints on a child after surgery for correction of strabismus.

4. _____ Feed a child with cleft lip and palate using a cup and straw to promote independence.

5. _____ Using the side of a spoon to feed a child after cleft palate repair.

6. _____ Teach parents of an infant being monitored for apnea to stimulate the child immediately if the monitor alarms, even if the child is pink.

7. _____ When a child informs you that his uncle is sexually abusing him, consider the age of the child and say nothing because young children are easily confused.

8. _____ Attempt to establish a supportive relationship with the caregivers of a suspected child abuse victim.

9. _____ Keep a child with glomerulonephritis on bed rest and away from people with URIs.

10. _____ Encourage parents to start introducing solid foods to infants at age 2 months.

11. _____ Teach children not to share combs, brushes, or hats with their friends.

12. _____ Monitor child's respiratory status during a gastric lavage.

13. _____ Feed FTT infants every 4 hours.

14. _____ Monitor the child with spina bifida for signs of urinary tract infections.

15. _____ Teach caregivers to administer all of the antibiotic therapy, even if the child appears better.

■ Sequencing

Number the following actions in the correct order for use of the apnea monitor. The first action should be number 1. Continue to number the items.

_____ Attach the belt to the infant.

_____ Wash hands, gather equipment, and explain procedure to caregivers.

_____ Insert the corresponding lead wire into the cable and insert the cable into the monitor.

_____ Insert lead wires.

_____ Settle the infant comfortably or allow caregivers to hold infant.

_____ Prepare the infant's skin by making sure it is clean and dry.

_____ Make sure monitor is plugged in, the cable is attached, and the alarms are properly set. Turn on the monitor.

▪ Labeling

Indicate the name of the defects in tetralogy of Fallot marked with lines in the illustration below.

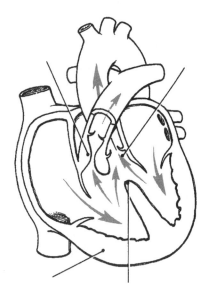

▪ Multiple Choice

Circle the best answer.

1. Which assessment findings most closely correlate with the diagnosis of tetrology of Fallot?
   a. Cyanosis
   b. Elevated blood pressure
   c. Normal weight
   d. Weak pulse in lower extremities

2. Which action would be most appropriate when caring for a child with idiopathic thrombocytopenic purpura?
   a. Administer enemas to promote bowel movements.
   b. Do not give intramuscular injections.
   c. Place child with head of bed elevated.
   d. Weigh daily at the same time.

3. When evaluating for side effects and adverse reaction of chemotherapy, the nurse would assess for:
   a. adequate urine volume.
   b. stable temperature.
   c. tolerating diet.
   d. vomiting.

4. The most common chronic childhood illness is:
   a. asthma.
   b. common cold.
   c. diabetes mellitus.
   d. mumps.

5. Which of the following is the number one cause of death in children older than the age of 1 year?
   a. Abuse
   b. Accidents
   c. Asthma
   d. SIDS

CHAPTER 72

Care of the School-Age Child or Adolescent

■ Terminology Review

Match the following definitions with the correct terms.

1. _____ infection caused by staphylococci, streptococci, or mixed bacteria that presents with reddened vesicles that break open and leave a sticky, honey-colored crust

2. _____ pain occurring with ovulation

3. _____ "kissing disease"

4. _____ tick-borne bacterial illness

5. _____ disorder characterized by extreme weight loss with no underlying physical cause

6. _____ chronic inflammation of the colon and rectum; is relatively common in adolescents and young adults

7. _____ difficulty falling asleep

8. _____ gorge–purge syndrome

9. _____ consists of blackheads, whiteheads, pimples, cysts, nodules, and scarring

10. _____ brief attack of irresistible sleep

11. _____ faulty tooth positioning

12. _____ uncontrollable urge to sleep, characterized by lengthy sleep periods of 12 to 18 hours

13. _____ surgical means of smoothing the skin

14. _____ painful menstruation

15. _____ attack of muscular weakness and lack of muscle tone; may accompany narcolepsy

a. acne vulgaris

b. anorexia nervosa

c. bulimia nervosa

d. cataplexy

e. chronic ulcerative colitis

f. dermabrasion

g. dysmenorrhea

h. hypersomnia

i. impetigo contagiosa

j. insomnia

k. Lyme disease

l. malocclusion

m. mittelschmerz

n. mononucleosis

o. narcolepsy

Match the following definitions with the correct terms.

16. _____ characterized by a slowly progressive, bilateral retinal degeneration that often causes blindness

17. _____ inflammatory bowel disease

18. _____ generalized systemic disease of the entire musculoskeletal system

19. _____ chronic ulcerative colitis

20. _____ retinitis pigmentosa

21. _____ sleep talking

22. _____ correction of tooth positioning and jaw deformities

23. _____ rapid eye movement

24. _____ type 2 diabetes mellitus

25. _____ sexually transmitted disease

26. _____ type 1 diabetes mellitus

27. _____ lateral curvature of the spine resulting in an S-shaped spinal appearance

28. _____ nonsteroidal anti-inflammatory drugs

29. _____ body mass index

30. _____ sleep walking

a. orthodontia
b. retinitis pigmentosa
c. scoliosis
d. somnambulism
e. somniloquism
f. BMI
g. CUC
h. IBD
i. IDDM
j. JRA
k. NIDDM
l. NSAIDs
m. REM
n. RP
o. STD

■ Nursing Actions

Indicate whether the following actions are appropriate (A) or inappropriate (I).

1. _____ Instruct a teen with acne to use gentle cleaning and to avoid scrubbing the face.

2. _____ Suggest that young people wear sandals and cotton socks if they have athlete's foot.

3. _____ Keep a child with Legg-Calvé-Perthes disease physically active to build the muscles in the legs.

4. _____ Administer nonsteroidal anti-inflammatory drugs and hot baths to a child with juvenile rheumatoid arthritis.

5. _____ Instruct a child with retinitis pigmentosa that sunglasses or shades should be avoided to prevent sensory deprivation to the eyes.

6. _____ Prepare to administer steroids to a teen with inflammatory bowel disease.

7. _____ Inform the parents of a child who experiences night terrors that noting spots of blood after an episode is expected and is nothing to worry about.

8. _____ Assist the family of a youngster who is a chronic lawbreaker in arranging for family counseling.

9. _____ Teach diabetic children and caregivers the signs and symptoms of both hypoglycemia and hyperglycemia

10. _____ Instruct adolescent girls to increase iron and calcium in their diets.

■ Labeling

Indicate which picture demonstrates the spinal deviation in A-scoliosis, B-kyphosis, C-lordosis, D-normal. (One letter will not be used.)

1.   2.   3.

■ Correct the False Statements

Circle the word True or False that follows the statement. If the word false has been circled, change the underlined word/words to make the statement true. Place your answer in the space provided.

1. Lyme disease is treated with <u>antibiotics such as doxycycline, amoxicillin, and erythromycin</u>.

   True   False   _____

2. Research indicates that <u>diets</u> accompanied by oversecretion of sebum are acne's underlying causes.

   True   False   _____

3. Juvenile rheumatoid arthritis <u>never has any long-term effects</u>.

   True   False   _____

4. <u>Osteogenic sarcoma</u> is a type of cancerous bone tumor, which frequently involves the long bones.

   True   False   _____

5. The three classic symptoms of diabetes mellitus are <u>polyuria, polydipsia, and polyphagia</u>.

   True   False   _____

6. Appendicitis is <u>frequently seen in children younger than 2 years of age</u>.

   True   False   _____

7. For the adolescent who is underdeveloped or overdeveloped, the nurse should <u>provide emotional support</u>.

   True   False   _____

8. <u>There are no known</u> underlying contributing factors to narcolepsy.

   True   False   _____

9. Most children <u>outgrow</u> nightmares.

   True   False   _____

10. Life-threatening complications associated with anorexia nervosa include <u>lowered blood pressure, hypokalemia, and death</u>.

    True   False   _____

■ Multiple Choice

Circle the best answer.

1. To assess for scoliosis, the examiner should:
   a. assist the child to look in a mirror for characteristic curing.
   b. have the child place the chin on the chest, place hands together, bend over, and let the hands hang freely.
   c. have the child turn sideways, and look for bulging in the thoracic region.
   d. palpate the spine for indentation in the lower back.

2. A client is admitted to the hospital with a diagnosis of chronic ulcerative colitis. When taking the client's history, which information would be most significant?
   a. Bloody diarrhea
   b. Cramping
   c. Food preferences
   d. Nausea

3. When evaluating the effectiveness of nonsteroidal anti-inflammatory drugs given before menses, the nurse would assess for:
   a. decreased cervical swelling.
   b. reduced blood flow.
   c. reduced discomfort.
   d. stable vital signs.

4. During an episode of somnambulism, which action would be most appropriate if taken by the nurse?
   a. Ask the child what he or she is doing.
   b. Immediately wake the child.
   c. Observe for safety measures to avoid injury.
   d. Pull the child back into bed.

5. Which instruction should the nurse provide the adolescent who is experiencing acne?
   a. Avoid chocolate in the diet.
   b. Inspect skin for adverse reactions to treatment.
   c. Pop pimples only when they are white with pus.
   d. Scrub skin twice a day with prescribed medication.

CHAPTER 73

The Child or Adolescent With Special Needs

■ Terminology Review

Match the following definitions with the correct terms.

1. _____ assorted groups of physical, cognitive, psychological, sensory, and speech impairments

2. _____ type of CP characterized by abnormal involuntary movements, such as twisting, grimacing, and sharp jerks

3. _____ results from a chromosomal abnormality and is the most common cause of mental retardation

4. _____ complex developmental disorder characterized by intellectual, social, and communication deficits

5. _____ most common learning disorder in which the person has difficulty with reading, spelling, or writing words

6. _____ most common degenerative muscular disorder in children

7. _____ symptom of muscular dystrophy

8. _____ study of heredity

9. _____ type of CP that results in tremors, unsteady gait, lack of coordination and balance, nystagmus, muscle weakness, and lack of leg movement during infancy

10. _____ genetic, sex-linked abnormality of the X chromosome that is carried by women

11. _____ interruption in the natural flow of speaking

12. _____ present at birth

13. _____ repeating words of other people

14. _____ speech impairment

15. _____ administration of medications that bind to lead to remove it from the body

a. ataxic cerebral palsy
b. autism
c. chelation
d. congenital
e. developmental disability
f. Down syndrome
g. Duchenne muscular dystrophy
h. dysfluency
i. dyskinetic cerebral palsy
j. dyslexia
k. dysphagia
l. echolalia
m. fragile X syndrome
n. genetics
o. Gower's sign

Match the following definitions with the correct terms.

16. _____ disorder in one or more of the processes involved in understanding or using language

17. _____ children of alcoholics

18. _____ attention deficit hyperactivity disorder

19. _____ individuals who demonstrate below-average intellectual abilities, accompanied by difficulty functioning independently

20. _____ most common type of CP that has increased muscle tone or spasticity, which may affect one or more limbs

21. _____ disorder in which the person loses contact with reality

22. _____ examples include alcohol, drugs, maternal diseases, and toxic substances

23. _____ autism spectrum disorders

24. _____ another name for Down syndrome

25. _____ medication given by deep intramuscular route to treat lead poisoning

26. _____ abnormal crease straight across the palms of children with Down syndrome

27. _____ blood lead levels

28. _____ increased levels measured in the amniotic fluid can indicate possible neural tube or ventral wall defects

29. _____ thoughts or ideas of suicide

30. _____ lead poisoning

a. intellectual or cognitive impairment
b. learning disability
c. plumbism
d. schizophrenia
e. simian line
f. spastic cerebral palsy
g. suicidal ideation
h. tertogen
i. trisomy 21
j. ADHD
k. AFP
l. ASD
m. BAL in oil
n. BLL
o. COAS

Match the following definitions with the correct terms.

31. _____ specific learning disabilities

32. _____ electroencephalogram

33. _____ general term used to describe movement and coordination disorders in children

34. _____ inherited neurologic disorder; chemical neurotransmitter abnormality is found

35. _____ intelligence quotient

36. _____ lysergic acid diethylamide

37. _____ obsessive-compulsive disorders

38. _____ level is elevated in children with muscular dystrophy

39. _____ fetal alcohol syndrome

a. CP
b. CPK
c. EEG
d. FAS
e. IQ
f. LSD
g. OCD
h. SLD
i. TS

■ Nursing Actions

Indication whether the nursing actions would be appropriate (A) or inappropriate (I).

1. _____ Instruct the parents of a child with AIDS that immunization and isolation from other sick children are critical.

2. _____ Use IQ scores to determine a child's abilities and plan education based on the scores.

3. _____ Focus nursing interventions for the child with Down syndrome on treatments to increase the child's IQ scores with age.

4. _____ When caring for a child with a specific learning disability (SLD), learn about the specific disability and set achievable goals.

5. _____ Provide a child with visual processing deficits with a tape recorder that reinforces information.

6. _____ Teach family caregivers of a child with attention deficit hyperactivity disorder to increase environmental stimuli to overcome the deficit.

7. _____ Keep the child with plumbism in the home and teach him or her not to eat the paint in the home or play with other items that contain lead.

8. _____ Help the child with cerebral palsy learn self-care activities.

9. _____ Encourage HIV-positive mothers to breastfeed.

10. _____ Instruct pregnant mothers that the incidence of Down syndrome decreases in women older than 35 years of age.

■ Correct the False Statements

Circle the word True *or* False *that follows the statement. If the word* false *has been circled, change the underlined word/words to make the statement true. Place your answer in the space provided.*

1. <u>Behavior modification</u> involves positive reinforcement, which encourages a child to repeat a desired behavior.

   True   False   _____

2. Substance abuse is one of the most common causes of <u>physical disabilities and cognitive impairment in children.</u>

   True   False   _____

3. Lead is contained in items such as <u>paint, leaded pottery, home remedies, shoes, and old eating utensils.</u>

   True   False   _____

4. Children taking stimulants should be assessed for <u>growth spurts.</u>

   True   False   _____

5. Drugs classified as <u>category A</u> have known teratogenic effects.

   True   False   _____

6. The lifetime consequences of <u>in utero alcohol exposure</u> include retardation, learning disabilities, and serious behavioral problems.

   True   False   _____

7. The use of zidovudine (AZT) by pregnant HIV-positive women and their newborns has resulted in <u>many more cases of pediatric HIV</u>.

   True   False   _____

8. A frequent complication of HIV in infants is <u>Kaposi's sarcoma</u>.

   True   False   _____

9. Autism affects more <u>boys than girls</u>.

   True   False   _____

■ Short Answers

Complete the following questions.

1. Compare differences between Down syndrome and fragile X syndrome relative to head, face, and ears.

2. What measures should a nurse take when assisting a child with long-term disability?

CHAPTER 74

Skin Disorders

■ Terminology Review

Match the following definitions with the correct terms and acronyms.

1. _____ staphylococcal infection starting around the hair follicle

2. _____ graft made from pigskin

3. _____ areas of skin that are completely lacking in pigmintation

4. _____ total parenteral nutrition

5. _____ venereal warts

6. _____ chronic, noncontagious proliferation of epidermal cells that form small, scaly patches of skin

7. _____ same as a heterograft

8. _____ cultured epithelial autografts

9. _____ swelling of deeper dermal and subcutaneous tissues, usually of the lips, eyelids, skin, GI tract, hands, feet, genitalia, tongue, or larynx

10. _____ thick, dry, black or dark brown dead tissue or skin

11. _____ growing new skin from a biopsy of unburned skin

12. _____ several interconnecting furuncles in a cluster

13. _____ graft using cadaver skin or skin from another person

14. _____ to remove loose skin, crusts, or denuded tissue

15. _____ treatment for warts that involves a short, high-frequency electrical current

16. _____ same as homograft

17. _____ boil

18. _____ inflammation of the skin

19. _____ vesicles formed by streptococcal or staphylococcal bacteria, usually in infants and young children

20. _____ abnormal shortening of muscles, tendons, or scar tissue that results in deformity and limited joint movement

21. _____ small flesh-colored, brown, or yellow papules caused by the human papillomavirus

22. _____ ultraviolet

23. _____ itching

24. _____ disease caused by mites burrowing under the outer layer of skin

25. _____ vascular skin tumors known as birthmarks

26. _____ form of dermatitis associated with heredity, allergy, and emotional stress

27. _____ removal of a skin tissue specimen for microscopic examination

28. _____ treatment of applying liquid nitrogen to remove warts

29. _____ graft using the client's own skin

30. _____ study of skin diseases

31. _____ hives

32. _____ painless, benign overgrowths that develop at the site of a scar or trauma

33. _____ means new growth

a. allograft

b. angioedema

c. angioma

d. autograft

e. biopsy

f. carbuncle

g. CEA

h. condylomata acuminate

i. contracture

j. cryosurgery

k. cultured epithelial autograft

l. débridement

m. dermatitis

n. dermatology

o. eczema

p. electrodessication

q. eschar

r. folliculitis

s. furuncle

t. heterograft

u. homograft

v. impetigo

w. keloid

x. neoplasm

y. pruritus

z. psoriasis

aa. scabies

bb. TPN

cc. uticaria

dd. UV

ee. vitiligo

ff. warts

gg. xenograft

a. Removal of skin sample for microscopic examination

b. Specimen shaved off the top of the lesion to diagnose scabies

c. Smear used to examine cells and fluids from vesicles

d. High-pressure mercury lamp that produces UV rays used to detect pigment abnormalities and skin infections

■ Short Answer

1. List the major functions of the skin and give an example of how the skin carries out each function.

2. Identify the type of primary or secondary lesion on each color plate located on page 599. Write a sample documentation entry for a patient's chart for each lesion, indicating your assessment findings.

   Figure 47-12

   Figure 47-13

   Figure 47-14

   Figure 47-15

3. State why boils should never be picked or squeezed.

■ Matching

Match the following diagnostic tests with the correct definition.

1. _____ Wood's light examination

2. _____ Tzanck's smear

3. _____ Tissue biopsy

4. _____ Scabies scraping

4. Discuss the differences and similarities between uticaria and angioedema.

5. What is the leading cause of death for people with burns? What nursing interventions can help to prevent this complication?

6. Complete the following table.

Disorder	Assessment Findings	How Disease Is Spread	Nursing Care
Venereal warts			
Impetigo			
Scabies			
Lice			

7. Why is eschar removed from burns and what methods are used to remove it?

10. Discuss methods to treat skin cancer.

8. List at least four types of dressing that may be used on burn victims.

■ Matching

Match the following nursing diagnoses and related to statements.

1. _____ Risk for Infection

2. _____ Fluid Volume Deficit

3. _____ Impaired Social Interaction

4. _____ Sexual Dysfunction

5. _____ Body Image Disturbance

9. For the following neoplasms, indicate which are malignant and which are benign.

_____ basal cell carcinoma

_____ pigmented nevi

_____ angiomas

_____ malignant melanoma

_____ keloids

_____ squamous cell carcinoma

a. related to burn trauma

b. related to pruritus, pain, lesions

c. related to laceration, rash, skin lesions, skin cancer, burn trauma

d. related to disfigurement

e. related to skin lesions disfigurement, pruritus, pain

■ Case Studies

1. A patient suffers from seborrheic dermatitis of the scalp, axillae, and groin.

   a. What assessment findings would the nurse expect to find?

   b. Outline nursing interventions that would minimize the patient's symptoms.

   c. Outline a patient teaching plan for the correct use of antihistamines and Selsun Blue shampoo.

2. A 76-year-old patient on oxygen therapy sustained a burn to the face and anterior chest while smoking. The patient was just admitted to the inpatient unit from the emergency department.

   a. What priority assessments would the nurse complete and why?

ASSESSMENT	RATIONALE

   b. Using the rule of nines, calculate the percentage of body surface area that was burned.

   c. The patient weighs 110 pounds. Calculate the total 24-hour fluid replacement using the Parkland formula.

   d. Outline potential complications that can occur during the resuscitative phase.

   e. What factors would the nurse need to consider that could have a detrimental effect on this patient's healing process and why?

■ Multiple Choice Questions

Circle the best answer.

1. To prevent disease transmission, the priority nursing intervention when caring for a patient with a skin disorder is to:

   a. wash hands before entering the room.

   b. adhere to Standard Precautions.

   c. always wear gloves when touching the patient's skin.

   d. encourage the patient to bathe daily.

2. Which of the following medications may be used to help minimize pruritus?

   a. Crotamiton (Eurax)

   b. Diphenhydramine (Benadryl)

   c. Silver sulfadiazine (Silvadene)

   d. Lindane (Kwell)

3. A patient receiving penicillin develops hives and dyspnea. The most appropriate nursing intervention would be to:

   a. continue to monitor the patient.

   b. place the patient in a low-Fowler's position.

   c. notify the RN or physician.

   d. obtain a set of vital signs.

4. Which of the following would provide the best source of protein for a burn victim during the acute phase?

   a. Add butter to hot foods like potatoes, cooked cereals, and soups.

   b. Substitute mayonnaise for salad dressing.

   c. Use double-strength milk (liquid milk fortified with skim milk powder).

   d. Use honey on toast, cereal, and in coffee.

5. Nursing care of the patient following a skin grafting should include all of the following. Which would be the immediate nursing priority?

   a. Assessment for fluid volume status

   b. Immobilizing the grafted area

   c. Instruction on turning, coughing, and deep breathing

   d. Providing a high-protein diet

6. Which of the following patients would need education to control the spread of his or her contagious disease?

   a. 21-year-old woman with eczema

   b. 36-year-old man with psoriasis

   c. 18-year-old young man with pubic lice

   d. 60-year-old woman with seborrheic dermatitis

7. The nurse is caring for a patient who has had plastic surgery involving the face. How should the nurse position the patient to reduce swelling?

   a. Trendelenburg

   b. Prone

   c. Side-lying

   d. Semi-Fowler's

8. A patient sustained burns to the buttocks, low back, and posterior legs. What is the percentage of body area that was burned?

   a. 18%

   b. 19%

   c. 27%

   d. 45%

9. An adult burn client's urine output was 25 mL for the past hour. What is the appropriate nursing action?

   a. Continue to monitor; this is expected in a burn patient.

   b. Notify the RN or MD immediately.

   c. Increase the IV flow rate.

   d. Encourage oral fluids.

10. A client has been diagnosed with psoriasis. The client asks the nurse about the disease. The nurse's most appropriate response would be that it is:

    a. a malignant form of skin cancer.

    b. severe scaling due to rapid cell division of the skin.

    c. an inflammation of the nerves.

    d. most commonly seen in childhood.

11. The nurse is caring for a client with severe pruritus and wants to promote the patient's comfort. Which intervention can the nurse perform without a physician's order?

    a. Administer an antihistamine.

    b. Apply a lubricant to unbroken skin.

    c. Apply a topical corticosteroid to the area.

    d. Give the patient a phototherapy treatment.

12. Which of the following statements indicates that the client with atopic dermatitis needs more education?

    a. "I should use my moisturizing cream as directed."

    b. "I should use antihistamines to relieve itching."

    c. "I should cleanse my skin using a gentle soap with lanolin."

    d. "I should avoid tension and anxiety."

13. A client has a severe burn, and the burned skin has lost the ability to produce oil and sweat, has lost sensation, and has lost the ability to develop piloerection. The nurse would expect to assess which type of burn?

    a. Superficial partial-thickness (first-degree)

    b. Superficial partial-thickness (second-degree)

    c. Deep dermal partial-thickness

    d. Full-thickness

14. A physician has ordered Accutane 0.5 mg/kg/day PO in two divided doses. The client weighs 60 kg. How many milligrams would the nurse give with each dose?

    a. 1.5
    b. 15
    c. 30
    d. 150

15. Which of the following would the nurse teach a client to do to prevent skin cancer?

    a. Use sun screen with a sun protective factor of at least 15.
    b. Use commercial tanning booths instead of natural sunlight.
    c. Keep skin moisturized.
    d. Cleanse the skin daily.

16. If a patient is receiving Silvadene cream to burn wounds, the nurse knows to monitor:

    a. respirations.
    b. complete blood counts.
    c. for headaches.
    d. for scarring.

17. The nurse must teach a patient with pediculosis to:

    a. avoid washing the hair for 12 hours.
    b. report the condition to the health department.
    c. wash all clothing and linens.
    d. wash the body with Kwell every day.

18. All of the following nursing diagnoses stems are appropriate for the patient with a burn. Which would be the nurse's priority in the first 24 hours?

    a. Fluid Volume Deficit
    b. Altered Body Image
    c. Altered Coping
    d. Risk for Infection

CHAPTER 75

Disorders in Fluid and Electrolyte Balance

■Terminology Review

Match the following definitions with the correct terms.

1. _____ swelling that does not indent when slight pressure is applied

2. _____ decrease in blood carbon dioxide caused by hyperventilation

3. _____ deficiency of fluid and electrolytes in the ECF

4. _____ when the blood is more basic than normal due to loss of body acids, or excessive retention of alkaline substances

5. _____ excess water in the extracellular spaces

6. _____ increase in blood carbon dioxide caused by hypoventilation

7. _____ decreased volume of water that does not occur without electrolyte changes

8. _____ elasticity or tonus of the skin

9. _____ caused by an excess of bicarbonate, often due to excess bicarbonate antacid administration or the loss of acids

10. _____ generalized body edema

11. _____ when the blood is more acidic than normal caused by a deficit of bicarbonate ions or an excess of hydrogen ions

12. _____ excessive accumulation of interstitial fluid

13. _____ excessive retention of water and sodium in the ECF

a. acidosis
b. alkalosis
c. anasarca
d. dehydration
e. edema
f. fluid volume deficit
g. fluid volume excess
h. metabolic alkalosis
i. nonpitting edema
j. overhydration
k. respiratory acidosis
l. respiratory alkalosis
m. turgor

Match the following definitions with the correct terms.

14. _____ bicarbonate ions

15. _____ form of energy

16. _____ blood test used to indicate acidosis or alkalosis

17. _____ liver function tests

18. _____ fluid within the cells

19. _____ milligrams per deciliter

20. _____ excessive retention of water and sodium in the ECF

21. _____ antidiuretic hormone

22. _____ total amount of water in the body expressed as a percentage of body weight

23. _____ unit of measurement of electrolytes that is milliequivalents per liter

24. _____ consists of the intravascular fluid and the interstitial fluid

25. _____ carbonic acid

26. _____ deficiency of fluid and electrolytes in the ECF

a. ABG
b. ADH
c. ATP
d. ECF
e. FVD
f. FVE
g. HCO_3^-

h. H_2CO_3

i. ICF

j. LFT

k. mEq/L

l. mg/dL

m. TBW

■ Assessment Review

For the following assessment data, mark the item with an E if the finding indicates a fluid balance excess and with a D if the finding indicates a fluid balance deficit.

1. _____ Increase in weight

2. _____ Pitting edema

3. _____ Hypotension

4. _____ Rales

5. _____ Thirst

6. _____ Intake < output

7. _____ Dry oral mucosa

8. _____ Poor skin turgor

9. _____ Decreased urine specific gravity

10. _____ Dependent edema

11. _____ Swelling in the sacral area

12. _____ Tenting

■ Short Answer

1. Identify causes of edema.

2. List the electrolytes and indicate the normal laboratory values.

3. Explain why imbalances in potassium levels are so dangerous.

■ Matching

Match the following.

1. _____ magnesium

2. _____ hyponatremia

3. _____ hyperkalemia

4. _____ amount of water in the human body

5. _____ potassium

6. _____ normal serum levels of magnesium

7. _____ sodium

8. _____ calcium

9. _____ normal serum levels of sodium

10. _____ chloride

11. _____ normal serum levels of phosphorus

12. _____ normal serum levels of potassium

13. _____ normal serum levels of calcium

14. _____ hypernatremia

15. _____ phosphorus

a. 50–70%

b. Na

c. 135–145 mEq/L

d. < 135 mEq/L

e. > 145 mEq/L

f. K

g. > 5.5 mEq/L

h. 3.5–5.5 mEq/L

i. Cl

j. Ca

k. 9–10.5 mg/dL

l. Mg

m. 1.5–2.5 mEq/L

n. P

o. 2.5–4.5 mg/dL

■ Correct the False Statements

Circle the word True *or* False *that follows the statement. If the word* false *has been circled, change the underlined word/words to make the statement true. Place your answer in the space provided.*

1. Potassium is the major electrolyte in the <u>intracellular fluid</u>.

   True   False   _____

2. Potassium <u>can</u> be stored in the body.

   True   False   _____

3. <u>Sodium</u> is the major electrolyte in the extracellular fluid.

   True   False   _____

4. <u>Potassium</u> may cause water retention and hypertension.

   True   False   _____

5. Calcium plays a role in <u>blood coagulation and maintaining a heartbeat</u>.

   True   False   _____

6. Hypermagnesemia is a <u>rare</u> condition.

   True   False   _____

7. <u>Hyperchloremia</u> is usually associated with a sodium and potassium deficit.

   True   False   _____

8. A client with <u>hypernatremia</u> may present with signs of dry mucous membranes and neurological changes.

   True   False   _____

9. A <u>potassium excess</u> can result from alcoholism.

   True   False   _____

10. Careful assessment of acidosis is essential to monitor for <u>worsening of the condition or overreaction to the treatment</u>.

    True   False   _____

■ Multiple Choice

Circle the best answer.

1. A deficit in bicarbonate ions or an excess of hydrogen ions causes a condition called:
   a. metabolic acidosis.
   b. metabolic alkalosis.
   c. respiratory acidosis.
   d. respiratory alkalosis.

2. Overhydration refers specifically to excess water in the:
   a. extracellular spaces.
   b. extrathecal spaces.
   c. intracellular spaces.
   d. interstitial spaces.

3. A dent that remains for some time after edematous tissue over a bone is pressed with a finger is called:
   a. dependent edema.
   b. pitting edema.
   c. pulmonary edema.
   d. sacral edema.

4. A deficit of plasma carbon dioxide or carbonic acid results in a condition called:
   a. metabolic acidosis.
   b. metabolic alkalosis.
   c. respiratory acidosis.
   d. respiratory alkalosis.

5. The term ascities describes the accumulation of fluid in the:
   a. abdominal cavity.
   b. interstitial spaces.
   c. lower extremities.
   d. renal pelvis.

CHAPTER 76

Musculoskeletal Disorders

■ Terminology Review

Match the following definitions with the correct terms.

1. _____ type of lumbar decompression that exposes the spinal canal and allows for relief of compression of the spinal cord and spinal nerve roots

2. _____ subluxation

3. _____ x-ray of a joint

4. _____ test of electrical conductivity of the client's muscles

5. _____ inflammation of the bursa

6. _____ humpback or hunchback

7. _____ joint inflammation

8. _____ invasive procedure using an endoscope designed to view joints

9. _____ scleroderma of the distal extremities and face

10. _____ swayback

11. _____ form of skeletal traction used for cervical fractures

12. _____ necrosis of tissue due to insufficient or lack of blood supply

13. _____ results from inadequate or obstructed blood flow to muscles, nerves, and tissue

a. acrosclerosis
b. arthritis
c. arthrogram
d. arthroscopy
e. bursitis
f. compartment syndrome
g. dislocation
h. electromyogram
i. gangrene
j. halo device
k. kyphosis
l. laminectomy
m. lordosis

Match the following definitions with the correct terms.

14. _____ metal pins or wires surgically inserted into the client's bones so that traction is applied directly to them

15. _____ adult vitamin D deficiency which results in softening of the bones

16. _____ bone infection

17. _____ narrowing of the intervertebral space

18. _____ inflammation of the tendon sheath

19. _____ pull of traction applied to the client's skin

20. _____ specialty in medicine that examines and treats diseases and injuries of the musculoskeletal system

21. _____ excision of the synovial membrane

22. _____ scleroderma of the fingers and toes

23. _____ side-to-side or lateral angulation of the spinal column

24. _____ fragments of dead bone loosen

25. _____ hard skin

26. _____ disease that results from a deficiency of vitamin D during childhood

a. orthopedics
b. osteomalacia
c. osteomyelitis
d. rickets
e. sclerodactyly
f. scleroderma
g. scoliosis
h. sequestration
i. skeletal traction
j. skin traction
k. spinal stenosis
l. synovectomy
m. tenosynovitis

■ Correct the False Statements

Circle the word True *or* False *that follows the statement. If the word* false *has been circled, change the underlined word/words to make the statement true. Place your answer in the space provided.*

1. Magnetic resonance imaging is <u>more expensive and invasive</u> than biopsy, surgery, or the use of radioactive isotopes or dyes.

   True   False   _____

2. During a <u>myelogram</u>, a contrast medium or air is injected into the spinal subarachnoid space, followed by x-ray examination.

   True   False   _____

3. Ultrasound uses <u>sound waves and their echoes</u> to display images to evaluate soft tissue masses, osteomyelitis, infection, and congenital and acquired pediatric disorders.

   True   False   _____

4. After an arthrocentesis, the client <u>will immediately be able to move the joint freely.</u>

   True   False   _____

5. The nurse should apply ice and elevate the client's joint following arthroscopy.

   True   False   _____

6. To hold a half-cast splint in place, the nurse uses <u>long strips of adhesive tape</u>.

   True   False   _____

7. Inflatable splints are often used in emergency first aid to support the <u>neck</u>.

   True   False   _____

8. A <u>benefit of using splints</u> is that they are light weight and do not need to be removed when x-rays are taken.

   True   False   _____

9. Plaster casts remain wet for <u>up to 3 or 4 days</u>.

   True   False   _____

10. Synthetic casts are more lightweight <u>but weaker</u> than plaster casts.

    True   False   _____

11. <u>Metastatic</u> bone tumors originate in the bone and are usually slow growing.

    True   False   _____

12. One of the most significant signs of a malignant bone tumor is <u>pathologic fracture.</u>

    True   False   _____

13. A <u>strain </u>is an injury to the ligaments around a joint causing the ligaments to stretch and tear.

    True   False   _____

■ Short Answer

1. Describe care and handling of a plaster cast during the drying phase.

2. Explain what petaling is and why is it done.

3. What should the nurse do to ensure safe cast removal?

4. What complications should the nurse watch for in clients with skeletal traction?

5. What type of diagnostic study is contraindicated in clients who have had internal fixation, and why?

6. What is arthroplasty and for which joints is it used?

7. Describe what CMS checks are. Why are they so important?

8. Discuss nursing interventions that can be used to relieve phantom limb pain.

9. Discuss nursing care following replantation.

10. Outline techniques used when positioning or moving a patient who has had lumbar decompression.

11. Why does the nurse need to assess carefully clients with arthritis?

12. What special instructions would you teach clients with gout who are taking anti-gout medications?

13. Which disorders result from repetitive motions or overuse?

■ Comparison Table

Complete the following table.

Complications Related to Musculoskeletal Disorder	Discription of Disorder	Nursing Care to Prevent Disorder
Neurovascular pressure		
Wound infection		
Osteomyelitis		
Hypostatic pneumonia and atelectasis		
Embolism		
Deep vein thrombosis		
Hemorrhage		
Compartment syndrome		

■ Matching

Match the following types of traction with the correct definition.

1. _____ Traction applied through a weight attached to a spreader bar below the foot.

2. _____ Skin traction applied by means of a head halter.

3. _____ Buck's traction with the addition of the leg supported by a sling.

4. _____ Traction applied by belt or sling.

5. _____ Traction that inserts skull tong device into the skull bone.

6. _____ Skeletal traction with device drilled through shaft of a bone and attached to the traction apparatus.

a. Skull or head traction

b. Steinmann pin or Kirschner wire

c. Buck's traction

d. Russell's traction

e. Cervical head halter traction

f. Pelvic traction

■ Fill-in-the-Blank

1. _____ _____ _____ is

    pain, pressure, or itching sensations that occur

    in the area of the amputation.

2. A _____ may be needed to relieve

    internal pressure for a patient with compartment

    syndrome.

3. An artificial device that replaces part or all of a

    missing extremity is a _____ .

4. _____ is the reattachment of a

    completely severed body part back to the body.

5. _____ _____ _____

    results from pressure on the spinal cord.

6. Osteoporosis is a condition in which bone mass

    _____ .

7. Most types of arthritis are more common in

    _____ .

8. _____ is a condition of an immovable

    joint.

9. People with gout may be placed on a diet low in

    _____ .

10. The two types of bone tumors are

    _____ and _____ .

11. A characteristic sign of systemic lupus

    erythematosus is a _____ ; however, a

    rash may appear over other body parts as well.

■ Case Studies

1. You are caring for a 77-year-old man who has
    had a right below-the-knee amputation. Your
    client is one day post-op.

    a. List the main complications that may occur
        after an amputation.

    b. Identify specific nursing measures to prevent
        the above complications.

    c. Identify three other potential postoperative
        problems that this client may develop.

2. You are caring for a 59-year-old woman with
    rheumatoid arthritis. She complains of fatigue
    and pain in her fingers, elbows, and knees. She is
    being treated with oral corticosteroids.

    a. What areas would you want to assess further?

    b. Your client states that she has given up
        socializing because of pain. She feels like the
        disease has caused her to become isolated.
        What nursing measures would you complete to
        provide emotional support?

    c. Which nursing diagnoses could apply to this
        client?

    d. Select one nursing diagnosis and write an
        appropriate goal.

    e. Outline nursing interventions related to your
        nursing diagnosis and goal.

■ Multiple Choice

Circle the best answer.

1. After repositioning a client in traction, the patient complains of some pain. Which of the following would be the nurse's priority?
   a. Perform a neurovascular check.
   b. Place call light within patient's reach.
   c. Provide pain medication.
   d. Take vital signs before giving patient narcotics.

2. Which laboratory value would the nurse expect to see in a client who has gout?
   a. Decreased hemoglobin
   b. Elevated white blood cell count
   c. Increased uric acid
   d. Increased creatinine

3. Which of the following nursing interventions would be appropriate for a client with scleroderma?
   a. Apply ice to the hands to prevent swelling.
   b. Encourage the client to join a support group.
   c. Encourage the client to take cold baths.
   d. Provide teaching about client's medications.

4. A patient experiencing low back pain is scheduled for an MRI. Nursing care before the test would include instructing the client that:
   a. fasting is required before and after the test.
   b. it is noisy and to remove all metallic objects.
   c. no strenuous activity can be done for 12 hours after the test.
   d. there will be some discomfort and the test will last 2 hours.

5. A patient fell and injured his wrist. He is told that the physician will need to do a closed reduction to reduce the fracture. Which statement demonstrates that the patient has an accurate understanding of the procedure?
   a. "A metal pin will be attached to the bone to stabilize it."
   b. "The bone ends will be aligned during a surgical procedure."
   c. "The bone ends will be manipulated manually into place."
   d. "There will be metal pins protruding from the skin surface."

6. A client is complaining of increased pain on the casted arm. The cast has been on for 2 weeks. The client also has a temperature of 100°F. What nursing action would be most appropriate?
   a. Advise the client that these symptoms are to be expected.
   b. Place a window in the cast.
   c. Remove the cast and assess the wound.
   d. Sniff the cast for foul odor.

7. During assessment of a patient's traction device, which of the following would require immediate nursing intervention?
   a. The body and traction are in alignment.
   b. The footpiece is touching pulleys at the end of the bed.
   c. The rope is positioned in the pulley.
   d. The weights are free hanging.

8. To prevent renal complications in a client with gout, the nurse instructs the client to:
   a. drink at least 12 glasses of fluid a day.
   b. eat a high-protein diet.
   c. start on bladder training exercises.
   d. strain all urine.

9. When giving a gold salt injection, the nurse would:
   a. advise the client that only one injection will be needed.
   b. advise the patient that this will cure the condition.
   c. call the physician to verify the route.
   d. give the injection deep IM using Z-track technique.

10. Which assessment finding is most important in determining nursing care for a client with rheumatoid arthritis?
    a. Client has disheveled appearance.
    b. Client's mother also had arthritis.
    c. Client takes nonsteroidal anti-inflammatory medications.
    d. Weight is stable.

CHAPTER 77

Nervous System Disorders

■ Terminology Review

Match the following definitions with the correct terms.

1. _____ chronic seizure disorder

2. _____ lack of tone

3. _____ difficulty swallowing

4. _____ sudden, dangerous hypertension

5. _____ surgical entry into the skull

6. _____ slowness of movement

7. _____ double vision

8. _____ abnormal involuntary movements

9. _____ pressure that the brain, blood, and cerebrospinal fluid exert inside the cerebrospinal cavity

10. _____ premonition or forewarning of an impending seizure

11. _____ defective muscular coordination, lack of coordination, difficulty in walking, or a progressive condition characterized by a marked spasticity

12. _____ headache

13. _____ difficulty in speaking

14. _____ injury without breaking the skin

15. _____ may not damage the brain structures, but may cause temporary unconsciousness

a. ataxia

b. aura

c. autonomic dysreflexia

d. bradykinesia

e. cephalalgia

f. chorea

g. concussion

h. contusion

i. craniotomy

j. diplopia

k. dysphagia

l. dysphasia

m. epilepsy

n. flaccidity

o. intracranial pressure

Match the following definitions with the correct terms.

16. _____ acute viral inflammation caused by the varicella zoster virus

17. _____ drooping eyelids

18. _____ tearing of brain tissue caused by direct impact or penetrating injury

19. _____ pain in a nerve

20. _____ slow forming below the dura

21. _____ paralysis of all four extremities

22. _____ acute spasm in which the body is bowed forward, with the head and heels bent backward

23. _____ medical specialty related to the nervous system

24. _____ sensation of rotation of self or one's surrounding

25. _____ spontaneous alteration in brain function resulting from abnormal discharge of neurons in the brain

26. _____ sensitivity to light

27. _____ second most common neurologic disease in older adults

28. _____ paralysis of the legs and lower body

29. _____ stiff neck

a. laceration
b. neuralgia
c. neurology
d. nuchal rigidity
e. opisthotonos
f. paraplegia
g. parkinsonism

h. photophobia
i. ptosis
j. quadriplegia
k. seizure
l. shingles
m. subdural hematoma
n. vertigo

■ Comparison Chart

Complete the following chart.

Diagnostic Test	Discription of Test	Nursing Care Before Test	Nursing Care After Test
CT scan			
MRI			
Cerebral angiography			
Lumbar Puncture			
EEG			

■ Short Answer

1. Outline patient teaching for the client undergoing a craniotomy.

2. Describe key components of a neurologic nursing assessment.

3. What is the earliest and most important sign of increased intracranial pressure?

4. Compare and contrast symptomatic, migraine, and cluster headaches.

5. Describe nursing care for the client experiencing a seizure.

6. Which people are most at risk to develop carpal tunnel syndrome and why?

7. For the following nerve disorders, list the involved nerves and associated symptoms.

                   NERVE INVOLVED   **SYMPTOMS**

  a. Trigeminal   _____   _____
     neuralgia

  b. Bell's   _____   _____
     palsy

  c. Shingles   _____   _____

8. What are the three categories of spinal cord problems?

9. Describe the difference between paraplegia and quadriplegia.

10. Describe nursing care that is common to multiple sclerosis, Parkinson's disease, and myasthenia gravis.

11. Outline patient teaching that would be specific for a female client who is paralyzed.

12. List at least three health problems that a paralyzed person may develop and indicate nursing interventions to prevent the problem.

    PROBLEM   **INTERVENTION**

■ Case Studies

1. You are the nurse assigned to a medical-neurologic unit. You are the nurse caring for the following clients:

  a. A 46-year-old woman who is 4 days status postcraniotomy and is complaining of moderate pain. Last medicated 2.5 hours ago.

  b. A 36-year-old male with bacterial meningitis. His temperature has increased to 103°F and has become confused.

  c. A 29-year-old woman with multiple sclerosis who is complaining of fatigue

  d. A 59-year-old man with ALS who is complaining of weakness and difficulty swallowing. It is currently mealtime.

Describe how you would prioritize your nursing care. Provide rationale for each intervention.

                 CARE   **RATIONALE**

First priority

Second priority

Third priority

Fourth priority

2. You are caring for a client who is 63 years old and diagnosed with Parkinson's disease. He has fine tremors of the hands and forearms and a masklike facial expression. He shuffles and stoops forward when walking. He also has some drooling. He has the following orders: l-dopa 100 mg PO b.i.d., regular high-calorie diet, ambulate with assistance t.i.d., range-of-motion exercises b.i.d. Vital signs q shift, CBC.

  a. What other findings would you assess for?

b. Based on the patient's orders, what other diseases or conditions would you assess and why?

c. Why are ambulation and range-of-motion exercises so important for this client?

d. Why would you monitor laboratory results?

3. A 40-year-old man is just admitted to the unit with Guillain-Barré syndrome. All of the following are appropriate nursing actions. In which order will the nurse prioritize care? Give rationales for your choices.

Obtain admitting history, assess neurologic status, orient client to room, inform client of MD orders

PRIORITY   **RATIONALE**

■ Matching Exercise

Match the following clients and assessment findings with the correct classification of seizure disorder.

1. _____ A 39-year-old man states he is having a seizure and begins to have tonic-clonic contractions of the lower extremity spreading the entire length of the extremity.

2. _____ A 56-year-old woman complains to her husband that the right side of her face and her right hand feels numb. Shortly after she begins smacking her lips and salivating. This is followed by clonic-type contractions of the hand.

3. _____ A 40-year-old woman falls to the floor in an unconscious state. She begins to have tonic-clonic movements of her entire body for 30 seconds.

4. _____ A 16-year-old boy is observed by his teacher staring vacantly at the blackboard. His eyes focus straight ahead, and he is unresponsive to verbal stimuli.

5. _____ A 6-month-old has rapid movement of the extremities with neck flexion and arm extension.

a. generalized tonic-clonic seizure
b. infantile seizure
c. complex partial seizure
d. absence seizure
e. simple partial seizure

■ Multiple Choice Questions

Circle the best answer.

1. If in the room when a client has a generalized tonic-clonic seizure, the nurse first:
   a. places a tongue depressor in the mouth.
   b. gives oxygen by mask.
   c. offers emotional support.
   d. turns client's head to the side.

2. Medications that cause drowsiness should not be given to a client with a head injury because they may:
   a. produce a coma.
   b. mask changes in LOC.
   c. increase the client's blood pressure.
   d. lead to cerebral hemorrhage.

3. The most important aspect of nursing care for patients with head injuries would be:
   a. turning the client frequently.
   b. administering narcotics.
   c. placing in Trendelenburg position.
   d. monitoring the patient's LOC and vital signs.

4. A patient with trigeminal neuralgia asks why shaving increases his facial pain. The nurse's best response would be:

   a. "Have you considered permanent hair removal?"

   b. "You should grow a beard."

   c. "Shaving stimulates the nerve of your face."

   d. "Warm water causes dilation of blood vessels."

5. L-Dopa is given to patients with Parkinson's disease to replenish:

   a. dopamine.

   b. epinephrine.

   c. norepinephrine.

   d. acetylcholine.

6. A client has an intraventricular catheter in place to monitor ICP. The system does not seem to be functioning properly. The nurse should:

   a. place the client in a side-lying position.

   b. elevate the head of the bed.

   c. notify the physician.

   d. obtain a blood sugar.

7. A client with a spinal cord injury and paraplegia has a sudden increase in blood pressure, has flushed skin, and is diaphoretic. The nurse's first intervention should be to:

   a. check client for bladder distention.

   b. nothing because the symptoms are temporary.

   c. call for the crash cart.

   d. call the physician immediately.

8. When caring for a client with a C-4 spinal injury, the priority nursing diagnosis should be:

   a. Risk for Constipation.

   b. Ineffective Breathing Pattern.

   c. Impaired Skin Integrity.

   d. Altered Self-Concept.

9. When providing discharge instructions for family members of a client who is a quadriplegic, the nurse teaches them about autonomic dysreflexia. Which of the following conditions does the nurse teach can cause this condition?

   a. Hypertension and immobility

   b. Decubitus ulcers and intermittent catheterization

   c. Bladder distention and fecal impaction

   d. Headaches and bladder distention

10. What is the most important goal of care for a client who is receiving ergot alkaloids?

    a. No seizure activity

    b. Relief of nausea and vomiting

    c. Decrease in tremors

    d. Relief of headache

11. In preparing a care plan for a person with a spinal cord injury, it is most important for the nurse to include a goal that addresses the need for:

    a. preventing disabilities.

    b. increasing family discussion.

    c. increasing appetite.

    d. decreasing temperature.

12. Regarding sexuality, paralyzed clients should be instructed that:

    a. their sex life is over.

    b. adaptation by the partner may be necessary.

    c. a paralyzed man cannot father a child.

    d. a paralyzed woman cannot bear a child.

CHAPTER 78

Endocrine Disorders

■ Terminology Review

Match the following definitions with the correct terms and acronyms.

1. _____ system that stimulates a target gland to produce a hormone and the hormone level rises, then the stimulus stops and the target gland stops the hormone release

2. _____ non–insulin-dependent diabetes mellitus

3. _____ overproduction of T_4, which increases the metabolic rate

4. _____ decreased tissue sensitivity to insulin

5. _____ overproduction of somatotropin in childhood

6. _____ ketones accumulate because of utilization of fats and proteins as a source of energy

7. _____ syndrome of inappropriate antidiuretic hormone in which clients cannot excrete dilute urine

8. _____ another name for hyperthyroidism

9. _____ bedtime insulin and daytime sulfonylureas

10. _____ excessive thirst

11. _____ deficiency of T_4, which slows down metabolic processes

12. _____ abnormally low blood sugar

13. _____ kidney disease caused by microvascular changes

14. _____ impaired fasting glucose

15. _____ nerve damage in long-term poorly controlled diabetes

16. _____ underproduction of ADH in which urine is copious

17. _____ propylthiouracil

18. _____ deficiency of PTH results in reduced amount of calcium available to the body

19. _____ excess of somatotropin in adults

20. _____ bulging eyes

21. _____ impaired glucose homeostasis

22. _____ loss of functional retinal tissue in the eye due to microvascular damage

23. _____ catecholamine-secreting adrenal tumor

24. _____ congenital form of hypothyroidism

25. _____ excessive hunger

26. _____ diabetic ketoacidosis

27. _____ hypoglycemia followed by a compensatory period of rebound hyperglycemia

28. _____ self-monitoring of blood glucose

29. _____ excessive urination

30. _____ surgical removal of the thyroid gland

31. _____ impaired glucose tolerance

32. _____ metabolic diseases characterized by hyperglycemia resulting from defects in insulin secretion, insulin action, or both

33. _____ advanced hypothyroidism in adults

34. _____ destruction or degeneration of the adrenal cortex

35. _____ gestational diabetes mellitus

36. _____ overproduction of hormones secreted by the adrenal cortex, overuse of corticosteroids, or tumors of adrenal glands or pituitary

37. _____ abnormally high blood sugar

38. _____ enlarged thyroid gland that does not cause toxic symptoms

39. _____ excess of PTH causing elevated calcium levels in the blood

40. _____ insulin-dependent diabetes mellitus

a. acromegaly
b. Addison's disease
c. BIDS
d. cretinism
e. Cushing's syndrome
f. diabetes insipidus
g. diabetes mellitus
h. DKA
i. exophthalmos
j. GDM
k. gigantism
l. goiter
m. Graves' disease
n. hyperglycemia
o. hyperparathyroidism
p. hyperthyroidism
q. hypoglycemia
r. hypoparathyroidism
s. hypothyroidism
t. IDDM
u. IFG
v. IGH
w. IGT
x. insulin resistance
y. ketoacidosis
z. myxedema
aa. negative feedback system
bb. nephropathy
cc. neuropathy
dd. NIDDM
ee. pheochromocytoma
ff. polydypsia
gg. polyphagia
hh. polyuria
ii. PTU
jj. retinopathy
kk. SIADH
ll. SMBG
mm. Somogyi phenomenon
nn. thyroidectomy

■ Assessment Review

For the following assessment findings of endocrine disorders, label each finding as indicated in each grouping:

G = gigantism; A= acromegaly

1. _____ unusually tall
2. _____ thick lips
3. _____ large hands and feet
4. _____ impotent

S = SIADH; DI= diabetes insipidus

5. _____ increased urinary output
6. _____ decreased urinary output
7. _____ large appetite
8. _____ increased thirst
9. _____ confusion and lethargy

HE = hyperthyroidism; HO = hypothyroidism

10. _____ excitable and overactive
11. _____ slowed physical and mental activity
12. _____ heart palpitations
13. _____ exophathlomos
14. _____ weight gain
15. _____ weight loss
16. _____dry skin

HE = hyperparathyroidism; HO = hypoparathyroidism

17. _____ elevated serum calcium
18. _____ pathologic fractures
19. _____ tremors and tetany
20. _____ positive Trousseau's sign

C= Cushing's syndrome; A = Addison's disease

21. _____ moon face
22. _____ darkening of skin
23. _____ anemia and weight loss
24. _____ hyperglycemia and hypertension

HE = hyperglycemia; HO = hypoglycemia

25. _____ flushed cheeks, dry skin

26. _____ weak, cold, tired

27. _____ sweetish smelling breath

28. _____ drowsy

29. _____ nausea and vomiting

30. _____ dehydration

■ Matching Diagnostic Tests

Match the following definitions with the correct diagnostic test.

1. _____ reflects the client's average blood glucose level over the previous 6 to 10 weeks

2. _____ serum levels used to assess thyroid function

3. _____ measures amount of radioactive uptake by the thyroid at various intervals

4. _____ client consumes large amount of glucose, and blood levels are checked at 1/2, 1, 2, and 3 hours

5. _____ intravenous pyelogram

6. _____ amount of glucose in the blood after client has fasted

7. _____ 24-hour urine test to detect catecholamine metabolites

8. _____ radioactive dye is administered and a scanogram determines the amount of radioactivity in the body and thyroid gland

9. _____ serum glucose levels taken 2 hours after a meal

a. 2hPP

b. fasting plasma glucose

c. glucose tolerance test

d. HbA$_{1c}$

e. IVP

f. Radioscan

g. RAIU

h. TFT

i. VMA

■ Case Studies

1. You are caring for the following clients on your medical/surgical unit:

   A.P. is a 76-year-old client with type 1 diabetes mellitus, complains of dizziness and shakiness

   B.R. is a 56-year-old client with hyperthyroidism who had a thyroidectomy yesterday am and is resting comfortably

   J.T. is a 44-year-old client with hypoparathyroidism who complains of muscle twitching

   G.S. is a 64-year-old client with pheochromocytoma who is currently obtaining a 24- hour urine for VMA

   Explain how you would prioritize your care and provide rationales for each action.

   ACTION   **RATIONALE**

2. A client has been diagnosed with type 1 diabetes mellitus. He has been in the hospital for 4 days to regulate his glucose levels. The client is being discharged tomorrow. He will be on Regular insulin 10 units and NPH insulin 10 units subcutaneously every am and pm. He will need to monitor glucose levels twice a day. He has expressed concern about following a diabetic diet.

   Outline discharge teaching that you would include.

3. You are caring for a client who is receiving the following insulin:

Ultra-lente NPH 25 units SQ q am (8 am)
Ultra-lente NPH 10 units SQ q pm (6 pm)
Calculate the times when this client is most at risk for experiencing hypoglycemic reactions.

■ Multiple Choice

Circle the best answer.

1. Which of the following nursing interventions would be the priority for a client returning to the hospital unit immediately after having a thyroidectomy?

   a. Assess for drainage on dressing and on pillow.

   b. Assess for respiratory distress and have a tracheostomy set at bedside.

   c. Place client in semi-Fowler's position.

   d. Assess for signs and symptoms of decreased calcium levels.

2. A client is started on levothyroxine (Levothroid), 50 mcg/day IM. The medication available is levothyroxine (Levothroid), 200 mcg/6 mL vial. How much medication would you administer?

   a. 0.25 mL

   b. 1.25 mL

   c. 1.5 mL

   d. 1.75 mL

3. A client is admitted with diabetes insipidus and has complaints of thirst, fast heart rate, and diuresis. Which nursing diagnosis stem is most appropriate for this client?

   a. Altered Body Image related to thirst

   b. Altered Skin Integrity related to increased heart rate

   c. Decreased Cardiac Output related to dizziness

   d. Fluid Volume Deficit related to diuresis

4. In preparing a care plan for a client with diabetes insipidus, it is most important for the nurse to include a goal that addresses the need for

   a. adequate gas exchange.

   b. adequate fluid balance.

   c. intact skin.

   d. positive self-image.

5. As part of the nursing care plan, the nurse explains that diabetes insipidus is caused by a deficiency of

   a. ACTH

   b. ADH

   c. FSH

   d. TSH

6. A client has type 1 diabetes mellitus. The nurse notices that the client is diaphoretic and lethargic and is complaining of a headache. The nurse suspects the client is having an insulin reaction. The priority nursing intervention is to

   a. check client's vital signs.

   b. check finger stick blood sugar.

   c. give foods high in fat.

   d. give 4 oz of orange juice.

7. Which of following instructions should be included in a preventative teaching plan on foot care for a diabetic client?

   a. Cut toenails straight across only with physician's permission.

   b. Go bare foot as much as possible to keep feet dry.

   c. Inspect feet weekly for cuts, sores, and foreign objects.

   d. Wash feet weekly with a strong soap.

8. Regular insulin has which of the following effects?

   a. Onset immediate, peaks in 15 minutes, and lasts 1 hour

   b. Onset in 30 minutes, peak 3 to 4 hours, duration 6 to 8 hours

   c. Onset in 4 to 6 hours, peak 8 to 14 hours, duration 16 to 24 hours

   d. Onset 8 to 14 hours, peak is minimal, duration 24 to 36 hours

9. A client is depressed about the changes in her personal appearance related to Cushing's syndrome. The nurse formulates the following nursing diagnosis: Altered Body Image related to physical changes caused by biochemical agents manifested by

   a. hand tremors and nervousness.

   b. muscle atrophy, bruising, and weight loss.

c. retracted eyelids and increased skin pigmentation.

d. weight gain, moon face, and increased facial hair.

10. A client should be assesses closely because Cushing's syndrome may mask signs and symptoms of

a. compression fractures.

b. infection.

c. hirsutism.

d. vascular changes.

11. Before an adrenal venogram, it is most important for the nurse to assess for

a. an allergy to dye.

b. a history of diabetes mellitus.

c. orientation level.

d. a smoking history.

12. Acarbose (Precose) is an alpha-glucosidase inhibitor that acts by

a. increasing insulin secretion.

b. increasing peripheral glucose uptake.

c. inhibiting glucose absorption.

d. inhibiting hepatic glucose output.

13. The nurse will closely monitor which two serum electrolytes in a client who has hyperparathyroidism?

a. Serum iron and calcium

b. Serum phosphate and calcium

c. Serum sodium and chloride

d. Serum sodium and phosphorus

14. Which of the following serum laboratory values would the nurse expect to see in a client with Addison's disease?

a. Decreased iron, decreased glucose, decreased cortisol

b. Decreased potassium, increased glucose, normal cortisol

c. Increased potassium decreased glucose, decreased cortisol

d. Increased potassium, increased glucose, increased cortisol

15. Which assessment data most directly relate to a diagnosis of diabetes mellitus?

a. Fasting glucose level of more than 126 mg/dL on two occasions.

b. Glucose level of 130 mg/dL at 2-hour point of a glucose tolerance test

c. Nausea and vomiting

d. Weight loss

16. Which of the following statements indicates that the client with hypothyroidism needs further teaching?

a. "I should increase the fiber in my diet."

b. "I should increase my calories in my diet."

c. "I should limit the fat and saturated fat in my diet."

d. "I should limit the sodium in my diet."

CHAPTER 79

Sensory System Disorders

■ Terminology Review

Match the following definitions with the correct terms.

1. _____ accumulation of blood in the eye's anterior chamber

2. _____ earwax

3. _____ condition of increased fluid pressure within the eye

4. _____ inflammation of the eyelid

5. _____ disturbance of the inner ear's semicircular canals

6. _____ double vision

7. _____ accumulation of lipid material

8. _____ inward turning of the lid margin

9. _____ pink eye

10. _____ corneal transplant

11. _____ opacity or cloudiness of the lens

12. _____ rapid, rhythmic eye movement

13. _____ removal of eyeball

14. _____ sense of taste

15. _____ outward turning of the eyelid due to the aging process

a. blepharitis
b. cataract
c. cerumen
d. chalazion
e. conjunctivitis
f. diplopia
g. ectropion
h. entropion
i. enucleation
j. glaucoma
k. gustation
l. hyphema
m. keratoplasty
n. Meniere's disease
o. nystagmus

Match the following definitions with the correct terms.

16. _____ sense of location in space

17. _____ drooping of the upper eyelid

18. _____ reconstruction of the middle ear to preserve vital parts, with less impairment of hearing

19. _____ instrument used to examine the ear

20. _____ ringing in the ear

21. _____ bony fixation of the stapes

22. _____ instrument that indirectly measures intraocular pressure

23. _____ inflammation of the middle ear

24. _____ sense of touch

25. _____ inflammation of the external ear

26. _____ instrument used to examine the outer and inner eye chambers

27. _____ drugs that are harmful to the inner ear

28. _____ sense of smell

29. _____ accurate testing for glasses

a. olfaction
b. ophthalmoscope
c. otitis externa
d. otitis media
e. otoscope
f. ototoxic

g. otosclerosis
h. tympanoplasty
i. proprioception
j. ptosis
k. refraction
l. tactile sense
m. tinnitus
n. tonometer

■ Fill-in-the-Blank

1. Myopia occurs when light rays focus at a point _____ of the retina.

2. Bifocals correct both _____ and _____ vision.

3. _____ is a system of raised dots that correspond to the alphabet.

4. Nonsighted people can use a _____ to help identify obstacles, curbs, and holes.

5. _____ can help people with sight or hearing problems obtain equipment that they cannot afford.

6. Hearing loss due to advanced aging is called _____.

7. _____ is the most common cause of conductive hearing loss.

8. Medications used to treat other diseases, which can harm the inner ear, are _____.

9. A _____ is removal of the stapes and is a treatment for otosclerosis.

10. Insertion of a _____ _____ is performed to allow for continuous drainage in clients with recurrent ear infections.

■ Matching

Match the following diagnostic tests with their uses.

1. _____ used to test the need for glasses

2. _____ allows viewing of the retina and other interior eye structures

3. _____ special microscope is used to view the eye's anterior structures

4. _____ indirectly measures intraocular pressure

5. _____ electrodes placed near the client's eyes to assess for alterations of the vestibular system

6. _____ records electrical impulses given off by the retina to determine whether the retina is functioning

7. _____ determines whether alterations exist in the vestibular origin of the acoustic nerve

8. _____ used to detect tumors of the eighth cranial nerve

9. _____ used to examine the external ear

a. slit lamp examination
b. tonometry
c. calorie test
d. refractive examination
e. electronystagmography
f. magnetic resonance imaging
g. ophthalmoscopic examination
h. electroretinogram
i. otoscope

■ Short Answer

1. Outline the procedure to insert and remove a prosthetic eye.

2. Describe what a cochlear implant is and how it works.

3. Why is patient teaching important for clients having ear or eye surgery?

4. Complete the following table.

	Preoperative Care	Postoperative Care
Eye Surgery		
Ear Surgery		

5. Describe differences when straightening the ear canal in an adult and a child.

6. Describe the differences between hard, soft, and extended-wear contact lenses.

7. What is the main complication that can result from wearing contact lenses?

8. Identify assessment data associated with the following disorders.

Chronic open angle glaucoma

Narrow (closed) angle glaucoma

Cataracts

Retinal detachment

9. List devices that can aid the hearing impaired.

10. You are caring for three clients. One has serous otitis media, one has acute purulent otitis media, and the last has chronic purulent otitis media. What assessment findings will be similar and what assessment findings will be different?

11. You are caring for the following clients on your medical-surgical unit:

a. A 76-year-old client who is preoperative for cataract surgery who complains of halos around lights and difficulty seeing

b. A 49-year-old woman with Meniere's disease who complains of dizziness and nausea. She is requesting her antiemetic medication

c. A 74-year-old client with chronic open-angle glaucoma whose timolol maleate (Timoptic) eye drops are due now

How would you prioritize your nursing assessments and interventions? Provide rationales for your responses.

12. The nurse had just completed the Weber and Rinne tests and determines that the test results are normal. Write a sample documentation for the results.

■ Case Study

You are caring for a 70-year-old man. His wife complains that he seems bored with her conversations and doesn't seem interested anymore in what she has to say. He is a retired factory worker. He seems to have lost interest in his usual activities.

1. What problem do you suspect this client has?

2. What additional assessment data would you obtain and why?

3. What information would you document and share with the RN and MD?

4. Outline a specific teaching plan to help the wife communicate with her husband.

■ Multiple Choice

Circle the best answer.

1. The nurse realizes that visual disturbances can be caused by systemic diseases such as:
   a. diabetes.
   b. congestive heart failure.
   c. lupus erythematosus.
   d. cancer.

2. To prevent injury after eye examinations that have included dilating the pupils, the nurse should instruct the patient to:
   a. wear a sunscreen while outdoors.
   b. wear sunglasses when going into brightly lit areas.
   c. go to sleep for several hours.
   d. no special instructions are needed.

3. To prevent injury after the eye is anesthetized, the nurse should instruct the patient:
   a. not to read for the remainder of the day.
   b. not to rub or press on the operative eyes.
   c. gently cleanse with warm soapy water.
   d. lay only on the affected side for the first 24 hours.

4. What is the safest way for the nurse to lead a patient who has both eyes patched?
   a. Walk slightly behind the patient.
   b. Lead the patient by the hand.
   c. Ask the patient to take the nurse's arm.
   d. Hold the patient around the waist.

5. A patient has just had surgery on the ear. The nurse observes ptosis on the operative side. The nurse's first action would be:
   a. elevate the head of bed.
   b. notify the RN or MD.
   c. gently cleanse the eye.
   d. change the dressing.

6. Following eye surgery, a client complains of nausea. The nurse's first action would be to:
   a. notify the RN or MD.
   b. elevate the head of bed.
   c. assess for bleeding at the operative site.
   d. medicate with ordered antiemetic.

7. Which of the following discharge instructions for a client with Meniere's disease should the nurse question?
   a. Instruct client to ask for assistance when needed.
   b. Take prescribed sedatives as ordered.
   c. Increase daily sodium chloride intake.
   d. During an attack, lie down and keep the head still.

8. Which of the following instructions can the nurse give to help a patient with Meniere's disease manage the vertigo?

   a. Avoid sudden movement.

   b. Listen to soft music.

   c. Increase fluid intake to 3 L/d.

   d. Rest on the involved side.

9. What is the most important goal for a client who is receiving acetazolamide (Diamox)?

   a. To decrease intraocular pressure

   b. To increase vision clarity

   c. To clear infection

   d. To prevent eye injury

10. A client who wears a hearing aid complains of background noises. What instruction is most important for the nurse to include in a teaching plan?

    a. Wash the earpiece every day.

    b. Wear the aid at all times.

    c. Turn the volume down.

    d. Discuss the matter with the physician.

CHAPTER 80

Cardiovascular Disorders

■ Terminology Review

Match the following definitions with the correct terms and acronyms.

1. _____ inflammation of the heart's muscular walls

2. _____ prolonged deficiency of oxygenated blood

3. _____ condition associated with many types of heart disease in which the heart contractions are weak and lack sufficient force to send blood from the atria into the ventricles

4. _____ excruciating pain in a limb with exercise which disappears with rest

5. _____ a wire coil used to keep an artery open

6. _____ enlarged

7. _____ outpouching of blood vessel

8. _____ inflammation of the heart's inner lining, usually involving the valves

9. _____ stroke or brain attack

10. _____ percutaneous transluminal coronary angioplasty

11. _____ blood clot that dislodges from its place of origin, moves through the circulatory system, and lodges in another place

12. _____ occurs when symptoms of stroke are present and stabilize over a period of time

13. _____ coronary artery bypass grafting in which a vein is grafted around the blockage in the coronary artery

14. _____ sudden, short-lived attack that is usually a warning that another, more serious stroke will occur later

15. _____ paralysis of one side of the body

16. _____ gradual worsening of symptoms of brain ischemia

17. _____ type of angioplasty that involves the use of a cutting device with a rotating shaver at the tip of the catheter

18. _____ unable to speak

19. _____ inflammation of a blood vessel without clot formation

20. _____ subacute bacterial endocarditis

21. _____ blindness in half of the visual field of one or both eyes

22. _____ procedure that uses high-energy lasers to create new channels through the heart muscle into the left ventricle

23. _____ pain in the chest

24. _____ premature ventricular contraction

25. _____ stage of CVA in which the symptoms last for as long as a week; is a warning sign that a more serious stroke is likely

26. _____ conversion of cardiac dysrhythmia with medications or electrically

27. _____ syndrome in which the heart is failing and unable to do its work—it has lost its pumping efficiency

28. _____ surgical procedure that widens the artery's lumen and improves blood flow to the heart muscle

29. _____ special hospital unit designed to care for people with heart disorders

30. _____ inflammation of the wall of a vein in which one or more clots form

31. _____ inflammation of the sac surrounding the heart

32. _____ elevated blood pressure

33. _____ complication of a CVA that includes symptoms of an elevated temperature,

lowered pulse, and lowered respiratory rate

34. _____ atrioventricular

35. _____ intensive care unit

36. _____ narrowing of an opening such as a vessel

37. _____ sudden blockage of one or more coronary arteries

38. _____ coronary artery disease

39. _____ blood clot that forms inside a deep blood vessel

40. _____ irregularity in the heartbeat's rhythm

41. _____ dissolves clots

42. _____ without heartbeat

43. _____ disorganized twitching of cardiac muscles

44. _____ implantable device used to manage ventricular dysrhythmias

45. _____ automatic implantable cardioverter-defibrillator

46. _____ to sever or cut pathways

a. ablation

b. aneurysm

c. angina pectoris

d. angioplasty

e. aphasia

f. arrhythmia

g. artherectomy

h. cardioversion

i. claudication

j. dysrhythmia

k. embolus

l. endocarditis

m. fibrillation

n. hemiplegia

o. hypertrophy

p. heart block

q. hemianopsia

r. ischemia

s. myocarditis

t. pericarditis

u. phlebitis

v. stenosis

w. stent

x. thrombolytic

y. thrombophlebitis

z. AICD

aa. AV

bb. CAD

cc. CCU/CICU

dd. CHF

ee. CABG

ff. CS

gg. CVA

hh. DVT

ii. HTN

jj. ICD

kk. ICU

ll. ICP

mm. MI

nn. PVC

oo. PTCA

pp. RIND

qq. SBE

rr. SGOT

ss. SIE

tt. TIA

uu. TMR

■ Assessment Review

For the following assessment data, indicate whether the finding is a normal assessment finding (N) or an abnormal assessment finding (A). Abnormal findings can be indicative of cardiovascular disorders.

1. _____ negative Homans' sign

2. _____ smokes ½ pack of cigarettes per day

3. _____ blood pressure of 120/80

4. _____ total cholesterol level of 130

5. _____ hemoptysis

6. _____ dizziness

7. _____ heart rate of 65 bpm

8. _____ mild swelling of the ankles

9. _____ ECG shows AV heart block

10. _____ decreased appetite

11. _____ chest pain relieved with rest

12. _____ exercises three times a week

13. _____ regular rate and rhythm of heart rate

14. _____ cold hands

15. _____ slurred speech that resolves within 24 hours

16. _____ heart murmur

17. _____ bounding pulse

18. _____ nonlabored respirations 16/minute

19. _____ tinnitus

20. _____ no coughing

■ Diagnostic Tests Review

Match the following diagnostic tests with the explanation of the test.

1. _____ good cholesterol

2. _____ prothrombin time used for monitoring of Coumadin

3. _____ serum glutamic oxaloacetic transaminase

4. _____ tissue plasminogen activator

5. _____ graphic record or tracing that represents the heart's electrical action

6. _____ sound waves used to produce a three-dimensional view of the heart and its blood flow with Doppler

7. _____ partial thromboplastin time

8. _____ blood screening for creatinine phosphokinase

9. _____ provides information about the function of the heart by locating the source of a dysthrthmia

10. _____ x-ray of the heart and major vessels after injection of a radiopaque dye into a vessel

11. _____ bad cholesterol

12. _____ blood screening for lactic dehydrogenase

13. _____ exercise test used to assess the severity of symptomatic and asymptomatic cardiac disease

14. _____ blood screening for aspartate aminotransferase

15. _____ hydroxybutyric dehydrogenase

16. _____ means of monitoring the heart by placing Doppler probe directly into the esophagus

17. _____ test used to obtain information about congenital or acquired heart defects, to measure oxygen concentration, to determine cardiac output, or to assess the status of the heart's structures and chambers

a. angiogram

b. cardiac catheterization

c. echocardiography

d. AST

e. CPK

f. ECG

g. EPS

h. HBD

i. HDL

j. LDH

k. LDL

l. PT

m. PTT

n. stress test

o. SGOT

p. TEE

q. t-PA

■ Case Studies

Complete the following case studies by providing the best answer.

1. You are assigned the following clients on your medical-surgical unit:

   Mr. Abe, an 80-year-old client admitted 3 days ago for an MI who is complaining of substernal pain

   Mrs. Garcia, a new admission with thrombophlebitis of the right lower extremity. She is having difficulty breathing.

   Ms. Crocker, who is being discharged on Coumadin and needs teaching before she leaves. Her ride will be arriving in 30 minutes.

Mr. Clooney, 53-year-old diabetic client with a venous stasis ulcer who is going to physical therapy for a whirlpool treatment and needs to medicated within the next 15 minutes.

a. How would you prioritize your care? Provide a rational for each intervention and the order you choose.

2. Mr. J is a 59-year-old client who has chronic peripheral vascular disease. During your assessment, he describes a pattern of pain that occurs when he walks and then disappears when he rests.

a. How would you document his symptoms?

b. When assessing Mr. J, what other findings would you expect to find?

c. What measures would you teach Mr. J to help arrest the disease process?

3. Mrs. Waters, 73 years of age, has been admitted to your unit with CHF. She began having dyspnea and orthopnea 3 days ago, and the symptoms have become progressively worse. She complains of restlessness, insomnia, and a productive cough with pink sputum. Your assessment reveals: temperature—98°F, pulse—114 beats/min and irregular, respirations—24 breaths/min; blood pressure—68/96 mmHg; weight, 152 pounds (a 7-pound increase in 1 week); skin is pale and diaphoretic; jugular vein distention is noted. She has bilateral crackles in the lower lobes. Abdomen is distended, 3+ pitting edema is present in both ankles. She has orders for a diuretic and a digitalis preparation.

a. What are two priority nursing diagnoses for this client? Provide rationale and assessment data to support your choices.

b. From the following list, indicate the order in which you would provide nursing care. Also include your rationale for the order you choose.

i. Document assessment findings.

ii. Prepare the client for an echocardiogram.

iii. Place client on intake and output.

iv. Administer medications as ordered.

v. Locate a Doppler to assess pedal pulses.

vi. Provide mattress and chair padding.

■ Multiple Choice

Circle the best answer.

1. A client asks, "What is the purpose of cardiac isoenzymes?" The nurses best response would be: "Cardiac isoenzymes:
   a. "determine how well the blood is being oxygenated."
   b. "determine the presence of myocardial tissue damage."
   c. "show the electrical activity of the heart."
   d. "allow the physician to view the inside of the ventricles."

2. A client has just returned from having an angiogram. All of the following are appropriate nursing interventions. Which would be the priority?

   a. Assess level of sedation.

   b. Encourage fluids and adequate diet.

   c. Enforce bed rest for 8 hours.

   d. Ensure that insertion site has no bleeding.

3. A 35-year-old female client is admitted to the hospital with a suspected myocardial infarction. Which information would be most important for the nurse to obtain before starting thrombolytic therapy?

   a. History of hypertension

   b. Family history of MI

   c. Pregnancy test

   d. Vital signs

4. What is the most important goal of a client who has undergone cardiac surgery?

   a. Maintain positive body image

   b. Maintain mobility

   c. Provide adequate tissue oxygenation

   d. Provide adequate sleep and rest

5. Which of following diets should the nurse recommend to the client who has arteriosclerosis?

   a. Diabetic diet

   b. Diet high in sodium

   c. Diet high in saturated fats

   d. Diet low in saturated fats

6. Which of the following are complications of hypertension?

   a. Kidney damage, MI, and CVA

   b. MI, asthma, and DM

   c. Rectal cancer, asthma, and MI

   d. Seizures, kidney damage, and CVA

7. The nurse is administering nitroglycerin sublingually to a client for angina. The client asks, "How does this medication work?" The nurse explains that the medication:

   a. causes dilation of the coronary arteries.

   b. causes vasoconstriction of the systemic arterial bed.

   c. increases the filling pressure.

   d. Increases the systemic blood pressure.

8. What is the expected outcome of a client who is taking thiazides?

   a. Increased blood pressure

   b. Increased heart rate

   c. Increased urinary output

   d. Increased weight

9. The nurse should advise a client with varicose veins to avoid:

   a. active exercise.

   b. leg elevation.

   c. loose clothing.

   d. prolonged standing.

10. A client is admitted with a complete stroke and is unresponsive. Which intervention is appropriate to ensure client safety?

    a. Position the client on the affected side.

    b. Position the client in a prone position.

    c. Positions the client in a supine position.

    d. Position the client on the unaffected side.

11. A client is admitted with a stroke and is unable to speak. The nurse would document this as:

    a. aphasia.

    b. dysphagia.

    c. dysphasia.

    d. hemiplegia.

12. A physician orders a potassium supplement for a client who is taking furosemide (Lasix). The rationale for ordering the potassium is to:

    a. control anxiety.

    b. control edema.

    c. dilate vessels.

    d. replace potassium.

13. An adult client who had rheumatic heart disease as a child is at risk for which of the following diseases in later life?

    a. Congestive heart failure

    b. Chronic pericarditis

    c. Myocardial infarction

    d. Valvular heart disease

CHAPTER 81

Blood and Lymph Disorders

■ Terminology Review

Match the following definitions with the correct terms.

1. _____ malignant hematologic disorder characterized by an abundance of abnormal WBCs

2. _____ medical specialty concerned with the hematologic and lymphatic systems

3. _____ occurs when a client's platelet count falls below 150,000/mm^3

4. _____ this procedure is done to evaluate the number, size, and shape of RBCs, WBCs, and megakaryocytes

5. _____ genetic disease in which the person's RBCs become crescent shaped when exposed to decreased oxygen

6. _____ most common type of cancer in young adults that presents with enlarged lymph nodes and accompanying pain, fever, fatigue, night sweats, itching, and weight loss

7. _____ decrease in the number of WBCs

8. _____ sex-linked genetic disorder in which the person's blood is slow to coagulate owing to lack of factor VIII or factor IX in the plasma

9. _____ bone marrow transplantation that uses the client's own bone marrow

10. _____ production of WBCs decreases, causing severe neutropenia

11. _____ cancer specialist

12. _____ bone marrow transplantation in which the client receives the bone marrow from someone else

a. agranulocytosis
b. allogeneic
c. autologous
d. bone marrow biopsy
e. hematology
f. hemophilia
g. Hodgkin's disease
h. leukemia
i. leukopenia
j. oncologist
k. sickle cell anemia
l. thrombocytopenia

Match the following definitions with the correct acronyms.

13. _____ type of chronic leukemia whose only cure is stem cell transplantation

14. _____ type of acute leukemia most commonly found in children

15. _____ complex test used to monitor the pathway of clot formation

16. _____ immune globulins

17. _____ type of chronic leukemia that appears to result from genetic influences and autoimmune diseases; it is incurable

18. _____ group of lymphatic neoplasms

19. _____ type of acute leukemia most commonly found in adults

20. _____ plasma protein fraction

21. _____ bone marrow transplantation

22. _____ blood test that can indicate the activity of certain factors found in the plasma that are important in blood clotting (factors V, VII, X, prothrombin, and fibrinogen)

23. _____ peripheral blood stem cell

24. _____ measures the speed at which RBCs settle to the bottom of a tube of unclotted blood that is used to detect inflammatory processes, neoplasms, and necrotic processes

25. _____ activated partial thromboplastin

26. _____ Hodgkin's disease

27. _____ condition in which the person develops antibodies to his or her own platelets

28. _____ iron dextran

a. ALL
b. AML
c. APTT
d. BMT
e. CLL
f. CML
g. ESR
h. HD
i. IG
j. InFeD
k. ITP
l. NHL
m. PBSC
n. PPF
o. PT
p. PTT

■ Anemia Comparison

Complete the following table.

Type of Anemia	Description	Nursing Care
Iron deficiency		
Acute hemorrhagic		
Aplastic		
Sickle cell		

■ Correct the False Statements

Circle the word True *or* False *that follows the statement. If the word* false *has been circled, change the underlined word/words to make the statement true. Place your answer in the space provided.*

1. Signs and symptoms of <u>neutropenia</u> include chills, fever, headache, and ulcers on the mucous membrane.

   True   False   _____

2. The most common symptoms of acute lymphocytic leukemia result from <u>changes in the shape of blood cells.</u>

   True   False   _____

3. Clients with <u>acute myelogenous leukemia</u> usually experience recurrent infections and fail to respond to antibiotics.

   True   False   _____

4. Chemotherapy is used to <u>cure</u> chronic lymphocytic leukemia.

   True   False   _____

5. Treatment of clients with thrombocytopenia includes the use of <u>corticosteroids and platelet transfusions.</u>

   True   False   _____

6. Disseminated intravascular coagulation is characterized by <u>clotting in the microvascular system and simultaneous hemorrhage.</u>

   True   False   _____

7. Treatment of hemophilia focuses on the prevention of <u>infection.</u>

   True   False   _____

8. <u>Hodgkin's disease and non-Hodgkin's lymphoma rarely</u> present with night sweats, fever, and weight loss.

   True   False   _____

9. Hodgkin's disease that is <u>stage IV</u> is present above and below the diaphragm.

   True   False   _____

10. <u>A single unit of blood should not be transfused over a period of time longer than</u> 4 hours.

    True   False   _____

11. <u>Blood should be transfused within</u> 30 minutes after removing from a monitored refrigerator.

    True   False   _____

12. Liquid iron preparations should be administered <u>using a straw.</u>

    True   False   _____

13. When administering blood to an unconscious client, <u>hypothermia</u> can indicate a transfusion reaction.

    True   False   _____

14. An <u>erythrocyte sedimentation rate</u> should be completed before administering antibiotics to determine if bacteria are present in the blood.

    True   False   _____

15. Most blood transfusion reactions occur <u>after the blood has infused.</u>

    True   False   _____

■ Multiple Choice

Circle the best answer.

1. When caring for a client with a diagnosis of neutropenia, which of the following is the most appropriate nursing action?
   a. Administer blood products.
   b. Avoid using razors during activities of daily living.
   c. Maintain the head of the bed at 90 degrees.
   d. Use proper handwashing and protect from infection.

2. When a client is admitted with thrombocytope-nia, which information is most important when obtaining a history?

    a. Bleeding from the nose or gums

    b. Family members available for support

    c. Recent infections

    d. When client was diagnosed with the disease

3. Which solution should be used when administer-ing blood?

    a. 0.45% saline

    b. 0.9% normal saline

    c. 5% dextrose water

    d. lactated Ringer's solution

4. One of the most common hematologic problems that affects people of all ages is:

    a. anemia.

    b. Hodgkin's disease.

    c. leukemia.

    d. leukopenia.

5. The two types of acute leukemia are lymphocytic and:

    a. hemophilic.

    b. lymphoblastic.

    c. myelogenous.

    d. thrombocytopenic.

6. The most common cancer in young adults, which is slightly more common in men, is:

    a. acute lymphocytic leukemia.

    b. Hodgkin's disease.

    c. non-Hodgkin's lymphoma.

    d. thalassemia.

7. The most frequent platelet complication of cancer and its treatment is:

    a. hemophilia.

    b. leukemia.

    c. leukopenia.

    d. thrombocytopenia.

CHAPTER 82

Cancer

■ Terminology Review

Match the following definitions with the correct terms.

1. _____ neoplasms not confined within a capsule that can spread to nearby tissues

2. _____ study of cells

3. _____ another name for cancer

4. _____ against cancer

5. _____ take a sample of a specimen

6. _____ diseases characterized by abnormal alterations in cell growth

7. _____ reduction in bone marrow function

8. _____ used after surgery to try to prevent metastases

9. _____ substances know to cause or promote cancer

10. _____ neoplasms that spread to other parts of the body through blood and lymphatic systems

11. _____ nonmalignant, self-contained, nonspreading

12. _____ use of chemical agents to destroy cancer cells

13. _____ type of chemotherapy that uses agents derived from biologic sources or agents that will affect biologic responses

a. adjuvant therapy
b. antineoplastic
c. benign
d. biotherapy
e. biopsy
f. cancer

g. carcinogen
h. carcinoma
i. chemotherapy
j. cytology
k. malignant
l. metastasis
m. myelosuppression

Match the following definitions with the correct terms.

14. _____ outlook for a cure

15. _____ medical specialty concerned with cancer and its treatment

16. _____ cancer that includes bone and muscle, arises in connective tissue

17. _____ reproduction

18. _____ test used to detect cancer of the cervix and uterus

19. _____ type of treatment used to provide relief to the client, not cure

20. _____ new growth

21. _____ decreased neutrophils

a. neoplasm
b. neutropenia
c. oncology
d. palliative
e. Pap test
f. prognosis
g. replication
h. sarcoma

Match the following definitions with the correct acronym.

22. _____ act as messengers that assist the immune defense activities

23. _____ tumor marker for prostate cancer

24. _____ interferon

25. _____ peripheral indwelling catheter

26. _____ substances that encourage growth and maturation of blood cell components

27. _____ tumor marker for testicular and certain types of ovarian cancers

28. _____ peripherally inserted central catheter

29. _____ National Cancer Institute

30. _____ tumor marker used with breast, colorectal, and lung cancers

31. _____ Oncology Nursing Society

32. _____ American Cancer Society

33. _____ tumor marker of germ cell tumors and liver cancers

a. ACS

b. CEA

c. PSA

d. HCG

e. AFP

f. IFN

g. IL

h. HGF

i. NCI

j. OONC

k. PIC

l. PICC

■ Short Answer

Complete the following.

1. List the five factors believed to contribute to cancer.

2. List the seven danger signals of cancer.

3. Describe the three methods that radiation therapy may be used to treat cancer.

4. What three factors are key to dealing safely with radiation therapy?

5. Describe signs and symptoms of cancer for which the nurse should be alert.

■ Medication Review

Match the following chemotherapy medications with the appropriate category.

1. _____ doxorubicin HCL (Adriamycin)

2. _____ carmustine (BCNU)

3. _____ cisplatin (Platinol)

4. _____ dexamethasone (Decadron)

5. _____ paclitaxel (Taxol)

6. _____ fluorouracil (Adrucil)

7. _____ vincristine sulfate (Oncovin)

8. _____ tamoxifen (Nolvadex)

9. _____ topotecan HCL (Hycamtin)

a. antimetabolites

b. alkylating agents

c. antitumor antibiotics

d. corticosteroids

e. hormonal agents

f. miscellaneous agents

g. nitrosureas

h. taxanes

i. vinca alkaloids

■ Correct the False Statements

Circle the word True *or* False *that follows the statement. If the word* false *has been circled, change the underlined word/words to make the statement true. Place your answer in the space provided.*

1. The place where cancer starts is called the <u>secondary site</u>.

   True   False   _____

2. A known <u>carcinogen associated with lung cancer</u> is cigarette smoking.

   True   False   _____

3. <u>Cell-cycle specific</u> agents are most effective against rapidly growing tumors.

   True   False   _____

4. Vascular access devices are used to <u>administer chemotherapy</u>.

   True   False   _____

5. <u>Interleukins</u> are substances that encourage growth and maturation of blood cell components.

   True   False   _____

6. Common side effects associated with tamoxifen include <u>amenorrhea, hot flashes, and insomnia</u>.

   True   False   _____

7. Cancer pain is controllable for <u>only some clients</u>.

   True   False   _____

8. <u>Fatigue</u> is the most common distressing symptom of cancer that clients report.

   True   False   _____

9. Alopecia can include hair loss on the <u>head, body, pubic area, and eyelashes</u>.

   True   False   _____

10. Clients receiving radiation or chemotherapy experience lowered blood counts and therefore have increased <u>risks for infection</u>.

   True   False   _____

■ Case Study

Prioritize your care and provide rationales for your actions when caring for the following clients.

- Mr. J with a new diagnosis of colon cancer is scheduled for surgery in the morning. He needs preoperative instructions and appears anxious.

- Mr. P has metastatic bone cancer with increasing confusion, high blood pressure, and poor muscle control.

- Mrs. L was admitted yesterday with unretractable pain and is currently resting comfortably.

- Ms. D is being discharged from the hospital; she has just finished a course of chemotherapy.

▪ Multiple Choice

Circle the best answer.

1. The leading cause of cancer deaths in both men and women is:

   a. brain cancer.

   b. colon cancer.

   c. lung cancer.

   d. pancreatic cancer.

2. Which of the following groups of food would the nurse teach a client to eat to reduce the risk for certain cancers?

   a. Bacon and lunch meats

   b. Broccoli and fruits

   c. Salt-cured pork and chicken

   d. Whole milk and cheeses

3. A client is receiving external-beam radiation therapy. Assessment findings include erythema, pain, and dry, peeling skin. Which action is most appropriate for the nurse to implement?

   a. Instruct client not to apply soap, powders, or lotion to the area.

   b. Instruct the client to wear natural-fiber wool clothing.

   c. Use ice packs to the area after treatment.

   d. Use a soft washcloth to scrub the area.

4. Which nursing action is appropriate for the client experiencing nausea and vomiting associated with chemotherapy?

   a. Administer antiemetics.

   b. Encourage client to avoid eating.

   c. Encourage large meals.

   d. Offer hot, spicy foods.

CHAPTER 83

Allergic, Immune, and Autoimmune Disorders

■ Terminology Review

Match the following definitions with the correct terms and acronyms.

1. _____ antigen that causes an immune response in the body

2. _____ treating symptoms as they occur, rather than treating the underlying condition

3. _____ allergic skin reaction characterized by wheals and often accompanied by itching

4. _____ autoimmune disorder that affects one or more organs

5. _____ foreign protein substance

6. _____ autoimmune disorders that affect the entire body

7. _____ allergic skin condition characterized by tiny blisters that cover the body and itch and ooze

8. _____ chemical mediator that is released during the antigen–antibody reaction

9. _____ autoimmune disorder that affects one organ

10. _____ antigen that causes a tissue reaction

11. _____ the body does not recognize itself as "self" and begins to produce antibodies against its own healthy cells or inhibit normal cell function

12. _____ hypersensitivity to one or more substances

13. _____ depression of the immune system

14. _____ allergic skin reaction, also known as urticaria

15. _____ the body's normal adaptive state designed to protect itself from disease

16. _____ hypersensitive reaction to an antigen

17. _____ desensitization by giving minute doses of allergens subcutaneously

18. _____ produced in the body to protect itself against antigens

19. _____ lump, wheal, or edema

20. _____ development of urticaria and edema in areas of skin and mucous membranes

a. allergen
b. allergy
c. anaphylaxis
d. angioedema
e. antibody
f. antigen
g. autoimmunity
h. eczema
i. histamine
j. hives
k. induration
l. immunity
m. immunogen
n. immunosuppression
o. immunotherapy
p. non–organ-specific
q. organ-specific
r. symptomatic
s. systemic
t. urticaria

■ Assessment Review

For the following manifestations of the allergic response, indicate whether the assessment findings are S—skin manifestations, R—respiratory manifestations, GI—gastrointestinal findings, or N—not a manifestation of allergic response.

1. _____ breath sounds clear

2. _____ nausea and vomiting

3. _____ skin reddened and itching

4. _____ cough

5. _____ abdominal pain

6. _____ skin warm to touch

7. _____ itching of the palate

8. _____ blisters in folds of the neck

9. _____ migraine headaches

10. _____ wheezing

11. _____ swelling of skin

12. _____ no change in appetite

13. _____ tenacious sputum

14. _____ profuse perspiration

15. _____ burping

■ Short Answer

Complete the following questions.

1. List three possible manifestations of allergic response that relate to drugs.

2. Describe three methods of treatment of multisystem allergy response. Provide an example of each method.

3. Why are women more at risk for developing autoimmunity than men?

4. Describe differences between organ-specific, non–organ-specific, and systemic autoimmune disorders. Give one example of each.

5. Describe what symptomatic treatment is and provide examples.

■ Case Studies

1. Ms. N is a 29-year-old client who has been referred to the allergy clinic for recurring allergy symptoms. She has had complaints of runny nose, watery eyes, and occasional cough with wheezing and mild chest tightness. She also relates having difficulty sleeping at night due to her symptoms. She is scheduled for evaluation at the clinic.

   a. Describe diagnostic procedures would you expect to be completed on Ms. N and indicate why they would be done.

   b. Skin testing is completed, and Ms. N is allergic to dust mites and several seasonal grasses. List three nursing diagnoses that would apply to Ms. N.

   c. Write outcomes for the nursing diagnoses listed in the previous question.

   d. Ms. N was started on cetirizime. Identify specific teaching for Ms. N regarding her medications and environment.

2. Your client is in the radiology department and is having a CT scan with radiopague dye containing iodine. Shortly after having the contrast dye injected, the client complains of severe shortness of breath. Anaphylaxis is suspected.

   a. Outline nursing interventions and rationales for each intervention.

   b. The client survives the anaphylactic reaction. What teaching would the client need to prevent any further reactions?

■ Multiple Choice

Circle the best answer.

1. When completing skin testing, which finding indicates a positive skin test?

   a. Coughing

   b. Erythema and induration

   c. Mild itching and edema

   d. Pallor

2. Before skin testing, which instructions should the nurse provide for the client?

   a. Avoid food for 6 hours before the appointment.

   b. Take analgesics 1 hour before the appointment.

   c. Wash the area thoroughly before the appointment.

   d. Withhold antihistamines before the appointment.

3. Which assessment relates most directly to a diagnosis of bronchial asthma?

   a. Dyspnea and chest tightness

   b. Erythema and uticaria

   c. Migraine headaches

   d. Swelling of the lips

4. After a desensitization treatment, it is most important for the nurse to document that the client:

   a. had no severe reaction after 20 minutes.

   b. reported improved symptoms.

   c. reported the injection hurt.

   d. was late to the appointment.

5. Which statement indicates that the client who has seasonal allergies has understood teaching provided by the nurse?

   a. "I need to bathe my dog each week."

   b. "I need to wear a mask when outside during allergy season."

   c. "I should avoid smoke-filled rooms."

   d. "I should get plenty of exercise outside each day."

6. What is the priority nursing diagnosis for a client experiencing anaphylaxis?

   a. Altered Thought Process related to loss of consciousness

   b. Anxiety related to inability to breathe

   c. Knowledge Deficit related to treatment

   d. Risk for Suffocation related to airway nonpatency

7. Which of the following statements indicates that the client needs further teaching regarding seasonal allergies and self-care?

   a. "After I start my allergy shots, I should be better in a week."

   b. "I need to avoid exposure to allergens."

   c. "I need to take my medications as directed."

   d. "My family understands how to help me manage my allergies."

8. An expected outcome for a client with allergies is that the client will make modifications in lifestyle, diet, and environment to avoid allergens. Which finding indicates that the outcome has been met?

   a. Client continues to be exposed to allergens.

   b. Client did not make any changes in lifestyle.

   c. Client experienced decreased allergic symptoms.

   d. Client experienced only one anaphylactic response.

9. A client was given a new medication 10 days ago. The client has returned to the clinic with complaints of skin rash, swollen joints, and general weakness. These findings most likely indicate:

a. adverse drug reaction.

b. drug allergy.

c. serum sickness.

d. severe sensitivity.

10. After the client undergoes organ transplantation, the nurse observes fever, chills, edema, and diaphoresis. The priority nursing action would be to:

a. administer antipyretic medication.

b. encourage turn, cough, and deep breathing exercises.

c. monitor pain level.

d. notify the RN or MD.

CHAPTER 84

HIV and AIDS

■ Terminology Review

Match the following definitions with the correct terms and acronyms.

1. _____ disease that affects global geographic areas

2. _____ *Mycobacterium avium* complex that causes fever, diarrhea, and other nonspecific symptoms

3. _____ viral load of HIV

4. _____ *Pneumocystis carinii* pneumonia

5. _____ virus that overtakes the biosynthesis of living cells to duplicate itself

6. _____ early treatment used to prevent infections

7. _____ occurs during the later stages of HIV infection in which the immune system is destroyed by HIV

8. _____ World Health Organization

9. _____ medications used to decrease the amount of circulating virus and to restore immune functions

10. _____ postexposure prophylaxis

11. _____ lymphocytes that mature in the thymus

12. _____ protozoan infection of the lungs

13. _____ AIDS dementia complex

14. _____ human immunodeficiency virus

15. _____ progressive decline of neurologic function as HIV/AIDS disease process progresses

16. _____ helper T lymphocytes

17. _____ progressive decline in cognition and memory, headache, difficulty with concentration, progressive confusion, psychomotor slowing, apathy, ataxia, depression, psychosis, hallucinations, tremors, seizures, and death

18. _____ infectious human retrovirus first seen in the early 1980s

19. _____ Centers for Disease Control and Prevention

20. _____ test used to measure how virulent the HIV virus is

21. _____ virus causing colitis, pneumonitis, and retinitis

22. _____ infections caused by organisms that do not usually cause disease in people with normal immune systems

23. _____ acquired immunodeficiency syndrome

24. _____ human papillomavirus

a. acquired immunodeficiency syndrome
b. ADC
c. AIDS
d. AIDS dementia complex
e. antiretroviral therapy
f. CD4
g. CDC
h. CMV
i. HIV
j. HIV encephalopathy
k. HIV-RNA
l. Human immunodeficiency virus
m. HPV
n. MAC
o. opportunistic infections
p. pandemic
q. PCP
r. PEP
s. *Pneumocystis carinii* pneumonia
t. prophylaxis
u. retrovirus
v. T cells
w. viral load
x. WHO

■ Assessment Review

For the following assessment data, indicate whether the finding is common to HIV (H), AIDS (A), or both HIV and AIDS (B), or is a normal (N) finding.

1. _____ positive Western blot

2. _____ abnormal pap smears

3. _____ less than 200 T cells

4. _____ night sweats

5. _____ negative ELISA

6. _____ Kaposi's sarcoma

7. _____ general malaise

8. _____ undetectable viral load

9. _____ weight loss

10. _____ regular menstrual periods

11. _____ persistent lymphadenophathy

12. _____ hallucinations

13. _____ toxoplasmosis

14. _____ herpes zoster

15. _____ candidiasis fungal infections

16. _____ cervical cancer

17. _____ fever

18. _____ diarrhea

19. _____ anorexia

20. _____ *Pneumocystis carinii* pneumonia

■ Correct the False Statements

Circle the word True *or* False *that follows the statement. If the word* false *has been circled, change the underlined word/words to make the statement true. Place your answer in the space provided.*

1. <u>Acyclovir</u> is a medication used to treat the opportunistic infections herpes simplex and shingles.

   True   False   _____

2. HIV was first seen in the <u>early 1980s</u> when several unusual infections were noted in young homosexual men.

   True   False   _____

3. <u>T cells</u> are lymphocytes that originate in the bone marrow, and <u>B cells</u> are lymphocytes that mature in the thymus.

   True   False   _____

4. The average time from acquisition of HIV until the diagnosis of AIDS is made is about <u>5 years</u>.

   True   False   _____

5. HIV is transmitted through <u>infected body fluids</u>.

   True   False   _____

6. HIV <u>cannot</u> be transferred by oral sex, from a woman to her newborn baby, or through breast milk.

   True   False   _____

7. Once a person is exposed to HIV, antibodies <u>develop immediately</u>.

   True   False   _____

8. The functions of T cells and B cells are to fight infection and to <u>produce antibodies for specific immune responses</u>.

   True   False   _____

9. AIDS occurs when the <u>immune system</u> is destroyed by HIV.

   True   False   _____

10. People with HIV and certain opportunistic infections or cancers meet the <u>case definition for AIDS</u>.

    True   False   _____

11. During data assessment, the nurse should assess for evidence of depression, anxiety, or other symptoms of <u>lack of coping mechanisms</u>.

    True   False   _____

12. HIV is <u>now curable</u> with the early use of anti-retroviral medications.

    True   False   _____

13. HIV testing can be done on a client <u>without his or her knowledge</u>.

    True   False   _____

14. Healthcare workers <u>can protect themselves</u> against HIV exposure by adhering to Standard Precautions.

    True   False   _____

15. <u>Respiratory problems</u> for the HIV-infected client can result from fungal infections, wasting syndrome, or side effects of medication.

    True   False   _____

■ Case Study

A 26-year-old man has been newly diagnosed with AIDS. He is currently a client on a medical unit and is scheduled to be discharged for home tomorrow. He and his partner have expressed concern about the progression of his illness and care needed once discharged from the hospital.

1. Outline a teaching plan, including categories of information that you will need to discuss with discharge teaching. For each category, provide at least one specific example.

2. What methods will you use to help ensure success of your teaching plan?

■ Multiple Choice

Circle the best answer.

1. A person diagnosed with AIDS would have a CD4 count of:
   a. less than 200
   b. 200 to 400
   c. 500
   d. 500 to 1,500

2. Which test is specific for the detection of HIV?
   a. ELISA
   b. Complete blood count
   c. Western blot
   d. Urinalysis

3. Which of the following are signs and symptoms of HIV that are often overlooked in women?
   a. Anorexia and weight loss
   b. Cervical cancer and recurrent vaginal candidiasis
   c. Diarrhea and general malaise
   d. Fever and persistent lymphadenopathy

4. A client is admitted to the hospital with a medical diagnosis of AIDS. When taking the client's history, which information would be most significant?
   a. Date of first exposure to HIV
   b. Family members also infected with HIV
   c. Sexual preference
   d. Signs and symptoms of opportunistic infections

5. The nurse knows that a client with AIDS susceptibility to infection is most likely related to:
   a. adherence to medication regime.
   b. CD4 counts.
   c. lifestyle.
   d. sexual partners.

6. A client was seen in the clinic for HIV testing and has returned to obtain the results of the test. The test is positive. In planning the client's care, which measure would be most essential?

   a. Date for follow-up appointment

   b. Financial resource information

   c. Knowledge of disease transmission

   d. Side effects of medications

7. A client is admitted to the unit with AIDS and a CD4 count of 150. Which nursing intervention would be the priority?

   a. Administer medications

   b. Obtain laboratory samples

   c. Orient to the unit

   d. Place in protective isolation

8. Which of the following statements by a client with AIDS indicates that further education is needed?

   a. "I can still clean out my cat's litter box."

   b. "I should not share my razor."

   c. "Protected sex does not guarantee that I won't transmit the disease."

   d. "Sharing bathroom facilities does not transmit the disease."

9. A client is admitted to the hospital with a diagnosis of *Pneumocystis carinii*. Which assessment data relates most closely with this diagnosis?

   a. Fever, weight loss, and diarrhea

   b. Headache, tremors, and chest pain

   c. SOB, fever, and cough

   d. Tremors, depression, and fever

10. A client is admitted to the hospital with a new diagnosis of AIDS dementia complex. Which nursing intervention would be most appropriate?

    a. Allow client to express his or her feelings.

    b. Assess neurologic status.

    c. Orient client to place, date, and time.

    d. Provide nutritional supplements between meals.

CHAPTER 85

Respiratory Disorders

■ Terminology Review

Match the following definitions with the correct terms and acronyms.

1. _____ puncturing of the chest wall to remove excess fluid or air from the pleural cavity

2. _____ inflammation of the nasal mucous membranes

3. _____ pulmonary function test; measures how much air a client inhales and exhales in one breath and assesses the client's general respiratory function

4. _____ inflammation of the pleura

5. _____ shortness of breath on exertion

6. _____ infectious disease caused by the tubercle bacillus, *Mycobacterium tuberculosis*

7. _____ abnormal, permanent enlargement of the alveoli and alveolar ducts with destruction of the alveolar walls

8. _____ partial pressure of oxygen; a measurement of the arterial blood gas

9. _____ stoppage of breathing and the asphyxia that results when breathing stops

10. _____ inflammation of one or more of the sinuses

11. _____ PPD appears to be negative because a person's body cannot respond appropriately to any antigen

12. _____ suffocation resulting from externally applied pressure to the throat

13. _____ inflammation of the lining of the bronchial airways in response to irritants and allergens

14. _____ plastic surgery of the nose for cosmetic reasons or to correct deformities resulting form injury

15. _____ adult respiratory distress syndrome

16. _____ nosebleed

17. _____ chest physiotherapy; uses position and gravity to drain secretions for lungs

18. _____ surgery to remove the entire larynx or tumorous part of the larynx

19. _____ invasive procedure in which a bronchoscope is passed through the mouth and pharynx and into the trachea and bronchi

20. _____ removal of an entire lung

21. _____ puncturing of a body cavity for aspiration of fluid

22. _____ procedure to provide an opening in the lower part of the anterior neck

23. _____ chronic obstructive pulmonary disease

24. _____ intermittent positive-pressure breathing

25. _____ within normal limits

26. _____ continuous positive airway pressure

27. _____ broad classification of disorders that includes bronchial asthma, bronchiectasis, chronic bronchitis, and pulmonary emphysema

28. _____ pyrazinamide that is used to treat tuberculosis

29. _____ partial pressure of carbon dioxide; a measurement of the arterial blood gas

30. _____ collapsed lung

31. _____ TB vaccine know as bacilli Calmette-Guérin

32. _____ condition in which the blood lacks oxygen and the blood and tissues contain excess carbon dioxide

33. _____ hemorrhage into the lung cavity

34. _____ uses position and gravity to drain secretions and mucus form the individual's lungs

35. _____ tuberculosis

36. _____ used to prevent atelectasis after surgery

37. _____ collection of air in the pleural cavity causing collapse of all or part of a lung

38. _____ *Pneumocystis carinii* pneumonia

39. _____ purified protein derivative; test that indicates whether a person has ever been exposed to tubercle bacillus

40. _____ collection of purulent exudate in the pleural cavity

41. _____ inflammation of the bronchial tubes

42. _____ shortness of breath, also called dyspnea

43. _____ inflammation of the lung with consolidation or solidification

44. _____ chest x-ray

45. _____ chronic dilation of the bronchi in which the walls become permanently distended

46. _____ removal of a lobe of a lung

47. _____ arterial blood gas

48. _____ medication used to treat tuberculosis that has few side effects

49. _____ person breathes abnormally fast or deeply

a. ABG
b. anergic
c. asphyxiation
d. ARDS
e. asthma
f. atelectasis
g. BCG
h. bronchiectasis
i. bronchitis
j. bronchoscopy
k. COLD
l. COPD
m. CPAP
n. CPT
o. CXR
p. empyema

q. epistaxis
r. hemothorax
s. hyperventilation
t. incentive spirometer
u. INH
v. IPPB
w. laryngectomy
x. lobectomy
y. $PaCO_2$
z. PaO_2
aa. PCP
bb. paracentesis
cc. PFT
dd. pleurisy
ee. pneumonia
ff. pneumonectomy
gg. pneumothorax
hh. postural drainage
ii. PPD
jj. pulmonary emphysema
kk. PZA
ll. rhinitis
mm. rhinoplasty
nn. sinusitis
oo. SOB
pp. SOBOE
qq. strangulation
rr. suffocation
ss. TB
tt. throracentesis
uu. tracheostomy
vv. tuberculosis
ww. WNL

■ Procedure Comparison

Fill in the following chart. Compare and contrast nursing care for the patient undergoing the following procedures.

Bronchoscopy	Thoracentesis	Thoracotomy
Before procedure	Before procedure	Before procedure
After procedure	After procedure	After procedure

1. What nursing care is common to all three before the procedures?

2. What nursing care is common to all three after the procedures?

■ Infectious Respiratory Disorders

In the figure below, identify the anatomic location and signs and symptoms of each of the following disorders: rhinitis, laryngitis, bronchitis, pneumonia, pleurisy, and streptococcal sore throat.

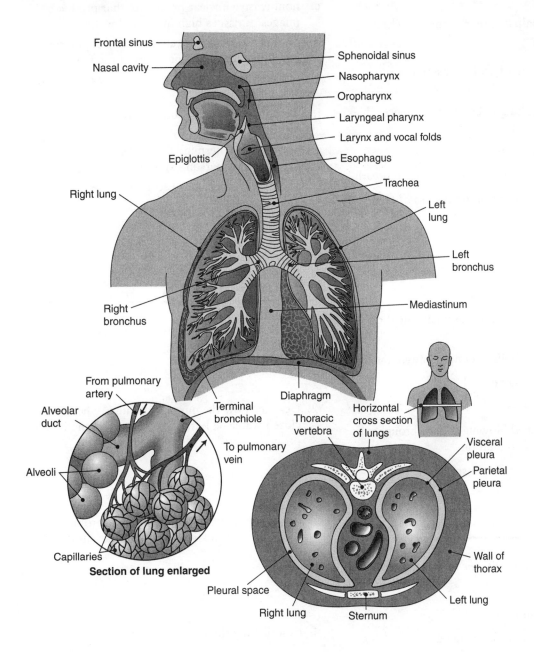

Frontal sinus
Nasal cavity
Sphenoidal sinus
Nasopharynx
Oropharynx
Laryngeal pharynx
Larynx and vocal folds
Epiglottis
Esophagus
Right lung
Trachea
Left lung
Left bronchus
Right bronchus
Mediastinum

From pulmonary artery
Alveolar duct
Terminal bronchiole
Diaphragm
Thoracic vertebra
Horizontal cross section of lungs
To pulmonary vein
Alveoli
Visceral pleura
Parietal pleura
Capillaries
Section of lung enlarged
Pleural space
Wall of thorax
Right lung
Sternum
Left lung

■ Assessment Review

Review Assessment of the Chest on pages 604 to 606. Indicate with an X which of the following assessment findings are abnormal.

_____ No complaints of pain when the chest is palpated

_____ Small mass palpated on the anterior chest

_____ Scoliosis

_____ Respiratory rate of 16 breaths/min, nonlabored

_____ Difficulty speaking in complete sentences due to SOB

_____ Barrel-shaped chest

_____ Chest rises and falls slightly with each breath

_____ Equal breath sounds on both sides of chest

_____ Cough

_____ Dyspnea

_____ Retractions

_____ Symmetric shape of chest

_____ High-pitched continuous musical sound on auscultation

_____ Low-pitched bubbling sound on auscultation

_____ Scapulae at the same level

_____ Relaxed breathing

_____ Low, soft-pitched blowing sound throughout lung fields on auscultation

_____ Expiration longer than inspiration

■ Matching

Match the diagnostic test with the correct definition or use.

1. _____ throat culture

2. _____ magnetic resonance imaging

3. _____ pulmonary function test

4. _____ lung perfusion scan

5. _____ arterial blood gas test

6. _____ PPD tuberculin test

7. _____ bronchoalveolar lavage

8. _____ throat culture

9. _____ sputum sample

a. measures how much a client inhales and exhales

b. determines relative amounts of arterial PaO_2, $PaCO_2$, and pH

c. noninvasive nuclear procedure that produces images of tissues high in fat and water

d. radioactive material lodges in lung capillaries and illustrates different views of the lungs

e. intradermal test used to determine exposure to TB

f. secretions that are incubated to determine the presence of organisms

g. test used to determine the presence of organisms or blood in a person's sputum

h. a sample of mucus and secretions are taken from the back of the throat

i. saline is pumped into a bronchus to obtain a sputum sample

■ Short Answers

1. List four reasons for having skin testing done.

2. Describe how the nurse determines whether a closed water-seal drainage system is functioning properly.

3. List nursing interventions that will promote respiration for a client who has had nasal surgery.

4. Describe the three types of tuberculosis.

5. Discuss nursing interventions to prevent the spread of tuberculosis.

6. What is sleep apnea?

7. How is sleep apnea treated?

8. Compare the symptoms, medical care, and nursing care for the following cancers.

   LARYNGEAL CANCER

   Signs and Symptoms

   Medical Care

   Nursing Care

   LUNG CANCER

   Signs and Symptoms

   Medical Care

   Nursing Care

9. What substances commonly cause allergic rhinitis?

10. Describe common causes of ARDS.

11. Describe three common causes of respiratory trauma and give an example of each.

12. Describe diagnostic methods used to differentiate between benign and malignant lung disorders.

13. List clients who would be at risk for epistaxis.

14. You arrive on the medical-surgical unit and are assigned to care for the following clients:

   • AJ is a 20-year-old man with a pneumothorax who complains of SOB.

   • PD is a 50-year-old woman who is 3 days post-op for a thoracotomy. She complains of pain with movement.

   • DK is a 77-year-old man with COPD who is requesting to speak to his doctor. He is resting comfortably.

   • TL is a 40-year-old woman with pneumonia and a temperature of 100.9°F. She was medicated with Tylenol 5 hours ago.

   How would you prioritize your nursing care? Give rationales for each action.

   NURSING CARE **RATIONALE**

■ Case Studies

For the following case studies, identify all abnormal assessment findings that pertain to the indicated diagnosis. Outline a teaching plan for each client.

CASE STUDY 1

Mrs. Wills is recovering from a thoracotomy for removal of a lung mass. She had surgery 3 days ago and was transferred from the surgical intensive care unit to the surgical unit. She ambulates to the bathroom with assistance but prefers to lie in bed. She complains of pain and states, "My chest hurts all the time, I can't take a breathe in." Your assessment reveals:

Mrs. Wills lying in bed with the HOB elevated.
Dressing over chest is dry and intact.
Chest tube is in place and connected to low continuous suction.
Oxygen is being delivered at 2 L/min per nasal cannula.
Skin is pink and moist.
Vital signs: T—98.8, R—24, P—88, B/P 128/70. You note that her respirations are shallow and irregular.
Client has mild retractions of the intercostal muscles.
Client raises her incentive spirometer to the 200 mL mark; her baseline was 750 mL.
ABGs were normal.
Client has morphine sulfate ordered for pain but does not request it often.

Nursing Diagnosis	Teaching Plan

Ineffective Breathing Pattern
  Subjective
 	
  Objective	

CASE STUDY 2

Mr. Appleton is a 77-year-old man who was admitted with an exacerbation of COPD yesterday. He is complaining of SOB at rest. He is in bed with the HOB elevated. Your assessment reveals that Mr. Appleton is changing position frequently, moving his legs and arms. He states, "Where is my dinner? I placed my order over an hour ago. It's hard to get service in this restaurant." You notice that he is able to only say a few words at time between breaths. His vital signs are: T—97, R—16, P—108, and B/P—150/80. He has a prolonged expiratory phase. His blood gases reveal a PaO_2 of -80. He uses Azmacort and Proventil inhalers at home but only when he needs them. He currently is receiving Decadron and aminophylline IV and is on Alupent nebulizer treatments every 4 hours.

Nursing Diagnosis	Teaching Plan

Ineffective Breathing Pattern
  Subjective
 	
  Objective	

■ Multiple Choice

Circle the best answer.

1. A client has just had a bronchoscopy. The nurse knows that the client is at risk for aspiration because the:
   a. ciliated cells have been damaged.
   b. client has just eaten.
   c. cough reflex is suppressed.
   d. lungs have been punctured.

Mrs. Powell is admitted to the medical unit with pneumonia. The next two questions relate to this scenario.

2. When you auscultate Mrs. Powell's lungs, you hear breath sounds that indicate the presence of fluid in the trachea and bronchi. You would document this as:
   a. coarse crackles.
   b. fine crackles.
   c. sonorous wheezing.
   d. wheezing.

3. Which one of the following describes the best technique for collecting a sputum specimen?
   a. Ask the client to cough up secretions from deep in the lungs.
   b. Collect saliva in a sterile culture tube.
   c. Swab the throat with a sterile cotton applicator.
   d. Wipe the inner mouth and tongue with a piece of gauze.

4. The physician orders *epinephrine 0.1 mg SQ now* for a client admitted with an allergic reaction. The medication available is in a 1:1,000 (1.0 mg/mL) solution. How much epinephrine would you administer?
   a. 0.1 mL
   b. 0.5 mL
   c. 1.0 mL
   d. 1.5 mL

This case study applies to the next four questions:

Mrs. Smith is a 43-year-old woman admitted to the medical unit with an acute asthma attack. Her vital signs are: T—98, R—28, P—102, and B/P—132/80.

She is currently sitting at the bedside, leaning on the bedside table. She has a weak productive cough.

5. When auscultating Mrs. Smith's lungs, which adventitious breath sound would you most like hear?
   a. Crackles
   b. Clear breath sounds
   c. Pleural friction rub
   d. Wheezing

6. Mrs. Smith's physician prescribes medication to treat her condition. Which asthma medication would not be appropriate for Mrs. Smith during this acute asthmas attack?
   a. albuterol by metered-dose inhaler
   b. aminophylline by oral or IV route
   c. cromolyn sodium by metered-dose inhaler
   d. corticosteroids by oral or IV route

7. Mrs. Smith becomes drowsy and lethargic, has diminished breath sounds, and is very quiet. Which of the following interventions would be your priority?
   a. Continue to monitor her respiratory status
   b. Encourage Mrs. Smith to rest
   c. Notify the RN and MD immediately
   d. Offer frequent oral fluids

8. After 2 days, Mrs. Smith's condition has improved and she is being discharged from the hospital. She has been prescribed two metered-dose inhalers; Proventil (bronchodialator) and Vanceril (glucocorticoid). Client teaching for use of the inhalers includes:
   a. use Proventil inhaler first and follow immediately with Vanceril.
   b. use Proventil inhaler first and wait 5 minutes; follow with Vanceril.
   c. use Vanceril first, wait 2 minutes, follow with Proventil.
   d. use Vanceril first, wait 5 minutes, follow with Proventil.

9. T.J. has emphysema and complains that he gets short of breath when performing his ADLs. The most appropriate intervention would be to:
   a. ensure bath water temperature is cool.
   b. increase oxygen to 6 L/min per nasal cannula while doing ADLs.

c. instruct T.J. to bathe only once a week.

d. teach T.J. to perform pursed-lip breathing before and during ADLs.

10. The nurse is assessing the respiratory pattern of Mr. Wallace, 75 years of age. When the nurse asks him to cough, he has difficulty. This most likely indicates:

   a. airway obstruction.

   b. crackles in both lungs.

   c. effects of aging.

   d. he has an infection in the lungs.

11. Your client has bronchiectasis. Which of the following would you include in your teaching plan?

   a. Avoid protein in the diet.

   b. Encourage client to stop smoking.

   c. Instruct client visit the physician only when very ill.

   d. Limit fluid intake to less than 1000 mL/d

12. Mr. Ling has just arrived on your unit with the diagnosis of active TB. Your priority nursing intervention would be to:

   a. administer prescribed medications.

   b. place client on airborne precautions.

   c. provide a diet high in protein and vitamins A and C.

   d. teach Mr. Ling about his disease.

13. Your client has sleep apnea syndrome. When completing your assessment, which data would you most likely find?

   a. Chronic cough

   b. Extreme tiredness all day

   c. Hoarse voice

   d. Runny nose

14. To prevent the spread of infection during naso-tracheal suctioning, the nurse should:

   a. flush the catheter between suctioning with normal saline.

   b. oxygenate the client before and after suctioning.

   c. wear sterile or clean gloves.

   d. withdraw the catheter with a rotating motion.

15. A client is diagnosed with tuberculosis. Which assessment findings would the nurse expect to see?

   a. Cough, gradual weight loss, nocturnal diaphoresis

   b. Flu symptoms, purulent drainage, weight gain

   c. High temperature, barrel chest, wheezing

   d. Sinus congestion, painful respirations, respiratory failure

16. What instructions would you give your client taking medications for tuberculosis?

   a. The medication must be inhaled deep into the lung.

   b. The medication will quickly cure the disease.

   c. The medication will need to be taken for a period of at least 6 months.

   d. You will need to check your pulse before taking the medication.

17. Which of the following assessment findings would be most consistent with the diagnosis of chronic bronchitis?

   a. Onset at age 40 years, peripheral edema, purulent sputum

   b. Onset at age 50 years, history of smoking, decreased breath sounds

   c. Onset at age 60 years, barrel chest, SOB

   d. Onset at age 70 years, "pink" appearance, SOB

18. A.L. was in an automobile accident and sustained blunt trauma to his chest. He has three fractured ribs and has difficulty breathing because of pain. His respirations are shallow and 26 per minute. The most immediate goal for A.L. is:

   a. client will ambulate without assistance.

   b. client will have respirations at less than 20 per minute with normal depth.

   c. client will state that he will attend driving school.

   d. client will verbalize the healing process of fractured ribs.

19. Assessment of lifestyle factors that can affect respiratory function should include:

    a. immunity to disease.

    b. marital status.

    c. number of children.

    d. smoking history.

20. Which of the following medication's action is to block the inflammatory biochemical pathway, making airways less sensitive to asthma triggers?

    a. metaproterenol (Alupent)

    b. montelukast (Singulair)

    c. salmeterol (Serevent)

    d. theophylline (Theo-Dur)

CHAPTER 86

Oxygen Therapy and Respiratory Care

■ Terminology Review

Match the following definitions with the correct terms and acronyms.

1. _____ taking oxygen into the body in concentrations higher than possible at normal atmospheric pressure because of a hyperbaric chamber

2. _____ intermittent positive-pressure breathing

3. _____ low-flow oxygen delivery system that has a bag attached

4. _____ effective and sanitary device used to provide high oxygen concentration for a client who is unable to breathe

5. _____ machine that forces air into the lungs

6. _____ chamber that simulates deep-sea diving, by increasing atmospheric pressure

7. _____ convenient monitor that measures the percentage of oxygen saturation in the blood

8. _____ another name for ventilator

9. _____ oxygen delivery system that has valves on the outside of the mask as well as valves between the mask and bag

10. _____ continuous positive airway pressure

11. _____ low-flow oxygen deliver system that fits over the client's nose, mouth, and chin

12. _____ adult respiratory distress syndrome

13. _____ chronic obstructive pulmonary disease

14. _____ high-flow oxygen delivery system that provides the most reliable and consistent oxygen enrichment

15. _____ per square inch

16. _____ liters per minute

17. _____ type of ventilation in which constant pressure is applied as the person inspires

18. _____ arterial blood gas

19. _____ tube inserted directly into a person's trachea as a lifesaving measure

20. _____ two short tubes that fit into each nostril to deliver low-flow oxygen

21. _____ type of ventilation that gives the client a preset number of mechanical breaths at a certain volume

a. ABG
b. ARDS
c. COPD
d. CPAP
e. HBO
f. hyperbaric
g. IPPB
h. LPM
i. manual breathing bag
j. nasal cannula
k. NRM
l. PRM
m. psi
n. PSV
o. pulse oximeter
p. respirator
q. simple mask
r. SIMV
s. tracheostomy
t. ventilator
u. Venturi mask

■ Correct the False Statements

Circle the word True *or* False *that follows the statement. If the word* false *has been circled, change the underlined word/words to make the statement true. Place your answer in the space provided.*

1. Therapeutic oxygen is necessary when a client is unable to obtain sufficient oxygen for the body's needs and <u>is always helpful</u>.

   True   False   _____

2. One goal of oxygen therapy is to <u>increase oxygen concentration</u> in the blood.

   True   False   _____

3. In the presence of oxygen, even a small spark can <u>ignite an explosion</u>.

   True   False   _____

4. Pulse oximeters <u>may be used</u> on fingernails with polish or fingernails with acrylic nails.

   True   False   _____

5. After inserting an adapter into an oxygen wall outlet, <u>you should check for oxygen leaks around the edges</u>.

   True   False   _____

6. A large oxygen cylinder has <u>a rectangular valve with no handle and three holes on one side</u>.

   True   False   _____

7. Cylinder oxygen tanks have a <u>regulator</u> to reduce pressure and a <u>flowmeter</u> to indicate oxygen flow.

   True   False   _____

8. <u>Oxygen strollers</u> are much safer and more convenient to use than oxygen tanks.

   True   False   _____

9. <u>Gowns and goggles</u> should always be worn when setting up oxygen therapy to prevent the transmission of disease.

   True   False   _____

10. <u>Volume ventilators</u> help support clients who are breathing on their own but are breathing inadequately.

    True   False   _____

■ Oxygen Table

Complete the following table on oxygen therapy.

Type of Therapy	Description	Concentration and Flow Rate	Use	Nursing Considerations
Nasal Cannula				
Simple Mask				
Partial rebreathing mask				

Continued

Oxygen Table (Continued)

Type of Therapy	Description	Concentration and Flow Rate	Use	Nursing Considerations
Non-rebreathing mask				
Venturi mask				

■ Multiple Choice

Circle the best answer.

1. A client is on oxygen therapy and the nurse notices a small amount of blood-tinged sputum. The most appropriate action would be to:
   a. elevate head of bed.
   b. encourage oral hygiene.
   c. monitor the sputum.
   d. report findings to RN or MD.

2. A client has oxygen administered through a partial rebreather. The bag completely deflates with each breath. The most appropriate nursing action would be to:
   a. change the oxygen delivery method.
   b. decrease the flow rate.
   c. increase the flow rate.
   d. notify the RN or MD.

3. When administering a medication that sedates a client, the nurse should assess for:
   a. decrease in respirations.
   b. increase in respirations.
   c. increase in sputum production.
   d. productive cough.

4. Which action is most appropriate when caring for a client on a ventilator in which the alarms sound and the nurse is unable to quickly identify the cause?
   a. Increase the oxygen to 100% through a nonrebreather mask.
   b. Notify the respiratory therapist.
   c. Suction the client.
   d. Support respirations with an Ambu bag.

5. Which assessment data relates most directly support a nursing diagnosis of Impaired Gas Exchange?
   a. Abnormal ABG
   b. Dyspnea
   c. Respiratory rate of 22 breaths/min
   d. Thick respiratory secretions

6. A client is being discharged to home on oxygen therapy. It is important for the nurse to instruct the family and client not to smoke around the oxygen because:
   a. oxygen can cause an explosive fire.
   b. oxygen would not work with smoke in the lungs.
   c. smoking causes lung cancer.
   d. smoking increases the risk for oxygen toxicity.

7. Which finding indicates that oxygen therapy is effective?
   a. Client breathes more easily, and pulse rate increases.
   b. Client breathes more easily and has decreased anxious attitude.
   c. Client's pulse rate increases, and client has decreased anxious attitude.
   d. Client's pulse rate decreases, and client remains anxious.

8. When performing tracheostomy care, which action would place the client at risk for injury?
   a. Assist to semi- or high-Fowler's position.
   b. Remove twill tapes prior to suctioning.
   c. Suction tracheostomy before removing inner cannula.
   d. Suction for no longer than 10-second intervals.

CHAPTER 87

Digestive Disorders

■ Terminology Review

Match the following definitions with the correct terms.

1. _____ inflamed appendix

2. _____ general ill health and malnutrition

3. _____ indigestion

4. _____ place where the two ends of the digestive system are joined together

5. _____ clenching the jaw or grinding the teeth

6. _____ motility disorder of the lower portions of the esophagus in which food cannot pass into the stomach

7. _____ liver is damaged and can no longer do its work; alcoholism is responsible for more than half of the cases

8. _____ accumulation of fluid in the peritoneal cavity

9. _____ tooth decay

10. _____ artificial opening of the colon for bowel elimination

11. _____ complication of gastrectomy in which immediate discomfort occurs when overeating or eating foods that are not recommended

12. _____ gallstones

13. _____ scars from previous surgeries

14. _____ condition in which inflammation occurs of outpouches along the intestinal wall

15. _____ examination of the colon with a special lighted instrument

a. achalasia

b. adhesions

c. anastomosis

d. appendicitis

e. ascites

f. bruxism

g. cachexia

h. caries

i. cholelithiasis

j. cirrhosis

k. colonoscopy

l. colostomy

m. diverticulitis

n. dumping syndrome

o. dyspepsia

Match the following definitions with the correct terms.

16. _____ inflammation of the stomach

17. _____ artificial opening of the ileum for bowel elimination

18. _____ occurs when abdominal muscle weakness causes a portion of the GI tract to protrude through muscle

19. _____ precancerous lesion that is a creamy white, nonsloughing patch on the mucous membranes

20. _____ inflammation of the liver

21. _____ procedure that visualizes the stomach and duodenum

22. _____ telescoping of the bowel

23. _____ black stool containing blood

24. _____ general term for the diseases of ulcerative colitis and Crohn's disease

25. _____ absence of intestinal peristalsis

26. _____ surgical removal of the stomach

27. _____ procedure that allows for the visualization of the esophagus

28. _____ swollen veins of the anus or rectum

29. _____ protrusion of abdominal contents out of the body through the suture line

30. _____ abnormal channeling between loops of bowel

a. esophagoscopy

b. evisceration

c. fistula

d. gastrectomy

e. gastritis

f. gastroscopy

g. hemorrhoids

h. hepatitis

i. hernia

j. ileostomy

k. inflammatory bowel disease

l. intussusception

m. leukoplakia buccalis

n. melena

o. paralytic ileus

Match the following definitions with the correct terms.

31. _____ inflammation of the serous membrane lining the walls of the pelvis and abdomen

32. _____ opening of the intestine through the abdominal wall

33. _____ removal of polyps during endoscopy

34. _____ inflammation of the gums and teeth

35. _____ twisting of the bowel

36. _____ painful abdominal cramps or spasms

37. _____ abdominal tap

38. _____ floating stools

39. _____ outpouching blood vessels

40. _____ closed fistula containing hair follicles; is located in the lower sacral or perineal area

41. _____ open sore in the skin or mucous membrane that is accompanied by sloughing of the inflamed and necrotic tissue

a. paracentesis

b. peritonitis

c. pilonidal cyst

d. polypectomy

e. pyorrhea

f. steatorrhea

g. stoma

h. tenesmus

i. ulcer

j. varices

k. volvulus

■ Sequencing

Number the following actions in the correct order for irrigating a nasogastric tube. The first action should be number 1. Continue to number the items.

_____ Put on gloves.

_____ Disconnect the nasogastric tube from suction and check placement.

_____ Reconnect the tube to suction as ordered.

_____ Dispose of glove, wash your hands, and properly dispose of equipment.

_____ Wash your hands, follow clean technique.

_____ Note amount, color, and consistency of any drainage.

_____ Document the procedure, noting the time, description of the drainage, and relevant client reactions.

_____ Slowly introduce the solution using the specified irrigating syringe.

_____ Pour the ordered solution into the irrigation bottle.

_____ Assemble the appropriate equipment and solutions at the client's bedside.

■ Correct the False Statements

Circle the word True *or* False *that follows the statement. If the word* false *has been circled, change the underlined word/words to make the statement true. Place your answer in the space provided.*

1. <u>Histamine receptor antagonists</u> reduce gastric acid secretions.

   True   False   _____

2. <u>Abdominal infection and hemorrhage</u> are serious complications of ulcers.

   True   False   _____

3. Most clients tolerate drinking GoLYTELY if it is first <u>warmed</u>.

   True   False   _____

4. Before a colonoscopy, the client should avoid <u>aspirin, ibuprofen, and anticoagulants for 5 to 7 days</u>.

   True   False   _____

5. During periods of abdominal pain associated with diverticulits, the client should eat a <u>fiber-rich diet</u>.

   True   False   _____

6. Obstructions of the <u>small bowel</u> tend to progress slowly.

   True   False   _____

7. Colon cancer is often treated with <u>5-fluorouracil, leucovorin, and interferon</u>.

   True   False   _____

8. Immediately after surgery, the stoma may be <u>swollen and bleed profusely</u>.

   True   False   _____

9. <u>Jaundice</u> results from an excessive concentration of bile salts in the bloodstream.

   True   False   _____

10. Vitamin K is usually given to clients with cirrhosis to prevent <u>muscle wasting</u>.

    True   False

11. <u>Hepatitis A and hepatitis E</u> are spread by the fecal-oral route.

    True   False   _____

12. Only individuals infected with HBV can contract <u>hepatitis D</u>.

    True   False   _____

13. The liver is <u>often</u> a site of primary cancer and <u>rarely</u> a site of metastasis.

    True   False   _____

14. Cholecystectomy is often done using <u>laparoscopy</u>.

    True   False   _____

15. Encourage rectal screening tests for clients <u>older than 40 years of age and those who are at risk</u>.

    True   False   _____

▪ Multiple Choice

Circle the best answer.

1. To verify a tube's placement in the stomach, the nurse should:
   a. aspirate all of the stomach contents into a syringe.
   b. gently pull the tube out and advance it back into place.
   c. inject a small amount of air while auscultating over the stomach.
   d. push 40 to 50 mL of water down the tube.

2. After oral surgery, which of the following is contraindicated?
   a. Coughing
   b. Deep breathing
   c. Elevated head of bed
   d. Use of incentive spirometer

3. Antacid preparations that contain aluminum hydroxide, such as Amphojel, may cause:
   a. acid reflux.
   b. constipation.
   c. diarrhea.
   d. vomiting.

4. The action of sucralfate (Carafate) is to:
   a. enhance gastric mucosal defenses.
   b. inhibit the secretion of gastric acid.
   c. provide a protective mucous coating to the lining of the stomach.
   d. reduce inflammation of the stomach lining.

5. After a gastrectomy, the nurse instructs the client that he or she must receive which of the following for life?

   a. Vitamin B_{12}

   b. Vitamin C

   c. Vitamin D

   d. Vitamin K

6. After any bowel surgery, a client should follow a low-fiber diet for approximately:

   a. 1 day.

   b. 1 week.

   c. 1 month.

   d. 3 months.

7. After a liver biopsy, the nurse should monitor closely for:

   a. bleeding.

   b. pain.

   c. vomiting.

   d. unconsciousness.

8. When monitoring for the effectiveness of lactulose (Cephulac), the nurse should assess for:

   a. absence of bleeding.

   b. absence of abdominal pain.

   c. decreased itching.

   d. decreasing ammonia levels.

9. Which nursing action should be performed when a client is receiving TPN?

   a. Administer the infusion intermittently.

   b. Change dressing only when it becomes bloody.

   c. Encourage oral liquids.

   d. Monitor blood glucose levels.

10. To enhance bowel movements in older adults, the nurse should:

    a. administer daily stool softeners.

    b. encourage regular use of laxative.

    c. order thickened liquid diets.

    d. promote water loss.

11. The nurse instructs the client taking steroids to:

    a. discontinue medication if symptoms improve.

    b. never abruptly stop taking the medication.

    c. stop taking the medication if client develops muscle aches.

    d. take the medication on an empty stomach.

CHAPTER 88

Urinary Disorders

■ Terminology Review

Match the following definitions with the correct terms.

1. _____ inflammation of the urinary bladder

2. _____ process that assumes the work of damaged, nonfunctioning kidneys

3. _____ crushing of stones

4. _____ painful urination

5. _____ urine forms, but its flow from the kidney is obstructed

6. _____ stones

7. _____ x-ray of the bladder and urethra made possible by instillation of dye directly in the bladder through a catheter

8. _____ urine output of less than 100 mL/d

9. _____ exercises used to manage incontinence by strengthening the perineal muscles

10. _____ group of diseases in which the kidneys are damaged and partly destroyed by inflammation of the glomeruli

11. _____ epithelial, fatty, or waxy material abnormally forced out of the renal tubules

12. _____ formation of stones

13. _____ normal condition in aging men in which the prostate continues to grow and narrow the urethra

14. _____ blood in the urine

15. _____ application of firm, gentle pressure to the bladder to help drain the bladder of urine

a. anuria
b. benign prostatic hypertrophy
c. calculi
d. casts
e. Credé maneuver
f. cystitis
g. cystogram
h. dialysis
i. dysuria
j. glomerulonephritis
k. hematuria
l. hydronephrosis
m. Kegel exercises
n. lithiasis
o. lithotripsy

Match the following definitions with the correct terms.

16. _____ kidneys lose ability to adapt to varying intakes of foods and fluids

17. _____ urine output of less than 400 mL per 24 hours

18. _____ inflammation of the kidney and renal pelvis

19. _____ amount of urine obtained from a straight catheterization immediately after a client has voided

20. _____ device inserted into blood vessels to facilitate repeated dialysis

21. _____ cancer of the kidney

22. _____ urine that stays in the bladder

23. _____ device that is inserted into the vagina to support the organs of the pelvis

24. _____ type of congenital or acquired disease that causes true or total incontinence

25. _____ hollow tube

26. _____ pus in the urine

27. _____ inability to empty the bladder completely

28. _____ removal of the kidney

29. _____ due to bladder instability as a result of upper motor lesions or neuropathies

30. _____ narrowing

a. nephrectomy
b. nephroma
c. neurogenic
d. oliguria
e. pessary
f. pyelonephritis
g. pyuria
h. reflex incontinence
i. renal failure
j. residual urine volume
k. retention
l. shunt
m. stasis
n. stent
o. stricture

Match the following definitions with the correct terms and acronyms.

31. _____ benign prostatic hyperplasia

32. _____ end-stage renal disease

33. _____ clients experience urgency before voiding that is caused by bladder spasm

34. _____ urinary leakage that is nearly continuous

35. _____ transurethral resection of a bladder tumor

36. _____ catheter inserted by a physician directly into the bladder through the abdomen

37. _____ continuous ambulatory peritoneal dialysis

38. _____ blood urea nitrogen

a. suprapubic
b. symphysis pubis
c. total incontinence
d. urge incontinence
e. BPH
f. BUN
g. CAPD
h. ESRD
i. TURPT

■ Diagnostic Comparison Chart

Complete the following chart.

Diagnostic Test	Description of Test	Nursing Care Before Test	Nursing Care After Test
Intravenous pyelogram			
Cytoscopy			
Needle biopsy			

■ Assessment Review

Indicate whether the following are normal (N) findings or abnormal (A) findings.

1. _____ nausea and vomiting
2. _____ flank discomfort
3. _____ 98.9°F
4. _____ Urinalysis with no WBCs
5. _____ casts
6. _____ heavy feeling in abdomen
7. _____ yellow-tinged urine
8. _____ nighttime voiding
9. _____ intake = output
10. _____ colic
11. _____ painless hematuria
12. _____ urine output of 400 mL per 24 hours

■ Short Answers

1. Explain why a culture and sensitivity are usually ordered together.

2. Provide the rationales for the following general nursing procedures when caring for a client with a urologic problem.

   a. Assess and provide attention to skin and mouth care.

   b. Measure weight daily.

   c. Monitor fluid intake and fluid restrictions.

   d. Encourage fluid intake (if not contraindicated).

   e. Encourage movement and activity.

3. Which medications are most effective at treating incontinence?

4. Describe nursing care after an ESWL.

5. Describe the purposes of dialysis.

6. Explain the difference between peritoneal dialysis and hemodialysis.

7. Identify at least three medications that may cause possible renal damage.

8. Describe two signs that indicate proper functioning of a cannula or fistula used for hemodialysis.

■ Correct the False Statements

Circle the word True *or* False *that follows the statement. If the word* false *has been circled, change the underlined word/words to make the statement true. Place your answer in the space provided.*

1. The <u>BUN</u> is the one of the most valuable tests to identify early kidney disease and is useful in following the renal function of clients with known kidney disease.

   True   False   _____

2. The <u>blood chemistry</u> determines how efficiently the glomeruli remove nitrogenous wastes from protein metabolism.

   True   False   _____

3. True incontinence occurs with a nearly continuous leakage of urine

   True   False   _____

4. Clients with reflex incontinence <u>can</u> usually stop their urinary stream once it starts.

   True   False   _____

5. Stress incontinence is usually treated with <u>Kegal exercises</u>.

   True   False   _____

6. <u>Men</u> are more susceptible to urinary tract infections than <u>women</u> because of the length of the urethra.

   True   False   _____

7. Signs of acute glomerulonephritis appear approximately <u>2 to 3 months</u> after an upper respiratory infection or scarlet fever.

   True   False   _____

8. A client usually experiences <u>urgency, frequency, pain, and bacteria-free urine</u> with interstitial cystitis.

   True   False   _____

9. <u>Urgency, frequency, and nocturia</u> are classic signs of BPH.

   True   False   _____

10. Kidney tumors are almost <u>always benign</u>.

    True   False   _____

11. Bladder removal for men is often associated with <u>permanent sexual dysfunction</u>.

    True   False   _____

12. A <u>Kock pouch</u> is the most commonly used method for excretion of urine after bladder removal.

    True   False   _____

13. In all types of <u>dialysis</u>, monitor and document the client's vital signs, daily weight, and level of consciousness.

    True   False   _____

14. The goal of Kegal exercises is to work up to <u>three to four sets of 10 squeezes held for 10 seconds each</u>.

    True   False   _____

15. Clients receiving dialysis <u>usually do not void</u>.

    True   False   _____

■ Multiple Choice

Circle the best answer.

1. Before the client undergoes intravenous pyelogram, the nurse must first:
   a. ask the client if he or she is allergic to iodine of shellfish.
   b. encourage fluids before the exam to ensure hydration.
   c. keep the client on a clear liquid diet for 3 days.
   d. prep the area on the back over the kidneys.

2. Transient incontinence usually resolves:

   a. once the precipitating cause is treated.

   b. spontaneously with time.

   c. with psychological counseling.

   d. with surgery.

3. The nurse should instruct a client taking phenaz-ophridine hydrochloride (Pyridium) that:

   a. fluids should be restricted to water while taking this medication.

   b. frequency is a common side effect.

   c. pain is normal with urination.

   d. urine may appear orange-red in color.

4. The most common site for urinary system cancer is the:

   a. bladder.

   b. kidney.

   c. urethra.

   d. ureters.

5. Which of the following are risk factors for the development of bladder cancer?

   a. Bladder infections and incontinence

   b. Cigarette smoking and occupational exposure to chemicals

   c. Lung cancer and bladder infections

   d. Urgency and frequency

6. In older adults, the only presenting sign of a urinary tract infection may be:

   a. fever.

   b. change in bladder habits.

   c. mental status change.

   d. pain during urination.

CHAPTER 89

Male Reproductive Disorders

■ Terminology Review

Match the following definitions with the correct terms and acronyms.

1. _____ abnormal dilation of the testicular veins in the scrotum

2. _____ surgical fixation of the testes

3. _____ stitching of folds or tucks in the hydocele wall to reduce its size

4. _____ inability to achieve or maintain an erection sufficient to complete sexual intercourse

5. _____ inflammation of the epididymis

6. _____ inflammation of the testes

7. _____ foreskin becomes so tight that it will not retract over the glans penis

8. _____ inflammation of the prostate gland

9. _____ urethral meatus located on the underside of the penis

10. _____ chronic bacterial prostatitis

11. _____ blood test that detects a glycoprotein that is found only in the prostate gland

12. _____ acute bacterial prostatitis

13. _____ enlargement

14. _____ benign prostatic hyperplasia

15. _____ prostate-specific antigen

16. _____ difficulty starting the urine stream

17. _____ testicles have not descended into their normal position in the scrotum

18. _____ accumulation of fluid in the space between the membrane covering the testicle and the testicle itself

19. _____ transurethral resection of the prostate

20. _____ used to evaluate the client to determine whether he is having nighttime erections

21. _____ removal of the excess or abnormal prostate tissue

22. _____ abnormal or persistent penile erection without sexual stimulation

23. _____ testicular self-examination

24. _____ more common type of testicular cancer

25. _____ urethral meatus located on the upper surface of the penis

26. _____ type of testicular cancer in which orchiectomy and retroperitoneal lymph node dissection are commonly performed

27. _____ erectile dysfunction

28. _____ examination that should be taught to all males starting at age 13 to 14 years

a. cryptorchidism
b. epididymitis
c. epispadias
d. hesitancy
e. hydrocele
f. hyperplasia
g. hypospadias
h. erectile dysfunction
i. nonseminoma
j. orchiopexy
k. orchitis
l. phimosis
m. plication
n. priapism
o. prostatectomy
p. prostate-specific antigen
q. prostatitis
r. seminoma

s. testicular self-examination

t. varicocele

u. ABP

v. BPH

w. CBP

x. ED

y. NPT

z. PSA

aa. TSE

bb. TURP

■ Assessment Review

For the following assessment data, indicate whether the finding is a normal assessment finding (N) or an abnormal assessment finding (A). Abnormal findings can be indicative of male reproductive disorders.

1. _____ impotent

2. _____ pubic hair is in diamond-shaped pattern

3. _____ penis is curved when erect

4. _____ complaints of scrotal fullness

5. _____ scrotal skin is loose

6. _____ pain with urination

7. _____ dribbling after voiding

8. _____ testes are slightly moveable within the scrotum

9. _____ hesitancy

10. _____ foreskin retracts fully

11. _____ blood-tinged urine

12. _____ testes are egg shaped and firm

13. _____ decrease in urinary stream

14. _____ urinary catheter

15. _____ PSA level of zero

16. _____ normal libido

17. _____ organism with sexual intercourse

18. _____ cordlike structure on the top and back of the testicle

19. _____ urgency

20. _____ fever

■ Short Answer

Complete the following questions.

1. State the difference between a PSA and free prostate-specific antigen.

2. When would a physician order a prostatic biopsy?

3. Outline teaching for a client who has just been prescribed Viagra to treat erectile dysfunction.

4. Identify medications that can cause priapism.

5. Identify the signs of symptoms of each of the following disorders:

   a. Peyronie's disease

   b. Torsion of the spermatic cord

   c. Varicocele

   d. Hydocele

6. Describe teaching regarding antibiotic therapy for a client with acute bacterial prostatitis.

7. Briefly describe the following types of surgery to remove the prostate.

   a. Suprapubic prostatectomy

   b. Perineal prostatectomy

   c. Nerve-sparing radical prostatectomy

   d. Radical prostatectomy

   e. Cryosurgery

8. Indicate whether the following clients would be at risk for prostate, testicular, or penile cancer.

   a. Age 25

   b. African American

   c. Poor hygiene

   d. Not sexually active

   e. Diet high in animal fat

■ Case Studies

Complete the following questions with the most appropriate answer.

1. Joe is a 22-year-old client who presents to the clinic with complaints of a lump on his left testicle. The lump is nontender and is smaller than the size of a pea.

   a. What additmional assessment data would you obtain?

   b. Joe is scheduled to have an ultrasound of the scrotum completed. What teaching should be done before the examination?

   c. The ultrasound reveals a solid mass, and Joe is scheduled for surgery. What preoperative teaching will you provide?

   d. What nursing diagnoses will be of concern for Joe postoperatively?

2. Mr. Smith is a 60-year-old man who presents to the clinic with complaints of difficulty starting the urine stream.

   a. The physician suspects benign prostatic hyperplasia. What diagnostic exams would you expect the physician to order and why?

   b. Mr. Smith asks you if he is going to die because he is worried that he has cancer. How would you respond?

■ Multiple Choice

Circle the best answer.

1. Which laboratory test should be completed annually on all men beginning at age 50 years?
   a. Free prostate-specific antigen
   b. Prostate-specific antigen
   c. Testosterone level
   d. Urinalysis

2. An 18-year-old male client is admitted to the hospital with torsion of the spermatic cord. Which of the following would be your priority nursing intervention?
   a. Discuss client's sexual history.
   b. Medicate with oral pain medications.
   c. Monitor intake and output.
   d. Prepare client for surgery.

3. Which of the following nursing interventions would be appropriate for the client with a hydrocele?
   a. Apply warm packs to the scrotum.
   b. Inform the client that he will be sterile.
   c. Provide a scrotal support.
   d. Provide continuous bladder irrigation.

4. A client had a TURP yesterday and is on continuous bladder irrigation. The client complains of flank pain. The most appropriate action would be to:
   a. medicate with Demerol.
   b. place client in a supine position.
   c. reduce the rate of the irrigation.
   d. shut off the irrigation and notify RN.

5. Contributing factors for erectile dysfunction include:
   a. diabetes mellitus.
   b. elective sterilization.
   c. emphysema.
   d. urinary frequency.

6. A client is scheduled for a nerve-sparing radical prostatectomy. The nurse knows this procedure causes less:
   a. erectile dysfunction.
   b. postoperative pain.
   c. respiratory complications.
   d. time needed for postoperative catheter.

7. The nurse understands that the most important use of the continuous bladder irrigation is to:
   a. assist the client to void.
   b. keep the catheter from being occluded with blood clots.
   c. maintain production of urine until healing can occur.
   d. stop bleeding in the bladder.

8. A male client who was treated for prostate cancer is being discharged on GnRH analog (Lupron). It is most important that the nurse include a referral:
   a. for follow-up testosterone levels.
   b. for radiation therapy.
   c. to a dietitian for nutritional counseling.
   d. to physical therapy for exercise training.

9. At which age should males be instructed to start performing self-testicular examinations?
   a. before 10 years
   b. 13 to 14 years
   c. 20 to 25 years
   d. after 30 years

10. A client is on continuous bladder irrigations. The client had a total of 500 mL of irrigation solution instilled and a total of 1,000 mL of output during your shift. How much urine output will you document?
    a. 500 mL
    b. 1,000 mL
    c. 1,500 mL
    d. 2,000 mL

CHAPTER 90

Female Reproductive Disorders

■ Terminology Review

Match the following definitions with the correct terms and acronyms.

1. _____ excessive menstrual flow

2. _____ uterus that sags or herniates in the vagina or even can fall outside the vagina

3. _____ inflammation of the vulva

4. _____ loop electrosurgical excision procedure

5. _____ inflammation of the vagina

6. _____ surgical removal of a breast

7. _____ whitish vaginal discharge

8. _____ test used to detect cervical cancer

9. _____ toxic shock syndrome

10. _____ upward displacement of the rectum toward the vaginal orifice

11. _____ absence of or abnormal stoppage of menses

12. _____ x-ray examination of the breasts used to detect breast cancer

13. _____ inflammation of the cervix

14. _____ tissue resembling endometrial tissue appears in various places in the pelvic cavity

15. _____ procedure in which the surgeon removes a cone-shaped piece of cervix for examination

16. _____ painful sexual intercourse

17. _____ infection of the ovaries, oviducts, uterus, or pelvic cavity

18. _____ direct visualization of the uterus and accessory organs under general or spinal anesthesia

19. _____ medical specialty that focuses on the female reproductive system

20. _____ painful menstruation

21. _____ lymph node that drains the area of the breast involved by tumor

22. _____ dilation and curettage

23. _____ American Cancer Society

24. _____ human papillomavirus

25. _____ direct visualization of the uterus, oviducts, broad ligaments, colon and small intestine by passing an instrument through the vaginal wall behind the cervix

26. _____ plastic surgery revision of the breast

27. _____ National Institutes of Health

28. _____ bacterial infection associated with the use of tampons

29. _____ time when a female's reproductive system becomes fully functional

30. _____ downward displacement of the bladder toward the vaginal orifice

31. _____ obstetrician/gynecologist

32. _____ onset of menstruation

33. _____ premenstrual syndrome

34. _____ breast pain

35. _____ bleeding between menses

36. _____ National Cancer Institute

37. _____ most frequently preformed gynecologic surgery in which the cervix is dilated and endometrial lining is scraped out

38. _____ hormone replacement therapy

39. _____ anteroposterior

40. _____ surgical removal of the uterus

41. _____ sexually transmitted disease

a. amenorrhea

b. cervicitis

c. conization

d. culdoscopy

e. cystocele

f. dilation and curettage

g. dyspareunia

h. dysmenorrhea

i. endometriosis

j. gynecology

k. hysterectomy

l. laparoscopy

m. leucorrhea

n. mammography

o. mammoplasty

p. mastalgia

q. mastectomy

r. menarche

s. menorrhagia

t. metorrhagia

u. Pap test

v. prolapse

w. puberty

x. rectocele

y. sentinel lymph node

z. toxic shock syndrome

aa. vaginitis

bb. vulvitis

cc. ACS

dd. AP

ee. D & C

ff. HPV

gg. HRT

hh. LEEP

ii. NCI

jj. NIH

kk. OB/GYN

ll. PID

mm. PMS

nn. STD

oo. TSS

■ Assessment Review

Indicate whether each of the following assessment findings is a normal (N) finding or an abnormal (A) finding for an adult female.

1. _____ no breast tenderness

2. _____ fever of 102°F

3. _____ negative Pap test

4. _____ women in menopause with vaginal dryness

5. _____ bleeding between menses

6. _____ vesicovaginal fistula

7. _____ performs breast self-examination every month

8. _____ history of a hysterectomy

9. _____ stress incontinence

10. _____ no pain during menstruation

11. _____ vaginal itching

12. _____ heaviness in the pelvic region

13. _____ clumpy white vaginal discharge

14. _____ 60-year-old woman with no menstrual cycle

15. _____ backache

16. _____ reddened vulva

17. _____ malodorous vaginal discharge

18. _____ areola is darker than the breast

19. _____ breast tenderness around the time of menses

20. _____ retraction of one breast nipple

■ Diagnostic Test Review

Complete the following chart.

Diagnostic Test	Description of Test	Nursing Care Before Test	Nursing Care After Test
Laparoscopy			
Culdoscopy			
Colposcopy			
Cervical biopsy			
Conization			

What nursing care is common to all procedures before the test?

What nursing care is common to all procedures after the test?

■ Case Studies

Complete the following questions.

1. Your patient assignment consists of the following four clients:
   - Client who has just returned from having a hysterectomy
   - New admission with diagnosis of PID
   - Preoperative client for lumpectomy
   - Client to be discharged who had a tubal ligation

   a. Indicate the order in which you would assess these clients and provide rationale.

   b. What would you assess with each client?

2. Mrs. Toddy has had a vaginal hysterectomy. She has an IV of 1,000 mL of D5RL infusing at 125 mL/hour, indwelling urinary catheter to bedside drainage, vaginal packing in place, and PCA pump infusing with morphine sulfate for pain

control and is NPO. Her VS are stable, and she has minimal bloody vaginal drainage.

a. What postoperative complications is this client at risk for?

b. The client complains of severe back pain. What actions would you take?

3. Lillie is a 25-year-old woman with recurrent vaginal infections. Outline a teaching plan to assist her.

■ Multiple Choice

Circle the best answer.

1. A 40-year-old client has had a panhysterosal pingo-oophorectomy. Which statement indicates the client understands this surgery?

a. "I am too young to have to worry about menopause symptoms."

b. "I will continue to have a menstrual period."

c. "I will have hot flashes due to surgically induced menopause."

d. "I won't have hot flashes after surgery."

2. A client is scheduled for a laparoscopy. The client asks if she will have pain after the procedure. The nurse's best response would be:

a. "Don't worry about that until later."

b. "This procedure is usually painless."

c. "You may have some severe pain in the vaginal area."

d. "You will probably have some shoulder pain."

3. A client has chronic cystic mastitis. Which instructions should the nurse include in the teaching plan?

a. Avoid excessive exercise

b. Instruct client to have biannual mammograms

c. Limit caffeine in the diet

d. Tell client to direct all questions to the physician

4. Which instructions should be provided to a mastectomy client?

a. Continue to assess the chest wall and scar area as well as the remaining breast.

b. Follow-up with a physician for examination of the remaining breast only.

c. No further breast self-examinations are needed.

d. Perform breast self-examination only on the remaining breast.

5. When a client is being discharged from the hospital with a mastectomy, it is most important that the nurse include a referral to:

a. a dietitian.

b. physical therapy.

c. Reach to Recovery.

d. Volunteers of America.

6. A client had a mastectomy and states, "I'm afraid my husband won't be able to look at me." Which nursing diagnosis would be most appropriate?

a. Altered Urinary Elimination

b. Altered Sexuality Patterns

c. Body Image Disturbance

d. Impaired Tissue Integrity

7. Which of the following medications would be used to treat endometriosis?

a. diazepam (Valium)

b. leuprolide (Lupron)

c. metronidazole (Flagyl)

d. paclitaxel (Taxol)

8. Which of the following is a correct technique for performing breast self-examination?

a. Lie flat on your back and use the opposite to hand to palpate each breast.

b. Palpate the axillae keeping the fingers flat.

c. Use a left-to-right motion when palpating the breast.

d. Use the tips of the fingers to palpate the breast.

CHAPTER 91

Gerontology: The Aging Adult

■ Terminology Review

Match the following definitions with the correct terms.

1. _____ bad breath

2. _____ without teeth

3. _____ emotional, physical, and sexual abuse, financial exploitation, or neglect of older people

4. _____ choking

5. _____ inability to use or understand speech

6. _____ branch of medicine concerned with problems and illnesses of aging and their treatment

7. _____ medications given to control behavior

8. _____ easily broken

9. _____ study of the effects of normal aging and age-related disease on the human

10. _____ exhaustion and frustration of daily obligations related to the care of an older person

a. aphasia
b. aspiration
c. caregiver stress
d. chemical restraint
e. edentulous
f. elder abuse
g. friable
h. geriatrics
i. gerontology
j. halitosis

Match the following definitions with the correct terms and acronym.

11. _____ specific hearing disorder of aging

12. _____ long-term care

13. _____ awareness of posture, movement, and changes in equilibrium in relation to other objects

14. _____ temporary relief and rest for caretakers

15. _____ many older people are considered this

16. _____ condition in depressed clients in which they give the impression of being demented and their behaviors actually are related to depression

17. _____ curvature of the spine that causes a hump-backed appearance

18. _____ facial hair

19. _____ autoimmune disease that includes dry eyes as a symptom

20. _____ anything that limits the client's free movement

21. _____ impaired vision that results from normal aging

a. hirsutism
b. kyphosis
c. presbycusis
d. presbyopia
e. proprioception
f. pseudodementia
g. respite
h. restraints
i. Sjögren's syndrome
j. vulnerable adult
k. LTC

■ Assessment Review

Indicate if the following findings are normal (N) or abnormal (A) for the older adult.

1. _____ stiff joints

2. _____ paranoia

3. _____ unsteady gait when walking

4. _____ incontinence

5. _____ presbycusis

6. _____ diarrhea

7. _____ increased total body fluid

8. _____ slower recovery from illness

9. _____ depression

10. _____ malnutrition

11. _____ decreased reaction time

12. _____ poor grooming

13. _____ excessive fear

14. _____ difficulty swallowing medications owing to dry oral mucosa

15. _____ decreased sense of balance

16. _____ donating large amounts of money

■ Correct the False Statements

Circle the word True *or* False *that follows the statement. If the word* false *has been circled, change the underlined word/words to make the statement true. Place your answer in the space provided.*

1. <u>Acute illnesses</u> are more common for older adults than for the rest of the population.

   True   False   _____

2. <u>Retirement complexes</u> offer older adults freedom and privacy while providing conveniences, security, and services.

   True   False   _____

3. A high-quality skilled long-term care facility has licensed nurses available <u>24 hours a day, 5 days a week</u>.

   True   False   _____

4. Protein requirements for older adults should be <u>5 grams of protein for each kilogram of body weight</u>.

   True   False   _____

5. A <u>chopped or pureed</u> diet is appropriate for an edentulous client.

   True   False   _____

6. <u>Daily bathing is not</u> necessary for all older adults.

   True   False   _____

7. Nails on older adults should be trimmed <u>in a curved manner that follows the shape of the finger</u>.

   True   False   _____

8. Older men often have difficulty voiding owing to <u>difficulty ambulating to the bathroom</u>.

   True   False   _____

9. Encouraging the older adult to keep mentally active can help prevent <u>feelings of boredom and depression</u>.

   True   False   _____

10. Relatives may thing an older adult is just confused, when he or she may be <u>under the influence of alcohol</u>.

    True   False   _____

■ Multiple Choice

Circle the best answer.

1. Which of the following phrases might an aging client with presbycusis have difficulty hearing?

   a. Don't add milk to the drug and don't drink milk until an hour after taking it.

   b. Mix the medication with water in a cup and drink it all.

   c. Never mix the two antibiotics unless the doctor tells you to.

   d. Shake the solution first, and then evenly pour it into two equal doses.

2. Which of the following would be an appropriate action for a client with Sjögren's syndrome?

   a. Asking the doctor to provide a prescription for artificial tears

   b. Instructing the client to rub eyes during the day to stimulate secretion of tears

   c. Limiting the client's fluid intake and intake of foods high in salt

   d. Suggesting the client wear glasses to decrease drying of eyes

3. Clients with presbyopia:

   a. may need speech therapy to resolve communication problems.

   b. may notice difficulty reading with bright light in the room.

   c. read better with bifocals to allow for far and near vision.

   d. require an antibiotic to cure the infection in each eye.

4. To prevent duplication of medications, older adults should be instructed to:

   a. not take pills that look alike.

   b. keep all medications in a cupboard.

   c. learn the generic and brand name of all medications.

   d. use a single pharmacy for all prescriptions.

5. What percentage of adverse drug reactions occurs in people older than 65 years?

   a. 25%

   b. 40%

   c. 50%

   d. 75%

CHAPTER 92

Dementias and Related Disorders

■ Terminology Review

Match the following definitions with the correct terms.

1. _____ fearfulness

2. _____ another name for dementia

3. _____ allows caregivers some time to themselves by having others care for clients on a short-term basis

4. _____ impairment of mental function; means poor judgment, impaired memory, and disorientation to person, place, situation, or time

5. _____ refusing to do things

6. _____ when clients with dementia become overly agitated when confronted with situations that are too overwhelming or difficult for them

7. _____ another name for dementia or senility

8. _____ has a sudden onset and is usually reversible

9. _____ debilitating confusion created when the client is physically present but psychologically absent

10. _____ chronic, irreversible condition that affects cognitive function

11. _____ problems carrying out purposeful movements

12. _____ condition in which a client has the appearance of dementia but whose confusion results from depression

13. _____ fabricating details of events

a. ambiguous loss
b. apraxia
c. balking
d. catastrophic reaction
e. confabulation
f. confusion
g. delirium
h. dementia
i. organic brain syndrome
j. paranoia
k. pseudodementia
l. respite care
m. senility

Match the following definitions with the acronyms.

14. _____ another name for Alzheimer's disease

15. _____ Cruetzfeldt-Jacob disease

16. _____ positron emission tomography

17. _____ multi-infarct dementia

18. _____ Huntington's disease

19. _____ serum glutamate pyruvate transaminase

20. _____ chronic, progressive, irreversible, fatal neurologic disorder

21. _____ diagnostic test that is helpful in evaluating blood perfusion to the brain and the brain's metabolic activity

22. _____ alanine aminotransferase

23. _____ diagnostic test that can be used to detect strokes

a. AD

b. ALT

c. CJD

d. HD

e. MID

f. MRI

g. PET

h. SDAT

i. SGPT

j. SPECT

▪ Assessment Review

Indicate whether the following assessment findings of Alzheimer's disease are found in the early (E), advanced (A), later (L), or final (F) stages of the disease.

1. _____ forgetfulness

2. _____ confuses day and night

3. _____ loss of sense of time

4. _____ incapable of self-care

5. _____ rambling, incoherent speech

6. _____ cannot remember facts, faces, names

7. _____ total memory loss

8. _____ decreased reaction time

9. _____ unable to recognize family, friends

10. _____ significant decline in memory

11. _____ difficulty with familiar tasks

12. _____ paranoid, great frustration, anger

13. _____ death

14. _____ has trouble with directions

15. _____ motor ability deteriorates

▪ Nursing Actions

Indicate whether the following actions are appropriate (A) or inappropriate (I).

1. _____ Including information such as the client's flu shots and Pneumovax immunizations in the nursing history and physical

2. _____ Determining whether an AD client's sleep problems are disruptive for family members

3. _____ Being firm and strong with AD clients who are physically aggressive and restraining these clients to help them see that they cannot overpower others

4. _____ Reasoning with an AD client who is paranoid and delusional and believes people on television are in the room by explaining that television is not real

5. _____ Monitoring an AD client closely for suicide, particularly in the early stages of AD

6. _____ Recognizing a history of falls or unsteady gait as danger signs of problems with walking without assistance

7. _____ Providing AD clients with daily baths in the morning with high levels of water to soak the body totally because body odor is distressing for the client with AD

8. _____ Maintaining hydration in the client with AD by providing fluids as requested to meet the more acute sense of thirst that older people experience

▪ Fill-in-the-Blank

Complete the following by writing in the correct word in each blank.

1. Three theories of the causes of Alzheimer's disease include _____, _____, and _____.

2. _____-_____ and _____-
   _____ memory impairment are symptoms
   in identification of dementia.

3. The three major physiologic changes that occur in
   the brain of a person with AD are _____
   _____ _____, _____
   _____ _____ , and _____
   _____ _____ _____.

4. Multi-infarct dementia can be distinguished from
   AD in the following ways: it has a _____
   onset; it progresses in a _____ fashion
   (not gradually); and it may coexist with other
   _____.

5. _____ dementias are related to drug
   overdoses; _____ dementias can occur
   after untreated end-stage renal disease or hepatic
   failure.

6. Pain control is important because clients with
   dementia may experience pain but may be unable
   to _____ it.

CHAPTER 93

Psychiatric Nursing

■ Terminology Review

Match the following definitions with the correct terms.

1. _____ inability to sit still, agitation, tapping, rocking, pacing and marching in place

2. _____ repetitive behavior

3. _____ fixed beliefs not shared by others

4. _____ writhing movements of the fingers, toes, and extremities

5. _____ reactions to stress that help individuals to resolve mental conflicts

6. _____ people who threaten to injure others or become physically violent

7. _____ outward manifestation of subjective emotions

8. _____ admitted for treatment involuntarily

9. _____ stupor, muscle rigidity

10. _____ common group of antianxiety medications

11. _____ fear of impending danger

12. _____ fear of being in a place from which escape may be difficult or embarrassing

13. _____ mild form of alternating between overactivity and underactivity

14. _____ specific side effect of neuroleptic medications that affect arm movements

15. _____ a person maintains body position in which he or she is placed

a. affect
b. agoraphobia
c. akathisia
d. anxiety
e. assaultive
f. athetoid
g. benzodiazepine
h. catalepsy
i. catatonia
j. cogwheeling movements
k. commitment
l. compulsion
m. cyclothymic
n. defense mechanism
o. delusion

Match the following definitions with the correct terms.

16. _____ feelings of invincibility and self-importance

17. _____ involuntary, coordinated rhythmic movements, jerking, tremors, twisting, tongue movements

18. _____ increased watchfulness

19. _____ mental illness combined with chemical dependency

20. _____ repetition of another person's movements

21. _____ internal, subjective emotional state

22. _____ feelings that everyone should wait on them

23. _____ characterized by agitation, elation, hyperactivity, and hyperexcitability

24. _____ interfering

25. _____ normal mood

26. _____ therapeutic environment

27. _____ depressed mood for most of the day, most days

28. _____ refusal to speak

29. _____ changes in behavior

30. _____ false sensory perceptions, without relevant external stimulation

a. dual diagnosis
b. dyskinesia
c. dysthymia
d. echopraxia
e. entitled
f. euthymia
g. grandiose
h. hallucination
i. hypervigilance
j. intrusive
k. labile
l. mania
m. milieu
n. mood
o. mutism

a. neologism
b. obsession
c. oculogyric crisis
d. opisthotonos
e. organic disorder
f. orthostatic hypotension
g. paranoid
h. phobia
i. psychiatrist
j. psychomethric
k. psychosis
l. rapport
m. regression
n. self-esteem
o. tardive dyskinesia

Match the following definitions with the correct terms.

31. _____ a thought disorder that interferes with one's ability to recognize and to deal with reality

32. _____ return to infantile or childish behavior

33. _____ testing that includes in-depth interview and various tests

34. _____ syndrome of involuntary movements that are serious and permanent

35. _____ recurrent, persistent, intrusive thought or belief that the person cannot ignore

36. _____ physical or organic cause of a client's mental disorder

37. _____ coin new words that are not really words

38. _____ severe head and neck extension

39. _____ self-value

40. _____ fall in blood pressure on standing

41. _____ pervasive distrust and suspiciousness of others

42. _____ harmonious relationship

43. _____ upward rolling of eyes

44. _____ excessive, unreasonable, and severe fear of a particular thing or event

45. _____ physician who has received advanced education in the treatment of mental disorders

■ Correct the False Statements

Circle the word True *or* False *that follows the statement. If the word* false *has been circled, change the underlined word/words to make the statement true. Place your answer in the space provided.*

1. <u>About 10% of all adults</u> will experience an alteration in mental health in their lifetime.

   True   False   _____

2. <u>Neuroleptic malignant syndrome</u> is a rare, life-threatening complication of neuroleptic medications.

   True   False   _____

3. The nurse would document difficulty speaking as <u>dystonia</u>.

   True   False   _____

4. <u>Oculogyric</u> conversation does not make sense, and the client returns to one subject or dwells on the subject.

   True   False   _____

5. <u>Schizophrenia</u> is a group of psychotic disorders that have two or more of the following positive symptoms: delusions, hallucinations, disorganized speech, grossly disorganized behavior, and catatonia.

   True   False   _____

6. <u>Neuroleptic drugs</u> (mood modifiers) include antipsychotics, antianxiety/sedative-hypnotics, mood stabilizers, and antidepressants.

   True   False   _____

7. The goal of psychiatric therapy is to <u>modify the client's behavior</u> so that he or she can meet life's demand and return to an optimum level of wellness.

   True   False   _____

8. <u>Punishment</u> as a form of behavior modification is usually effective.

   True   False   _____

9. <u>Negative symptoms</u> of psychosis include apathy, emotional withdrawal, and poor judgment.

   True   False   _____

10. Clozapine should not be given with medications that <u>cause respiratory failure</u>.

   True   False   _____

■ Completion

Complete the following sentences by filling in the blanks.

1. About 50% of all suicides can be attributed to a _____ disorder.

2. Diagnosis of a major depressive episode includes five or more symptoms, and at least one symptom must be _____.

3. The mood disorder in which broad mood variations range from mania to major depression is _____.

4. Give an example of a personality disorder, anxiety disorder, and psychosis. _____

   _____

   _____

5. Many mental health and geriatric units use _____ technique or reality orientation.

6. _____ therapy involves having a client interact with a kitten or puppy.

7. Psychotropic drugs such as antipsychotic or neuroleptic drugs may have side effects such as parkinsonism or general dyskinesia. These adverse effects are called _____ side effects.

8. The rights of the client are protected through _____ rights legislation, _____ adult legislation, and _____.

9. The program of nursing care for the very mentally ill client involves _____ care, _____ _____ skills, and building _____ skills.

10. If a client is admitted to a mental health unit under a _____ _____ _____ , the nurse cannot give out information regarding the person or that the person is even in the facility.

■ Matching

Match the nursing action in part A with the client in Part B for whom it would be most appropriate.

PART A

1. _____ Know whereabouts and condition of each resident at all times; 15-minute checks are a minimum.

2. _____ Maintaining a quiet atmosphere is important.

3. _____ Care includes physical protection; allow active clients a wide scope of activity for their surplus energy.

4. _____ Recognize the person's feelings without judgment; defensiveness is ineffective and dangerous.

5. _____ Be firm but kind, avoid familiarity and arguments, keep such clients from irritating others, and try to keep them occupied.

PART B

a. Overactive person
b. Hyponmanic or manic person
c. Hostile person or combative person
d. Suicidal person
e. Highly disturbed person

CHAPTER 94

Substance Abuse

■ Terminology Review

Match the following definitions with the correct terms.

1. _____ medical emergency that occurs during the third stage of alcohol withdrawal in which symptoms include delusions and hallucinations

2. _____ medications that are used in blocking the opioid's effects

3. _____ includes substance abuse plus other criteria such as tolerance, withdrawal, or other factors over a 12-month period

4. _____ tearing of the eyes

5. _____ memory loss during alcohol withdrawal

6. _____ maladaptive pattern of substance use leading to clinical significant impairment or distress

7. _____ occur during delirium tremens and can be auditory, visual, and tactile

8. _____ chronic interstitial inflammation

9. _____ medications such as disulfiram (Antabuse) are used during this treatment

10. _____ process of removing a drug and its physiologic effects from the addicted person's body

11. _____ also called an enabler

12. _____ one who has let someone else's behavior affect him or her

13. _____ mentally ill and chemically dependent

a. agonist therapy
b. alcohol hallucinosis
c. aversion therapy
d. blackout
e. chemical or substance abuse
f. chemical or substance dependence
g. cirrhosis
h. co-dependent
i. delirium tremens
j. detoxification
k. dual disorder
l. enabler
m. lacrimation

Match the following definitions with the correct terms.

14. _____ rapid eyeball movement

15. _____ fainting

16. _____ abuse of more than one substance

17. _____ maladaptive pattern of substance use for a 12-month period including one or more of the following: failure to fulfill role obligations; use that presents a danger; recurrent use-related legal problems; continued use despite related interpersonal problems

18. _____ symptoms that occur when a person stops using the drug, or the person must take the same or related substance to avoid the symptoms

19. _____ objects appear smaller

20. _____ neurologic disorder found in alcoholics due to thiamine deficiency

21. _____ the person needs more of the drug to cause intoxication or the person experiences decreased effects from previously sufficient amounts

22. _____ relapse

23. _____ runny nose

24. _____ life-threatening situation in which a starving person receives carbohydrates too quickly

25. _____ objects appear larger

a. macropsia

b. micropsia

c. nystagmus

d. polysubstance abuse

e. refeeding syndrome

f. remission

g. rhinorrhea

h. substance abuse

i. syncope

j. tolerance

k. Wernicke-Korsakoff syndrome

l. withdrawal

Match the following definitions with the correct acronyms.

26. _____ weed

27. _____ angle dust

28. _____ ecstasy

29. _____ Mothers Against Drunk Drivers

30. _____ withdrawal

31. _____ Addiction Severity Index

32. _____ driving while under the influence or while intoxicated

33. _____ Narcotics Anonymous

34. _____ alcohol

35. _____ American Psychiatric Association

36. _____ type of hallucinogenic drug

37. _____ Alcoholics Anonymous

a. AA

b. APA

c. ASI

d. DUI/DWI

e. ETOH

f. LSD

g. MADD

h. MDA/MDMA

i. MJ

j. NA

k. PCP

l. W/D

■ Assessment Findings

Indicate whether the following withdrawal signs and symptoms are associated with alcohol (A), cocaine (C), heroin/narcotics (H), or sedative-hypnotics/anxiolytics (S). More than one category may apply to each sign or symptom.

1. _____ tremors

2. _____ gooseflesh

3. _____ seizures

4. _____ tactile hallucinations

5. _____ runny nose

6. _____ nausea and vomiting

7. _____ paranoia

8. _____ blackouts

9. _____ sleep disturbance

10. _____ muscle and joint pain

11. _____ constant yawning

12. _____ low urine output

13. _____ dilated pupils

14. _____ lowered temperature

15. _____ hypoglycemia

■ Short Answer

Complete the following by supplying the correct answer.

1. List a criterion that according to the APA defines substance abuse.

2. List possible contributing factors that can lead to the development of chemical dependency.

3. List the four steps in managing all dependencies.

4. What are the most important goals in detoxification management?

5. Describe the type of diet that would be appropriate in a severely malnourished client.

6. Discuss why alcoholics often have dietary deficiencies.

7. List the stages of alcohol withdrawal.

■ Multiple Choice

Circle the best answer.

1. When evaluating the effectiveness of chlordiazepoxide (Librium), the nurse would assess for:

   a. absence of diaphoresis.

   b. absence of seizures.

   c. adequate nutrition.

   d. stable heart rate.

2. A client is admitted to the hospital who has abused cocaine in the past year. Which of the following would the nurse include in the plan of care?

   a. Encourage the client to walk around the hospital unit to promote socialization.

   b. Maintain a steady noise in the environment to prevent depression during withdrawal.

   c. Monitor pulse for a decreased rate because of the depressant effect of cocaine withdrawal.

   d. Monitor respirations and prepare to give respiratory stimulants to counteract respiratory depression.

3. A client is admitted to the hospital for barbiturate abuse. Her husband inquires about drug abuse and the use of programs. Which of the following would the nurse include in a teaching plan?

   a. Getting the client to reduce her abuse of barbiturates is a sign that she will soon become drug free.

   b. Physical abuse cannot occur unless psychological dependence is present; hence, both must be treated.

   c. The 12-step program has been effective in curing people who abuse drugs.

   d. Treating the substance abuser alone in not enough; the family also needs intensive counseling.

4. A client is scheduled to receive Antabuse therapy. Which of the following should the nurse communicate immediately to the physician?

   a. The client had his last drink of alcohol about 35 hours ago.

   b. The client had a recent experience of left-sided weakness.

   c. The client has a strong family history of alcohol abuse.

   d. The client's wife is pregnant and in her second trimester.

5. How long must a client who has been drinking in the past few days be monitored for life-threatening withdrawal symptoms?

   a. 12 hours

   b. 24 hours

   c. 48 hours

   d. 72 hours

CHAPTER 95

Extended Care

■ Terminology Review

Match the following definitions with the correct terms.

1. _____ person who receives the client's monthly check and disbursing the funds appropriately if the client is unable to do so

2. _____ facilities that provide "in-between" level of care

3. _____ are protected by law from abuse or neglect

4. _____ care for clients who require more specialized and high-tech care than is provided in the traditional skilled nursing facility

5. _____ known as Section 8 housing in some states

6. _____ person in LTC who provides assistance and information to residents and families

7. _____ special high-rise or other building that is designated for a specific group

a. assisted living
b. congregate housing
c. medically complex nursing unit
d. ombudsperson
e. payee
f. subacute care
g. vulnerable adult

Match the following definitions with the acronyms.

8. _____ person who oversees the client's care

9. _____ activities of daily living

10. _____ also called a nursing home

11. _____ facilities that continue care that was started in the hospital

12. _____ National Association for Home Care

13. _____ Citizens for Long Term Care

14. _____ intermediate care facility

15. _____ Centers of Excellence

16. _____ skilled nursing facility

17. _____ American Association of Retired Persons

18. _____ unlicensed assistive personnel

a. AARP
b. ADL
c. CLTC
d. COE
e. CM
f. ECF
g. ICF
h. LTC
i. NAHC
j. SNF
k. UAP

■ Correct the False Statements

Circle the word True *or* False *that follows the statement. If the word* false *has been circled, change the underlined word/words to make the statement true. Place your answer in the space provided.*

1. Within facilities, there is usually only one level of care.

   True   False   _____

2. Transitional care or continual care facilities are other names for assisted living facilities.

   True   False   _____

3. A client may be classified as subacute for <u>20 days</u> under Medicare, and then this status must be reevaluated.

   True   False   _____

4. The two types of long-term care facilities are <u>the skilled nursing facility and the intermediate care facility</u>.

   True   False   _____

5. Residents of LTC facilities <u>may have a choice of meal plans</u>.

   True   False   _____

6. <u>Therapeutic dance</u> programs play a part in rehabilitation by providing safer exercises.

   True   False   _____

7. Payment for long-term care <u>is always paid directly by the family</u>.

   True   False   _____

8. The goal of the coalition of the AARP, NAHC, Alzheimer's Association, and CLTC was to <u>review long-term care financing in the United States and make recommendations for improvement</u>.

   True   False   _____

9. The benefit of medical day care programs is that it provides <u>time for shopping</u> for families.

   True   False   _____

10. Skilled nursing facilities must <u>always have a licensed nurse on duty</u>.

    True   False   _____

▪ Short Answer

Complete the following by supplying the best answer.

1. List the various types of facilities that make up extended care facilities.

2. How long do clients usually spend in a subacute care facility?

3. Describe nursing functions usually performed in a subacute care facility.

4. What type of clients would be in a medically complex nursing unit?

5. Describe the services that LTC facilities provide.

6. List common recreational activities that may be provided in LTC facilities.

7. Describe the role of the case manager in LTC.

8. Describe how clients are cared for and kept safe since starting "restraint-free" policies.

9. Describe benefits of intermediate care facilities.

10. Describe the type of clients who would be well suited to live at a board-and-care home or supervised group home.

CHAPTER 96

Rehabilitation Nursing

■ Terminology Review

Match the following definitions with the correct terms.

1. _____ lower limb paralysis

2. _____ lacking nerve stimulation

3. _____ physician who specialize in rehabilitation

4. _____ paralysis of one side of the body

5. _____ medical specialty involved in the fabrication of braces and splints

6. _____ fabrication and adjustment of artificial limbs

7. _____ placing young people who are mentally or physically challenged into regular classes in school

8. _____ restoring a person who becomes physically or mentally challenged to his or her former abilities as much as possible

9. _____ paralysis of all four extremities and possibly the trunk

10. _____ structural items that prevent easy access to buildings

11. _____ inflatable trousers that help maintain an upright position and prevent vascular collapse

a. architectural barriers
b. exoskeleton
c. hemiplegia
d. mainstreaming
e. neurogenic
f. orthotics
g. paraplegia
h. physiatrist
i. prosthetics
j. quadriplegia
k. rehabilitation

Match the following definitions with the acronyms.

12. _____ includes aspects of self-care such as dressing, bathing, toileting and continence, transfer, mobility, and eating

13. _____ muscular dystrophy

14. _____ traumatic brain injuries

15. _____ test that determines electrical activity and potential of muscles

16. _____ Huntington's disease

17. _____ cystic fibrosis

18. _____ sends a stimulus to the nerves to move muscles

19. _____ multiple sclerosis

20. _____ includes more complex living skills, such as food preparation, laundry, and money management

21. _____ physical medicine and rehabilitation

22. _____ prospective payment system

23. _____ stroke

24. _____ amyotrophic lateral sclerosis

a. ALS
b. CF
c. CVA
d. EMG
e. FADL
f. FES
g. HD
h. IADL
i. MD
j. MS
k. PPS
l. PM&R
m. TBI

■ Nursing Actions

Indicate whether the following nursing actions are appropriate (A) or inappropriate (I).

1. _____ Referring the client for rehabilitation who is physically challenged owing to an injury with no possibility of complete recovery

2. _____ Expecting the client who is adjusting to a physical or mental challenge to undergo shock, denial, anger, bargaining, depression, and then acceptance reactions

3. _____ Encouraging the client in rehabilitation to relax and become dependent on staff for a short time to rest and recuperate

4. _____ Suggesting clients get electrical outlets installed higher off the floor to promote easy reach

5. _____ Instructing clients who are wheelchair bound to take tub baths instead of showers

6. _____ Suggesting that the hemiplegic client place clothing on the unaffected arm or leg first and to undress the affected are or leg first.

7. _____ Assist the client in the acute stage to prepare meals.

8. _____ Encourage clients to perform as much self-care as possible during rehabilitation.

9. _____ Teach clients to use adaptive equipment, such as Velcro closures, as needed to maintain independence.

10. _____ Instruct the client who needs maximum support when ambulating to us a half-circle cane.

11. _____ Use alcohol to cleanse the skin of a wheelchair-bound client.

12. _____ Administer high-protein diet and dietary supplements as ordered by the physician.

13. _____ Assist in bladder and bowel retraining for a client with quadriplegia.

14. _____ Discourage manual disimpaction of bowel as part of a bowel elimination program.

15. _____ Encourage clients with neurogenic bladders to drink 1,000 mL/d.

16. _____ Instruct the client who is incontinent to restrict fluids.

17. _____ Provide pets for diversion and companionship for residents of long-term care facilities.

18. _____ Provide emotional support for clients who have been severely burned.

19. _____ Do not ask clients about complementary therapies because they do not interfere with rehabilitation.

20. _____ Introduce talking books to clients who have limited vision.

■ Multiple Choice

Circle the best answer.

1. Which action would be appropriate to help a client establish regular patterns of voiding?
   a. Assist the client to void every 2 hours.
   b. Complete manual disimpaction every day.
   c. Teach the client how to perform the Credé maneuver.
   d. Teach the client to drink 2,000 mL of fluid a day.

2. Which of the following is an example of instrumental activities of daily living?
   a. Bathing
   b. Communicating
   c. Managing money
   d. Walking with use of cane

3. A woman has recently become a quadriplegic as a result of an automobile accident. Which instructions should the nurse provide to the client regarding sexuality?
   a. Instruct the client that if she becomes pregnant, she will need a cesarean section.
   b. Instruct the client to use a form of birth control if she does not want to become pregnant.
   c. Instruct client that sexual intercourse will be painful.
   d. Instruct client that she should not have sexual intercourse.

4. A client's skin is becoming irritated owing to incontinence. Which action can the nurse implement without a physician's order?

   a. Apply barrier ointment.

   b. Place a dressing such as Duo-Derm over the area.

   c. Order a high-protein diet to encourage healing.

   d. Use adult protective undergarments (diapers).

CHAPTER 97

Ambulatory Nursing

■ Terminology Review

Match the following definitions with the correct terms or acronym.

1. _____ call-in services that may be in the form of crisis lines or nurse lines

2. _____ room where clients are triaged and stabilized for transfer to operating rooms or other areas

3. _____ established guidelines for providers based on national criteria that detail the required management of specific disorders

4. _____ defibrillation

5. _____ employee health service

6. _____ clients with noncritical conditions treated at free-standing clinics

7. _____ chronic disorders in which providers are required to follow specific managed care protocols

8. _____ health maintenance organizations

9. _____ entry points when using endoscopic surgery

10. _____ single-room occupancy hotel

11. _____ free-standing center not attached to hospitals

12. _____ use of small scopes to visualize and manipulate internal structures

13. _____ community health center

14. _____ primary care provider

15. _____ family health center

16. _____ crisis intervention centers

a. cardioversion
b. emerge-center
c. endoscopy
d. managed care protocol
e. port
f. stabilization room
g. telehealth
h. vertical clients
i. ACS
j. CHC
k. CIC
l. EHS
m. FHC
n. HMO
o. PCP
p. SRO

■ Nursing Actions

Indicate whether the following nursing actions are appropriate (A) or inappropriate (I).

1. _____ Performing special nonnursing procedures, such as laboratory procedures or electrocardiograms, when working in an ambulatory healthcare site

2. _____ Encouraging clients with underlying disorders to complete paperwork and laboratory tests so that they will be prepared for day surgery instead of inpatient surgery

3. _____ Giving instructions to clients verbally by telephone and in writing and at the last preoperative office visit when the client is scheduled for day surgery

4. _____ Performing specific preparations, such as preoperative scrub and shaving or drawing of blood the day before the procedure

5. _____ Instructing the client to drive in early and park close to the building so that there is less walking needed before driving home after the procedure

6. _____ Triaging clients (if in scope of practice) in the ambulatory care setting

7. _____ Taking vital signs, measuring blood sugar levels, and performing gross vision or hearing screenings while working in a mobile clinic

8. _____ Performing complete physical exams for children when working in a school-based health service setting

9. _____ Diagnosing physical health problems and addressing client's concerns when working in a telehealth setting

10. _____ Assist with cardioversion and stabilizing clients when working in the emergency department

■ Short Answer

Complete the following.

1. List the three classes for criteria for outpatient surgery. Briefly describe the type of client eligible for each category. Include one type of surgery that is performed in each category.

    CATEGORY

    DESCRIPTION

    EXAMPLE OF SURGERY

2. Describe at least two types of equipment that have made same-day surgery possible.

3. Describe benefits of having surgery in an outpatient or same-day surgery setting.

4. Describe teaching for the client and family that the nurse is responsible for in the day surgery center.

5. Describe interventions that the nurse can complete to help the client relax when having surgery at the day surgery center.

CHAPTER 98

Home Care Nursing

■ Terminology Review

Match the following definitions with the acronyms.

1. _____ group a client is assigned to for a given episode of care, usually is a 60-day period

2. _____ system in which third-party payers try to control medical costs and to improve efficiency in delivery of home care

3. _____ healthcare assistants

4. _____ Community Nursing Organization

5. _____ certified home health aides

6. _____ standardized data collection tool used to assess the case mix, according to clinical functional and service needs

7. _____ National Association for Home Care

8. _____ personal care attendants

a. CNO
b. HCA
c. (C) HHA
d. HHRG
e. NAHC
f. OASIS
g. PCA
h. PPS

■ Nursing Action

Indicate whether the following action is appropriate (A) or inappropriate (I).

1. _____ Instruct caregivers to plan some recreational activity each day.

2. _____ Recommend caregivers read intense books to keep their mind off caring for the family member.

3. _____ Encourage caregivers to have friends and family members visit.

4. _____ Encourage the caregiver to listen to lively music when at the bedside to stimulate the client and to provide energy for both caregiver and client.

5. _____ Teach caregivers to rest only at night to maintain a normal sleep–wake cycle.

6. _____ Telephone home care clients before visiting and informing them of your approximate arrival time.

7. _____ If confronted with an aggressive dog at a client's home, slowly back away and then run quickly to your car.

8. _____ Carry a charged cell phone at all times when at work as a home care nurse.

9. _____ When visiting clients at their home, park in an area that is not obvious to neighbors, to protect the client's privacy.

10. _____ Walk in a casual manner when approaching a client's home.

11. _____ Avoid eye contact when passing groups of strangers on the way to a home visit.

12. _____ Always wear a name badge when providing nursing care.

■ Correct the False Statements

Circle the word True *or* False *that follows the statement. If the word* false *has been circled, change the underlined word/words to make the statement true. Place your answer in the space provided.*

1. One of the reasons for an increase in home care is <u>that people are discharged from hospitals with complicated equipment</u>.

   True   False   _____

2. Home care is <u>always given on</u> <u>short-term basis</u>.

   True   False   _____

3. Hospital-based agencies <u>are the only agencies that provide</u> home care.

   True   False   _____

4. A client who needs total physical care <u>is an appropriate client</u> for home care.

   True   False   _____

5. <u>Urinary disorders</u> make up the highest percentage of caseloads in many comprehensive home care agencies.

   True   False   _____

6. An example of <u>long-term home care</u> is having the nurse visit once a week to assist in setting up medications for the next week.

   True   False   _____

7. A Center of Excellence team may provide <u>assistance with high-technology care</u>.

   True   False   _____

8. Center of Excellence nurses <u>may not</u> make actual home visits.

   True   False   _____

9. A role of the home care nurse is to educate the client and family to <u>understand, learn about, and manage the client's care</u>.

   True   False   _____

10. A <u>physician</u> is required to visit the client at certain intervals to determine whether the client's healthcare goals are being met and if requirements of the funding agency are being satisfied.

   True   False   _____

■ Multiple Choice

Circle the best answer.

1. While on a home visit, you notice that your client complains of having difficulty preparing meals. When planning care, it would be most important to make a referral to:
   a. escort services.
   b. Meals on Wheels.
   c. senior center.
   d. volunteer services.

2. In many states, the case manager is a:
   a. dietitian.
   b. physical therapist.
   c. physician.
   d. registered nurse.

3. Which of the following is a standard duty of the LVN/LPN in home care?
   a. Complete initial assessment and evaluate adequacy of available family caregivers.
   b. Initially evaluate safety of the client's living environment.
   c. Prepare clinical and progress notes.
   d. Stabilize critically ill clients so that they may remain in their home to receive care.

4. One advantage of working in home healthcare is:
   a. caring for only one or two clients.
   b. increased wages.
   c. structured work day.
   d. working in a safe, carefree environment.

CHAPTER 99

Hospice Nursing

■ Terminology Review

Match the following definitions with the correct terms and acronyms.

1. _____ program based on philosophy of care and quality of life for terminally ill clients

2. _____ caregivers taking a break from client care

3. _____ hospice team members who work together to provide a multitude of services

4. _____ neurosurgery to cut the pain pathway

5. _____ durable medical equipment

6. _____ gradually increasing a narcotic's dose

7. _____ symptom control, not curative measures

8. _____ medications used to potentiate the effect of opioid medication or for other symptoms

9. _____ certified registered nurse, hospice

10. _____ bedside commode

11. _____ significant others who care for hospice clients

12. _____ very difficult or impossible to arouse

13. _____ part of the process of dealing with a loved one's death

14. _____ before receiving Medicare and Medicaid assistance, client must meet these requirements

15. _____ palliative surgery done to relieve pressure or obstruction by removing part of a tumor

a. ablative surgery
b. adjuvant
c. bereavement
d. debulking
e. hospice
f. interdisciplinary care
g. palliative care
h. primary caregivers
i. respite
j. somnolent
k. titration
l. BSC
m. CRNH
n. COPs
o. DME

Match the following definitions with the correct acronyms.

16. _____ medical social worker

17. _____ do not resuscitate

18. _____ passed by Congress in 1991; allows people more say regarding their end-of-life care

19. _____ patient-controlled anesthesia

20. _____ established for each client to guide care for all interdisciplinary team members

21. _____ do not intubate

22. _____ founded in 1978 and established criteria for hospices; offers information and education to healthcare professionals and the public

23. _____ suicidal ideation

24. _____ consists of physicians, nurses, MSWs, therapists, clergy, bereavement coordinators, dietitians, pharmacologists, HHAs, homemakers, and volunteers

25. _____ overbed table

26. _____ applies electrical stimulation directly to nerves and interrupts transmission of pain sensations

27. _____ do not hospitalize

28. _____ interdisciplinary group

a. DNH
b. DNI
c. DNR
d. IDG
e. IDT
f. MSW
g. NHPCO
h. OBT
i. PCA
j. POC
k. PSDA
l. SI
m. TENS

■ Correct the False Statements

Circle the word True *or* False *that follows the statement. If the word* false *has been circled, change the underlined word/words to make the statement true. Place your answer in the space provided.*

1. The goal of hospice care is <u>intensive palliative care</u>.

   True   False   _____

2. Upon admission to hospice, the initial family visit evaluates <u>the willingness and intelligence of the primary caregiver</u>.

   True   False   _____

3. A client must have <u>no more than 1 year</u> to live in order to be entered into a hospice program.

   True   False   _____

4. A hospice must have an <u>interdisciplinary approach</u>.

   True   False   _____

5. Hospice nurses <u>assist caregivers</u> by setting up medications, answering questions, and performing functions.

   True   False   _____

6. <u>Nurses</u> compose more than 80% of all people involved in hospice.

   True   False   _____

7. Hospice staff members <u>rarely need</u> emotional support when working with dying people.

   True   False   _____

8. To relieve constipation, a <u>colon cocktail</u> may be administered twice daily.

   True   False   _____

9. Many clients <u>become dehydrated</u> shortly before death.

   True   False   _____

10. <u>More medication</u> is often needed if clients self-administer their medications and if they are taken around the clock.

    True   False   _____

11. Fentanyl (Duragesic) is administered <u>transdermally</u>.

    True   False   _____

12. It is not unusual for hospice clients to have a bowel movement <u>every 4 to 5 days</u>

    True   False   _____

13. Children in hospice programs should be <u>encouraged to ask questions</u>.

    True   False   _____

14. When a client dies at home, the coroner is <u>not required to come to the home</u> of a registered hospice client.

    True   False   _____

■ Multiple Choice

Circle the best answer.

1. A client is enrolled in the hospice program. The client experiences remission. A family member asks you what will happen. The best response would be:
   a. "No change in the current care is needed."
   b. "The doctor will see how the family member does and will possibly remove him or her from hospice."
   c. "The family member will be discharged from hospice to resume aggressive medical care."
   d. "What do you think the family member would want to do?"

2. The following clients are being discharged from the hospital. It is most important for the nurse to include a referral to hospice for which client?
   a. A 30-year-old man who is HIV positive and in relatively good health
   b. A 60-year-old man with lung cancer with an estimated 6 months life expectancy
   c. A 74-year-old woman with mild congestive heart failure
   d. An 80-year-old woman after surgery for a fractured hip

3. The greatest feat of most hospice clients is that:
   a. family members will no longer love them.
   b. nausea and vomiting will prevent them from eating.
   c. they will be left alone to die.
   d. they will experience pain.

4. The focus of the hospice nurse is:
   a. on identifying the needs of the client and family.
   b. on providing client care.
   c. to help the family cope.
   d. to process necessary insurance forms.

5. A client is experiencing nausea. Which nursing action is most appropriate?
   a. Administer increased doses of narcotics.
   b. Administer antiemetics 1/2 hour after meals.
   c. Offer one large meal per day.
   d. Position client on right side

6. A client is newly admitted to the hospice program. Which of the following is a goal regarding sleep and rest?
   a. Maintain normal sleep patterns taking a sleeping pill every night.
   b. Maintain 10 hours of sleep every night.
   c. Sleep adequately at night and maintain normal daytime activities.
   d. Take frequent short naps throughout the day to build strength and ensure adequate rest.

7. The occurrence of which condition would warrant the nurse discontinuing a hospice client's infusion of morphine sulfate?
   a. Constipation
   b. Sedation
   c. Slightly lowered blood pressure
   d. Somnolence

CHAPTER 100

From Student to Graduate Nurse

■ Terminology Review

Match the following definitions with the correct terms and acronyms.

1. _____ examination that must be passed in order to practice nursing

2. _____ World Wide Web

3. _____ reading the physician's order sheet and carrying out necessary actions so that the client receives and benefits from the treatment

4. _____ period of time for a new employee that is an opportunity to determine whether the job placement is appropriate

5. _____ format of the NCLEX

6. _____ education requirement for renewal of nursing license

7. _____ competencies that the LVN/LPN needs to demonstrate

8. _____ enormous source of information regarding medications, diseases, legislation, or new nursing procedures from many sources

a. entry-level skills
b. probationary status
c. transcribing orders
d. Internet
e. CAT
f. CEU
g. NCLEX
h. WWW

■ License Revocation Review

Indicate with an X which of the following examples are just cause to revoke or suspend a nurse's license.

1. _____ conviction of a felony

2. _____ traffic violation

3. _____ stealing medications

4. _____ mental illness

5. _____ sexual activity with consenting adult

6. _____ negligence in nursing practice

7. _____ neglecting a client

8. _____ revoked license in another state

9. _____ history of addictive behavior, now controlled

10. _____ fraudulent acquisition of a nursing license

■ Nursing Action

Indicate whether the following actions are appropriate (A) or inappropriate (I).

1. _____ Planning to work a night shift, but keeping regular day hours on your off days to maintain a social life

2. _____ Taking a nap when you get a break during your night shifts

3. _____ Bringing something interesting to do during your night shift to help you stay alert

4. _____ Keeping nursing records in different locations in the home so that all records will not be lost if a fire occurs in one room

5. _____ Placing a copy of professional documents in a file and keeping the originals in a safe deposit box

6. _____ Serving a period as a nurse intern to help the transition from student to practicing nurse

7. _____ Terminating all learning experiences with graduation from school; concentrating on practice

8. _____ Obtaining a permit to practice as a graduate nurse, if allowed in your state, before taking the nursing examination

■ Correct the False Statements

Circle the word True *or* False *that follows the statement. If the word* false *has been circled, change the underlined word/words to make the statement true. Place your answer in the space provided.*

1. The graduate nurse must obtain a license in order to <u>work as a nurse</u>.

   True   False   _____

2. Each examination question represents a <u>phase of the nursing process</u>.

   True   False   _____

3. NCLEX examination questions about medication administration would fit under the client need category of <u>psychosocial integrity</u>.

   True   False   _____

4. NCLEX examination questions include all <u>three phases of the nursing process</u>.

   True   False   _____

5. The NCLEX examination includes <u>application of nursing knowledge</u> by using critical thinking skills.

   True   False   _____

6. The best way to prepare for the NCLEX-PN is to <u>review all nursing school content during the two weeks before the examination</u>.

   True   False   _____

7. <u>Each nurse</u> is responsible for obtaining and maintaining the required CEUs for the state in which she or he practices.

   True   False   _____

8. <u>Organizational skills</u> are the key to providing efficient and safe care for all clients.

   True   False   _____

9. Computers can be used in the hospital setting to <u>forward physician's orders to pharmacy and the laboratory</u>.

   True   False   _____

10. An <u>advantage of working the night shift</u> is that the work is physically less demanding.

    True   False   _____

11. When working the night shift, the nurse should <u>keep the work area darkened</u> to enhance the body's biorhythms.

    True   False   _____

12. When transcribing orders, always complete <u>procedures first</u>.

    True   False   _____

■ Multiple Choice

Circle the best answer.

1. NCLEX examination questions about early detection of breast cancer would fit under which category of client need?
   a. Health promotion and maintenance
   b. Physiologic integrity
   c. Psychosocial integrity
   d. Safe, effective care environment

2. Which of the following is recommended before taking the NCLEX-PN?

    a. Eat a large meal the night before the examination.

    b. Get plenty of sleep the night before the examination.

    c. Spend time reviewing basic nursing care on the evening before the examination.

    d. Wear your school uniform to the examination.

3. Which full-time work schedule allows for the most time off from work?

    a. 8 hour shifts

    b. 10 hour shifts

    c. 12 hour shifts

    d. 13 hour shifts

4. When working the night shift, which of the following might the nurse expect?

    a. Drop in temperature

    b. Decrease in pain

    c. Increase in the number of procedures

    d. Increase in client confusion and acting out

5. To enhance sleep during the day when working the night shift, the nurse should:

    a. avoid exercise during the evenings.

    b. eat a large breakfast before sleeping.

    c. limit caffeine after about 3 am.

    d. take a sleeping pill.

CHAPTER 101

Career Opportunities and Job-Seeking Skills

■ Terminology Review

Match the following definitions with the correct terms and acronyms.

1. _____ growing area of nursing employment in which clients call with symptoms and questions and the nurse performs assessments over the phone

2. _____ unlicensed assistive personnel

3. _____ letter of application that accompanies a resume

4. _____ delivers oxygen under pressure to clients with carbon dioxide poisoning, some types of cancer chemotherapy, near drowning, and rapid reentry into the earth's atmosphere

5. _____ Employee Health Service

6. _____ works with physicians and other healthcare professional to ensure that quality care is given in the most cost-effective manner

7. _____ recruits nurses to work in facilities that need extra help for special-duty clients, during busy periods, or during maternity, illness, or vacation coverage

8. _____ agency that provides free job information, both in private industry and government positions

a. claims analyst
b. cover letter
c. employment services
d. registry
e. telehealth
f. EHS
g. HBO
h. UAP

■ Correct the False Statements

Circle the word True *or* False *that follows the statement. If the word* false *has been circled, change the underlined word/words to make the statement true. Place your answer in the space provided.*

1. <u>Extended care facilities</u> are a major source of new jobs for LVNs and LPNs.

   True   False   _____

2. An <u>advantage of hospital nursing</u> is that it gives the nurse the opportunity to practice basic bedside and teaching skills and to meet one client's total needs.

   True   False   _____

3. The nurse who works in a physician's office needs to be skilled in <u>crisis intervention</u>.

   True   False   _____

4. The nurse who works in occupation health is interested in the welfare of employees <u>as well as promoting minimal absenteeism</u>.

   True   False   _____

5. A <u>parish nurse</u> may provide support to terminally ill clients and their families.

   True   False   _____

6. A nurse working in <u>pharmaceutical sales</u> is often required to travel and provide a professional wardrobe.

   True   False   _____

7. It is important for the graduate nurse to build <u>agency pools</u> to learn about positions that are not advertised.

   True   False   _____

8. A <u>disadvantage</u> of working for a registry is that sometimes there are no benefits but there is a higher hourly wage.

   True   False   _____

9. When preparing for a job search, it is important to <u>complete a self-evaluation</u>.

   True   False   _____

10. A prospective employee should show up <u>1 hour</u> before an interview.

    True   False   _____

11. When resigning from a position, the employee should give <u>1 week's notice</u>.

    True   False   _____

12. About 90% of all positions <u>are filled based on personal contact</u>.

    True   False   _____

■ Short Answer

Complete the following questions.

1. List six types of healthcare facilities or related agencies in which the LVN or LPN might seek employment.

2. List at least five specialized areas of nursing available to the LPN and LVN.

3. Describe the role of the nurse in correctional facilities.

4. Describe how the Internet can be used to apply for and obtain a job.

5. Review Box 101-1, Factors to Consider When Looking for a Place of Employment. Prioritize *your* top six considerations for choosing a place of employment as well as the top six professional considerations when choosing job.

   CONSIDERATIONS

   1.

   2.

   3.

   4.

   5.

   6.

   PROFESSIONAL CONSIDERATIONS

   1.

   2.

   3.

   4.

   5.

   6.

6. Describe the components of a well-written cover letter.

7. List items that should be included in your resume.

8. Review Box 101-3, Guidelines for the Job Interview. Identify five items that you feel will be easy to accomplish when going for a job interview and five items that you will have to work hard to accomplish when going for a job interview.

ITEMS THAT ARE EASY TO COMPLETE

1.

2.

3.

4.

5.

ITEMS TO WORK ON

1.

2.

3.

4.

5.

CHAPTER 102

Advancement and Leadership in Nursing

■ Terminology Review

Match the following definitions with the correct terms.

1. _____ Omnibus Budget Reconciliation Act

2. _____ written evaluations of staff members' ability to complete their jobs

3. _____ people-oriented style that tries to guide staff in the right direction

4. _____ written statement of deficiencies of an employee, actions needed to correct deficiencies, time line, and consequences if plan fails

5. _____ centers for Medicare and Medicaid services

6. _____ least-structured style that has loosely structured goals with no firm guidelines

7. _____ self-directed style that calls for little or no input from staff

8. _____ Health Care Financing Administration

9. _____ coordinates and controls the work of others

10. _____ procedure to inform employee that his or her performance is not acceptable and measures taken to assist the employee. If the performance does not improve, the employee can have various consequences or be terminated.

11. _____ certification for LPNs in long-term care

12. _____ verbal or written means of informing an employee of a deficiency

13. _____ person who uses specific skills such as role modeling to influence others to accomplish a task or do the work

14. _____ policy-minded style that relies on established protocols for decision making

a. autocratic leadership
b. bureaucratic leadership
c. democratic leadership
d. due process
e. laissez-faire leadership
f. leader
g. manager
h. performance review
i. plan of assistance
j. oral or written reprimand
k. CLTC
l. CMMS
m. HCFA
n. OBRA

■ Nursing Action

Indicate whether the following actions are appropriate (A) or inappropriate (I).

1. _____ Taking the examination to qualify for certification in LTC after 2,000 hours of clinical practice within 3 years in LTC

2. _____ Completing a refresher course after not working as a nurse for several years

3. _____ Being a manager who seeks guidance from others before working

4. _____ Being a good leader by providing support to those being led

5. _____ Using a democratic leadership style with a new graduate to make the new employee feel a part of the team

6. _____ Using a laissez-faire style to promote independence in experienced employees

7. _____ Make client and staff assignments when working as a team leader in the skilled nursing facility

8. _____ Counting narcotics at the beginning and end of the shift when working as a charge nurse

9. _____ Accepting a position as a charge nurse with 6 months' experience

10. _____ Triaging telephone calls when working in a leadership role in a clinic setting

11. _____ When working as a charge nurse, instructing staff members to write their own performance evaluations to gain insight on their perspective

12. _____ Allowing an open-ended time line for a plan of assistance

13. _____ Using basic problem-solving methods when functioning as a leader

■ Multiple Choice

Circle the best answer.

1. A question regarding a resident's potential for aspiration would be under which category of the LTC certification examination?
   a. Leadership and management
   b. Physiologic integrity
   c. Psychosocial integrity
   d. Specialty practice issues

2. A question regarding a resident's care plan would be under which category of the LTC certification examination?
   a. Leadership and management
   b. Physiologic integrity
   c. Psychosocial integrity
   d. Specialty practice issues

3. The usual length of the mobility programs from LPN or LVN to RN licensure at community colleges is:
   a. 6 months.
   b. 1 year.
   c. 2 years.
   d. 3 years.

4. A nurse is working in LTC, and a client goes into cardiac arrest. Which leadership style would be most appropriate?
   a. Autocratic
   b. Bureaucratic
   c. Democratic
   d. Laissez-faire

5. Which type of leadership style would be most appropriate to use when formulating a new nursing unit documentation sheet?
   a. Autocratic
   b. Bureaucratic
   c. Democratic
   d. Laissez-faire

Answers

Chapter 1
The History of Nursing

TERMINOLOGY REVIEW

1. k	4. d	7. h	10. j
2. f	5. a	8. l	11. e
3. g	6. i	9. b	12. c

FILL IN THE BLANKS

1. nourish
2. medicine man
3. demonic possession
4. Hippocrates
5. monastic or religious orders
6. Crusades
7. Pastor Theodor Fliedner
8. Pittsburgh Infirmary
9. Mary Adelaide Nutting
10. 1892
11. Smith-Hughes Act
12. Ann Goodrich
13. Katherine Densford
14. name tag

SHORT ANSWERS

1. Hippocrates was the first to emphasize many concepts of care, including holistic healthcare. This concept helped lay the foundations for nursing.
2. Phoebe—first deaconess and visiting nurse, Fabiola—construction of the first free hospital, St. Marcella—first nursing educator, St. Paula—established inns to care for travelers, and St. Helena established the first geriatric facility.
3. Nursing was considered the most menial of all tasks and least desirable; women who cared for the sick were prisoners or prostitutes.
4. She would make rounds on her patients during the night using an oil lamp.
5. Answers will vary.
6. Child care, cooking, light housekeeping, and care of the sick at home
7. Ballard School, Thompson Practical Nursing School, and Household Nursing School
8. Higher client acuity in hospital and long-term settings. This requires all nurses to have higher levels of skill, additional education, and more specialization.

   Shift to community-based care. Nursing care is delivered in a much wider range of settings.

   Technology. Nurses must know how to use technology and teach to clients.

   Social factors. The nurse must be familiar with social factors, and this increases the need for more nurses in the public sector.

   Lifestyle factors and greater life expectancy. More nurses will be needed to care for aging population in areas of extended, long-term, and home care.

   Changes in nursing education. Nurses are obtaining more education.

   Autonomy. Nurses' roles are more collaborative versus subservient to physicians.
9. cross, Star of David, Nightingale lamp
10. See table below.

Historical Timeline	Role of the Nurse
Ancient times	Medicine man or shaman cared for the sick. Women were not involved, except to help with childbirth.
500 BC, advanced Greek civilization	Illness believed to be caused by disease, not sins or demonic possessions. Female priestesses sometimes administered therapies.
First century	First recorded history of nursing begins with women who cared for sick and injured. Monastic orders were established to care for the sick.

(continues)

(Continued)

Historical Timeline	Role of the Nurse
Crusades (1096–1291)	Female religious orders in Europe were nearly eliminated.
Reformation (1500s)	Monastaries closed and work of women in religious orders nearly ended. Prisoners or prostitutes cared for the sick.
1800s	First school of nursing established in Germany. Nightingale's influence elevated nursing to a respected profession. Nursing schools were established in the United States.
1900s	Nursing rapidly evolves. Nursing schools move from hospital base to educational and technical institutions Expanse in LVN and RN schools. Expanse of nurses in the military.

MATCHING

1. f	3. d	5. a	7. c
2. h	4. g	6. e	8. b

MULTIPLE CHOICE

1. b
2. a
3. c
4. b
5. d

Chapter 2
Beginning a Nursing Career

TERMINOLOGY REVIEW

1. e	4. b	7. g	10. h
2. d	5. k	8. j	11. f
3. i	6. c	9. a	

SHORT ANSWERS

1. Associate degree in nursing obtained at a 2-year program at the community or junior college. A 3-year program is usually associated with community and state colleges. A 4-year program (bachelor's) prepares professional nurses to teach, administrate, or enter advanced-degree programs.
2. Curricula are designed to include classroom theory and to practice clinical skills. Most programs are 12 to 18 months and exist under a high school, vocational institute, or community college.

3. Both provide nursing care to persons who are ill. The RN can also teach, supervise, and work independently. RNs may also advance their level of nursing care with advanced education. LVNs may supervise nursing assistants and aides.
4. Answers will vary.
5. Practice nursing professionally, maintain confidentiality, raise standards of nursing, fulfill physicians orders, not administer harmful drugs
6. Each represents himself or herself, the school, the healthcare facility for which he or she works and the entire healthcare system
7. Answers will vary
8. Roles include care provider, communicator, teacher, advocate, leader, and team member. Examples will vary.

FILL IN THE BLANKS

1. technical nurse
2. California, Texas
3. career ladder or one-plus-one
4. approved, accredited
5. nursing practice
6. illness
7. nursing assistants, aides
8. ethically
9. health
10. home, family, outside job

MATCHING

1. b
2. a
3. e
4. c
5. d

MULTIPLE CHOICE

1. c
2. a
3. d
4. b
5. c

Chapter 3
The Healthcare Delivery System

TERMINOLOGY REVIEW

1. t	10. m	19. aa	28. r
2. b	11. ii	20. w	29. a
3. ee	12. q	21. f	30. c
4. z	13. gg	22. j	31. y
5. dd	14. v	23. h	32. i
6. n	15. bb	24. k	33. s
7. x	16. u	25. l	34. p
8. hh	17. cc	26. e	35. o
9. g	18. ff	27. d	

SHORT ANSWERS

1. a. Both terms are used for prospective payment based on categories. DRGs are used in hospital or home care, and RUGs are used in nursing homes and ECFs.

   b. Both are federal programs. Medicaid states can individually regulate, whereas Medicare is federally managed.

   c. In an SNF, 24-hour nursing care is provided under the supervision of an RN; in an ICF, 24-hour services are provided under the supervision of an LPN with an RN as a consultant.
2. Answers will vary. See Box 3-1 for list of trends.
3. Answers will vary. See Educating the Client 3-1: Detecting Fraud.

CORRECT THE FALSE STATEMENTS

1. False; emphasis on wellness and individuals assuming more responsibility for their own health.
2. True
3. False; state and federally
4. True
5. True
6. False; resource utilization
7. False; Occupational therapy
8. False; absence of disease and meeting of basic needs and avoidance of hazardous situations and the ability to cope with stress.
9. True
10. True

Chapter 4
Legal and Ethical Aspects of Nursing

TERMINOLOGY REVIEW

1. t	6. q	11. f	16. g
2. d	7. s	12. k	17. c
3. l	8. p	13. o	18. a
4. j	9. h	14. b	19. r
5. n	10. e	15. i	20. m

ACRONYM REVIEW

1. c	5. f	9. a	13. e
2. j	6. l	10. b	
3. i	7. h	11. g	
4. k	8. m	12. d	

SHORT ANSWERS

1. The nurse would be liable for a crime of omission by failing to administer the ordered medication.
2. Standards of practice are defined by the state's Nurse Practice Act, written agency policies, documented standards of care such as NCPs, and the testimony of expert witnesses.
3. The nurses could be liable for slander and defamation.
4. Proper notification of the nurse's supervisor should have been done. Also, ensuring that someone was assigned to take care of your assigned clients and then reporting off to that person.
5. The purpose of the Nurse Practice Act is to define and regulate the practice of nursing.
6. The Nurse Practice Act regulates length of program, curricula, and admission requirements.
7. The nurse should thank the client for his thoughtfulness but graciously decline to accept the gift.
8. The three types of advance directives are living will, which goes into effect only if the person becomes unable to make his or hew own decisions; directives to physicians, which direct the physician to be the client's decision maker; and durable power of attorney for healthcare, which names another person to make healthcare decisions if the patient is unable to do so.
9. Answers will vary.

CORRECT THE FALSE STATEMENTS

1. True
2. False; should not determine
3. False; are different from those in other situations
4. True
5. True
6. False; State Board of Nursing
7. False; can pass the examination with entry-level knowledge and who cannot

8. False; All nurses
9. True
10. True

MULTIPLE CHOICE

1. b
2. c
3. a
4. b
5. a
6. d

Chapter 5
Basic Human Needs

TERMINOLOGY REVIEW

1. b	4. i	7. l	10. j
2. c	5. g	8. d	11. h
3. k	6. a	9. e	12. f

SHORT ANSWERS

1. Both are levels in Maslow's hierarchy. Primary needs take precedence over higher level needs, without them an individual will die. Secondary needs are met after primary needs are met.

2. Oxygen; a person will die within a matter minutes if deprived of oxygen.

3. Lungs—carbon dioxide and water, skin—water and sodium, kidneys—fluids and electrolytes, intestines—solid wastes and fluid

4. Predictability, stability, familiarity, feeling safe and comfortable, trusting other people, financial security

5. Legally, the nurse must report suspected abuse.

6. Individuals who are homeless are unable to plan for healthcare. They must find food and shelter for themselves and their children. It is difficult to protect themselves and children. It is also difficult to find a permanent job.

7. 37° Centigrade or 98.6° Fahrenheit

8. Survival and security needs

9. Encourage visitors, cards, and telephone calls. Assist clients to worship services. Contact client's clergy or healthcare facility chaplain. See Box 5-1.

10. Encourage independence, reward progress, allow as much self-care as possible, observe for depression, overdependency, or refusal to cooperate. See Box 5-1.

11. A self-actualized individual copes with life's situations, deals with failure, is free of anxiety, has a sense of humor, is self-controlled, and deals with stress productively.

12. Public health measures, access to healthcare, maintenance services, environmental concerns, safely, and emergency services

Table

Basic Physiologic Need	Description of Need	Nursing Interventions Used to Meet Need
Oxygen	Most essential basic survival need. Person will die within minutes without oxygen.	Evaluate oxygenation status of clients. Evaluate circulation. Evaluate emotional status. Administer oxygen.
Water and fluids	Necessary to sustain life.	Assist individuals who are unconscious, unable to swallow, or severely mentally ill. Measure intake and output. Weigh client daily. Observe IV infusion
Food and nutrients	Necessary for life. Body can survive for several days without nutrients.	Encourage good nutrition. Monitor ability to chew or swallow, nausea, vomiting, allergies, refusal to eat, and overeating.
Elimination of waste products	Needed for life and comfort.	Administer enema. Catheterize client. Assist with dialysis. Administer medications. Administer oxygen.

(continues)

(Continued)

Basic Physiologic Need	Description of Need	Nursing Interventions Used to Meet Need
Sleep and rest	Maintains health, but not immediately life-threatening.	Provide safe, confortable, quiet environment. Provide back rub, warm bath, warm milk, medications.
Activity and exercise	Stimulates the mind and body. Enhances circulation and respiration. Not essential for survival.but needed for optimum health.	Ambulate after surgery. Teach client to walk with crutches. Provide passive range of motion. Turn client.
Sexual gratification	May be subliminated and is not vital to the survival of the individual, but is vital to the survival of the species.	Help client feel comfortable with care. Allow client to discuss sexual problems. Refer client to professional counselor if needed.

MATCHING

1. d
2. c
3. b
4. a
5. e

MULTIPLE CHOICE

1. d
2. c
3. b
4. a
5. a

Chapter 6
Health and Wellness

TERMINOLOGY REVIEW

1. n	12. v	23. g	34. dd
2. qq	13. f	24. ee	35. b
3. ll	14. w	25. mm	36. o
4. oo	15. jj	26. y	37. k
5. c	16. p	27. x	38. z
6. nn	17. hh	28. pp	39. aa
7. rr	18. j	29. i	40. t
8. kk	19. q	30. u	41. bb
9. ii	20. cc	31. gg	42. m
10. a	21. s	32. e	43. ff
11. l	22. d	33. r	44. h

CORRECT THE FALSE STATEMENTS

1. True
2. False; mortality
3. False; preventative measures
4. True
5. False; physical activity, overweight and obesity, and tobacco use
6. False; one pack of cigarettes
7. True
8. False; engage in inadequate
9. True
10. False; Smoking
11. True
12. False; just as dangerous
13. True
14. True
15. True

CASE STUDIES

1. The young women should be encouraged to seek prenatal care to prevent complications for her pregnancy. Many problems for the infant can be prevented by adequate prenatal education and care. The nurse should assist her in finding available resources and transportation, if needed.

2. The nurse should discuss with the mother and child the child's activity level. The child should be encouraged to increase physical play activities. The nurse should also discuss healthy eating and nutritious snacks. The nurse should inform the mother and child that health risks developed as a child can increase health risks that stay with them throughout a lifetime.

3. The nurse should discuss the risks of sexual activity, i.e., STDs, HIV/AIDS, unwanted pregnancy, emotional distress. The nurse should discuss safe sex and abstinence. The nurse should be aware of state laws regarding providing information to minors.

4. Discuss the man's risk factors for heart disease, hypertension, CVA, and cancer. Discuss choices he can make to decrease his risks of these disorders. Review benefits of stopping smoking, exercising, and eating healthier.

MULTIPLE CHOICE

1. a
2. b
3. c
4. d

Chapter 7
Community Health

TERMINOLOGY REVIEW

1. s	10. x	19. w	28. c
2. h	11. e	20. f	29. ff
3. ee	12. bb	21. z	30. i
4. a	13. n	22. v	31. d
5. aa	14. dd	23. cc	32. g
6. hh	15. p	24. y	33. l
7. gg	16. u	25. b	34. r
8. q	17. o	26. j	
9. m	18. k	27. t	

SHORT ANSWERS

1. Family, school, place of employment, town, city, state, province, nation, world
2. Goals of UNICEF include nutrition instruction, development of low-cost food supplements, support of general education, childhood immunization programs, procedures for supplying safe water, and infant rehydration programs.
3. Vaccinations, motor-vehicle safety, safer workplaces, control of infectious diseases, declines in deaths from coronary heart disease and stroke, safer and healthier foods, healthier mothers and babies, recognition of tobacco use as a health hazard
4. Roles of the CDC include investigating disease outbreaks at the local, national, or international level; providing current and accurate health-related information to the public; and fostering cooperative relationships with national, state, and local organizations to combat dangerous environmental exposures such as what might occur in the air, the water, and the workplace.
5. Answers will vary.
6. Two functions of the SSA include providing retirement income for many people and financial assistance for healthcare to special populations.

7. Functions of the Red Cross include providing help to victims of disaster and to help people prevent, prepare for, and respond to emergencies.
8. Answers will vary.
9. Causes of air pollution include exhaust, indoor pollution, and smoke. Causes of water pollution include mercury in water, unsafe recycled water, and sewers infecting rivers and lakes. Causes of land pollution include garbage and trash in large cities, overfilled landfills, and radon. Causes of noise pollution include loud noises and music associated with work or recreation.

CORRECT THE FALSE ANSWERS

1. True
2. False; FDA
3. True
4. False; is to uncover new knowledge that will lead to better health for everyone.
5. False; The mission of OSHA
6. True
7. True
8. True
9. False; VNA
10. False; specific disorders

Chapter 8
Transcultural Healthcare

TERMINOLOGY REVIEW

1. c	7. j	13. e	19. p
2. q	8. s	14. v	20. t
3. a	9. o	15. n	21. b
4. u	10. f	16. k	22. h
5. m	11. d	17. g	
6. l	12. r	18. i	

SHORT ANSWERS

1. Three barriers to providing culturally competent nursing care include prejudice, ethnocentrism, and stereotyping.
2. Refer to Box 8-3.
3. An interpreter understands the culture of the person as well as the language. The professional interpreter can explain nonverbal cues.
4. a. Magicoreligious believe that the supernatural forces dominate.
   b. Scientific/biomedical system believes that physical and biomedical processes can be studied and manipulated to control life.
   c. Holistic medicine system believes that the forces of nature must be kept balanced.

d. Yin-Yang theories belief that illness develops when life forces are out of balance.

5. a. Magicoreligious may view mental illness as angels, involvement of deity, or spirits talking.

b. Scientific/biomedical view mental illness as chemical imbalances in the brain.

c. Holistic medicine views mental illness as an imbalance in the forces of nature.

d. Yin-Yang theories view mental illness as an imbalance in life forces.

CASE STUDIES

1. a. Cultural assessment should include traditional healers and practices, traditional family roles and practices in healthcare, and traditional group or societal practices. Assessment should include use of a medicine man and traditional care of wounds.

b. Determine what the herbs are and what purpose they have. Discuss with the client and medicine man if the herbs could be used in a different manner and different placement. Review the information with other staff and the physician.

c. The nurse could have completed a thorough cultural assessment during the initial assessment. The nurse could practice transcultural nursing.

2. a. Completion of a cultural assessment would be needed. The nurse should discuss the decision with the family member.

b. The nurse should respect the client's culture and respect her wishes to allow the family member to make the decision.

3. a. The client's and families' wishes should be respected. The nurse should use nursing measures to provide comfort for the client.

b. Answers will vary.

MULTIPLE CHOICE

1. a. Women of East Indian culture often consider touching a member of the opposite sex other than their husband unacceptable.

2. b. The family members should be allowed to exercise their cultural practices. The candelabra should be examined by appropriate personnel to determine if it is working properly and not a safety hazard.

3. c. During times of stress, such as illness, clients may revert to their native language and an interpreter may be needed.

4. a. This action would help the client exercise cultural practices related to his kosher diet.

Chapter 9
The Family

TERMINOLOGY REVIEW

1. r	6. p	11. j	16. g
2. q	7. c	12. k	17. m
3. b	8. e	13. i	18. h
4. n	9. l	14. a	
5. o	10. f	15. d	

ASSESSMENT REVIEW

1. E	4. E	7. I	10. E
2. E	5. I	8. E	
3. I	6. I	9. E	

CORRECT THE FALSE STATEMENTS

1. True
2. False; childrearing phase
3. False; Parents
4. False; Birth order
5. True
6. True
7. False; Division of labor
8. True
9. True
10. False; child launching, postparenting, and aging.

MULTIPLE CHOICE

1. d. During the finalization stage of divorce the developmental tasks include letting go of the idea of "reunion" and staying connected with extended families.

2. a. See Table 9-1 for description of all developmental tasks.

3. b. Arranging for child care is a major issue when both parents work. Daycare services are a common option.

4. c. All changes in a family have a potential to be stressors; however, a promotion tends to have a positive affect on the family finances.

5. c. Establishing and maintaining a routine can help a child to improve his or her self-esteem and independence.

Chapter 10
Infancy and Childhood

TERMINOLOGY REVIEW

1. h	6. l	11. q	16. o
2. k	7. b	12. e	17. a
3. n	8. c	13. p	
4. f	9. m	14. g	
5. i	10. d	15. j	

THEORIST REVIEW

1. Havighurst theorizes that each life stage has its own group of developmental tasks that a person must accomplish to become a mature, fully functioning individual. As a person accomplishes each task, he or she is ready to take on the next task.
2. a. 2, b. 3, c. 1, d. 4
3. a. hope, b. self-control and will-power, c. direction and purpose, d. self-esteem and competence
4. a. 4, b. 2, c. 1, d. 3

SHORT ANSWERS

1. Growth and development occurs in an orderly sequence: simple to complex; cephalocaudal; and proximodistal.
2. Play is important to a child's development because it helps the child learn about the world, peer cooperation, interaction, and sharing. It promotes muscle coordination and strengthens muscles.
3. Solitary play occurs when children play alone without interaction between each other. This is most common in infants. Parallel play occurs when two children play side by side with the same or similar toys but do not interact with each other or the other's toy. This occurs with toddlers.

4. The nurse should explain to the parent that normal growth and development occurs with in a wide range.

MULTIPLE CHOICE

1. c. Learning to get along with age mates is a developmental task of middle childhood. The other tasks are developmental tasks of the toddler and preschool.
2. a. The deciduous teeth erupt after the principle of center to outside with the central incisors erupting first.
3. a. Motor vehicle accidents are the number one cause of death, and parents should know how to use car seats correctly.
4. c. During a temper tantrum, the family should remove the child from a public setting or ignore the behavior if it occurs at home. The adults should avoid giving in to the child's demands to prevent encouraging continued behavior.
5. a. Children become aware of sexual roles through fantasies and games.
6. b. Assigning simple household chores such as cleaning the bedroom or washing dishes help the child learn responsibility.

Developmental Stage	Age	Physical Development	Cognitive and Motor Development	Key Areas of Concern
Infancy	1–12 months	Gain 1–2 lbs/month Doubled weight by 6 months Teeth erupt at 6–7 months	1–3 months expect someone to comfort them; differentiate pleasant and unpleasant; sleep 18–20 hrs/day; social smile. 4–8 months coo and babble; sleep all night and nap; distinguish between good and bad voices. 9–12 months crawl; know meaning of "no"; take a few steps; hold bottles; say simple words; stranger anxiety	Feedings include breast milk or infant formula the first year; solids may be introduced at 6 months. Bottle mouth Weaning begins when babies can sit upright, support head and neck and grasp object with fingers and put them into mouths. Sucking provides comfort and relieves tension. Day care; difficult decision for parents.
Toddlerhood	1–3 years	Gain 4–6 lbs/year. Grow 2–3 inches/year. 20 deciduous teeth by age 2½.	Verbal skills improve; begin to sense they can control aspects of environment; move with more sureness; emotions are close to the surface.	Toilet training. Accident prevention. Limit setting; must know what behaviors are expected. Thumb sucking and security blanket. Temper trantrums.

Developmental Stage	Age	Physical Development	Cognitive and Motor Development	Key Areas of Concern
Preschool	3–6 years	By age 3 are half their adult height; gain less than 6 lbs/year; grow 3 inches/year.	Dress and undress by themselves; 3-year-olds desire to be independent; 4-year-olds have increased vocabulary, counting, print own name; 5-year-olds know address and phone number.	Sibling rivalry for parental attention; phobias and nightmares; masturbation; enuresis.
School age	6–10 years	Lose deciduous teeth; gain 5–7 lbs/year; grows 2.5 inches/year.	Begin to earn that they must abide by rules; reasoning and conceptual powers expand; produce all language sounds, use simple logic; grasp basics of mathematics; learn handwriting. friends are important.	Sibling rivaly may lead to jealousy, trauma, verbal arguments and physical fights; Responsibilities in the home Sex education.

Chapter 11
Adolescence

TERMINOLOGY REVIEW

1. h   3. b   5. c   7. a
2. d   4. g   6. f   8. e

SHORT ANSWERS

1. Heredity, environment, culture, determination, self-perceptions
2. See Box 11-1.
3. Provide privacy, encourage activities, support decisions, allow independence, give recognition and acceptance, maintain a good family atmosphere, facilitate information gathering
4. Gymnastics, photography, writing, carpentry, auto mechanics, dancing, student government, debate, religious groups, cooking, sports, computer use
5. See table on following page.
6. The adolescent reaches adult height. Hormonal changes occur. Glandular changes can cause acne. Body hair grows and reproductive organs mature. Secondary sex characteristics develop.
7. Boys: testicles and penis enlarge; scrotum changes appearance, pubic hair grows, spontaneous erections, nocturnal emission, and changes in voice and chin whiskers. Girls: breast and hips develop, pubic hair grows, menarche.
8. a. Can be delicate and fluctuate but can influence lifetime interpersonal success by fostering self-esteem and respect. b. Alternate between protectiveness and annoyance. c. Are important in the development of future identity as an adult and are very important to foster feelings of acceptance and belonging. d. Friendships are important in emotional preparation for more intimate and romantic relationships in later life. e. First experience of steady relationship and first love.
9. Noncompliance with medical regimen, school truancy, sexual promiscuity, dangerous activities
10. An unhealthy diet can lead to fatigue, unhealthy appearance, and susceptibility to illness.

FILL IN THE BLANKS

1. emotional
2. parental, individual responsibility
3. identity
4. Skill development
5. abstractly
6. lesbians
7. sexually transmitted diseases (STDs)
8. abstinence
9. firm, fairly

THEORIST REVIEW

1. H
2. E
3. P
4. P
5. H

MULTIPLE CHOICE

1. a
2. d
3. c
4. a

Adolescent Stage	When Stage Occurs	Characteristics of Stage
Pubescence, preadolescence, or early adolescence; sometimes referred to as the awkward stage.	11–14 years	Waver between desire for independence and trust; rebel against authority; quarrel with siblings; start to control emotions and see situations in perspective; begin psychological awareness and objectivity; are enthusiastic; may be seclusive and moody; reflective; verbalize ideas.
Middle adolescence	15–17 years	Introspective, fluctuations in self-assurance, physical alterations, loud-self-assertion, self-preoccupation, mood swings, shifts between dependence and independence, start to plan for the future, concerned with appearance, many friendships.
Late adolescence	18–20 years	Begin to deal with everyday mature issues; move away and become responsible for themselves; may go to college; enter work force or join the military; reflective; relationships are important.

Chapter 12
Early and Middle Adulthood

TERMINOLOGY REVIEW

1. b
2. a
3. d
4. c

ADULTHOOD REVIEW

1. M	4. M	7. M	10. M
2. M	5. E	8. M	
3. E	6. E	9. E	

MATCHING

1. g	4. b	7. k	10. f
2. c	5. h	8. j	11. d
3. i	6. a	9. e	

MULTIPLE CHOICE

1. b. Sheehy's focuses on women's views of adulthood.
2. c. The middle adult must accomplish the challenge of generativity versus self-absorption. The other options are challenges of early adulthood.
3. d. The middle adult focuses on self-awareness and personal fulfillment, although relationships and careers continue to be important.
4. d. All of the factors influence meeting developmental challenges.
5. b. This situation may become more prevalent as the older adult population expands and grown children move back with their families of origin.

Chapter 13
Older Adulthood and Aging

TERMINOLOGY REVIEW

1. d
2. c
3. b
4. a

THEORIST REVIEW

1. E	4. S	7. L	10. S
2. H	5. E	8. E	
3. H	6. L	9. H	

NURSING ACTIONS

1. I	4. I	7. A	10. A
2. A	5. I	8. I	
3. I	6. A	9. I	

MULTIPLE CHOICE

1. b. The older adult needs to prepare for his or her own mortality, but not by withdrawing from society.
2. d. Older adults are often discriminated against by not receiving standard diagnostic tests as younger adults, which reflects ageism.
3. b. Older adults achieve ego integrity if they sense that their lives have meaning and have been worthwhile.
4. d. The fastest growing segment of older adults is older than 85 years of age.
5. a. Older adults have been shown to value religion and spirituality as they age.

Chapter 14
Death and Dying

TERMINOLOGY REVIEW

1. b
2. a
3. d
4. c

CORRECT THE FALSE STATEMENTS

1. True
2. False; in some cultures
3. False; second level of spiritual support
4. True
5. True
6. False; second stage
7. False; may be a very short phase.
8. True
9. True
10. False; may confuse
11. True
12. False; the feeling of sudden helplessness.

MATCHING

1. e, j
2. d, l
3. f, k
4. c, g
5. a, h
6. b, i

MULTIPLE CHOICE

1. b. Spiritual beliefs and practices of Buddhist individuals include the priest performing last rites, chanting rituals, and cremation (common).

2. a. The nurse should assist clients with their spiritual needs whenever possible to help them with the dying process.
3. c. The nurse should continue to interact and provide attention and concern for the client who is dying in the context of the professional relationship.
4. a. Often when a client is in the acceptance and peace stage of dying, the family members feel as if the individual has rejected life or them.
5. b. People are often unresponsive during the detachment stage of dying, and care for others focuses on physical needs.

Chapter 15
Organization of the Body

TERMINOLOGY REVIEW

1. q	13. l	25. e	37. f
2. k	14. i	26. a	38. a
3. m	15. j	27. g	39. d
4. g	16. p	28. h	40. g
5. n	17. d	29. j	41. e
6. a	18. f	30. i	42. h
7. e	19. b	31. k	43. c
8. b	20. h	32. b	44. b
9. c	21. g	33. c	45.
10. h	22. c	34. d	
11. o	23. d	35. a	
12. f	24. i	36. e	

CORRECT THE FALSE STATEMENTS

1. False; Cholecystectomy
2. False; white blood cell
3. True
4. True
5. False; inflammation of the liver
6. True
7. False; pertaining to within a vein
8. False; Tracheostomy
9. True
10. False; wasting or diminution

SHORT ANSWERS

1. a. C, b. N, c. E, d. C, e. M, f. E, g. C, h. C
2. a. distal, b. proximal, c. parietal, d. deep, e. external, d. anterior, e. lateral
3. The brain and spinal cord
4. The heart, lungs, large blood vessels, trachea, esophagus, and thymus gland
5. The liver, gallbladder, part of the large intestine
6. cells, tissues, organs, systems
7. areolar, fibrous, and adipose

8. Membranes function to cover or line surfaces, separate organs or lobes, and some produce secretions.

9. During mitosis the cell replicates itself into two separate cells exactly as the original cell. During meiosis, each egg or sperm cell has half the number of chromosomes needed to form a complete new cell (fertilization). When the egg and sperm are fused during fertilization, a new organism has a full complement of chromosomes.

10. Systems function by groups of organs working together to do specialized work in the body.

MULTIPLE CHOICE

1. d
2. b
3. a
4. a
5. a
6. d
7. b

Chapter 16
The Integumentary System

TERMINOLOGY REVIEW

1. n	9. l	17. f	25. e
2. k	10. o	18. b	26. n
3. c	11. d	19. k	27. h
4. b	12. h	20. d	28. p
5. f	13. g	21. m	29. c
6. j	14. i	22. a	30. j
7. a	15. e	23. i	31. o
8. m	16. g	24. l	

ANATOMY REVIEW

1. nerve endings
2. sebaceous gland
3. papilla
4. stratum germinativum
5. pore of sweat gland
6. stratum corneum
7. muscle (arrector pili)
8. sudoriferous gland
9. fibrous connective tissue
10. adipose cells
11. vein
12. artery
13. pressure receptor
14. hair follicle
15. nerve
16. subcutaneous layer
17. dermis
18. epidermis

CORRECT THE FALSE STATEMENTS

1. False; Langerhans cells in the epidermis
2. False; nail root
3. True
4. True
5. False; the same number
6. True
7. False; of at least 15
8. True
9. False; Eccrine sweat glands
10. True
11. True
12. False; vitamin D deficiency
13. False; gray, brittle, and flaky cerumen
14. False; melanin production
15. True

MULTIPLE CHOICE

1. b	3. d	5. c	7. a
2. d	4. c	6. b	8. a

Chapter 17
Fluid and Electrolyte Balance

TERMINOLOGY REVIEW

1. n	8. p	15. g	22. h
2. w	9. z	16. l	23. m
3. o	10. r	17. d	24. i
4. t	11. v	18. c	25. j
5. s	12. q	19. e	26. f
6. y	13. u	20. k	
7. x	14. a	21. b	

MATCHING

1. f	7. l	13. b
2. m	8. e	14. k
3. i	9. j	15. h
4. d	10. g	16. p
5. n	11. c	
6. a	12. o	

SHORT ANSWERS

1. The three mechanisms of action are the thirst center, which stimulates or depresses the desire for a person to drink; ADH, which regulates the amount of water the kidneys absorb; and the RAA system in which aldosterone controls the reabsorption of sodium by the kidneys.

2. Third spacing occurs when body fluids are not available for use and have accumulated in the interstitial spaces.

3. See Box 17-1: Causes of Edema.

4. See Box 17-2: Functions of Water.

5. Sodium, potassium, calcium, and magnesium are responsible for normal neuron and muscle cell functioning.

6. Answers will vary. Encourage adequate nutrition, encourage balanced nutrition. Avoid excessive sodium in the diet.

7. Diffusion, filtration, and osmosis are passive transport mechanisms and do not required energy or assistance. Active transport requires an energy source.

8. Heat makes molecules move faster and thus the molecules will move across the membrane faster to equalize the number of molecules on both sides of the membrane.

9. The ABGs will indicate the extent of compensation by a buffer system in our clients.

10. Infants have more body fluids than adults as well as immature kidney function.

MULTIPLE CHOICE

1. b	5. b	9. d	13. a
2. d	6. c	10. d	
3. a	7. c	11. b	
4. a	8. a	12. d	

Chapter 18
The Musculoskeletal System

TERMINOLOGY REVIEW

1. c	11. i	21. h	31. g
2. g	12. h	22. e	32. h
3. k	13. a	23. a	33. j
4. m	14. f	24. d	34. a
5. l	15. e	25. b	35. f
6. b	16. l	26. c	36. i
7. j	17. g	27. i	37. e
8. d	18. n	28. k	38. b
9. o	19. j	29. o	39. d
10. n	20. f	30. m	40. c

ANATOMY AND PHYSIOLOGY REVIEW

1. S	5. F	9. S	13. S
2. S	6. S	10. S	14. S
3. F	7. S	11. F	15. F
4. S	8. F	12. F	

NUMBERS GAME

1. 25	4. 90, 90	7. 206	10. 3
2. 40	5. 28	8. 3	
3. 1,000	6. 12	9. 7	

ANATOMY IDENTIFICATION
1. clavicle
2. scapula
3. humerus
4. ribs
5. radius
6. carpals
7. ulna
8. metacarpals
9. phalanges
10. femur
11. patella
12. fibula
13. tibia
14. tarsals
15. phalanges
16. metatarsals
17. calcaneus
18. sacrum
19. pelvis
20. ilium
21. vertebral column
22. costal cartilage
23. sternum
24. mandible
25. facial bones
26. cranium

MULTIPLE CHOICE

1. b	4. d	7. c
2. c	5. a	8. c
3. b	6. b	9. a

Chapter 19
The Nervous System

TERMINOLOGY REVIEW

1. h	9. f	17. f	25. d
2. n	10. i	18. i	26. j
3. d	11. k	19. h	27. l
4. m	12. c	20. c	28. m
5. g	13. a	21. o	29. k
6. e	14. j	22. e	
7. b	15. b	23. a	
8. l	16. n	24. g	

ANATOMY REVIEW
1. Frontal lobe directs body movement.
2. Parietal lobe controls sensations of touch and spatial ability.
3. Gyri are elevations in the cerebrum that increase the brain's surface area.
4. Occipital lobe directs visual experiences.

5. Cerebellum's functions are concerned with movement, coordination, muscle tone, posture, and equilibrium.
6. Spinal cord functions as a major pathway to carry information between the body and the brain.
7. Medulla oblongata contains centers for many vital body functions, including cardiac, vasomotor, and respiratory centers.
8. Pons carry messages between the cerebrum and the medulla. It also acts as a center to produce normal breathing patterns.
9. Temporal lobe controls the sensations of hearing and auditory interpretation, and smell.

CORRECT THE FALSE STATEMENTS

1. True
2. True
3. False; The sympathetic nervous system
4. False; on the opposite side of the body
5. False; only milliseconds.
6. False; involuntary control
7. True
8. True
9. False; pia mater
10. False; cannot be

MATCHING

1. e	4. h	7. k	10. d
2. a	5. j	8. f	11. i
3. g	6. b	9. l	12. c

MULTIPLE CHOICE

1. c
2. b
3. b
4. a
5. c

Chapter 20
The Endocrine System

TERMINOLOGY REVIEW

1. j	5. i	9. d	13. k
2. g	6. a	10. c	14. f
3. m	7. l	11. o	15. h
4. e	8. b	12. n	

ACRONYM REVIEW

1. e	5. c	9. k	13. h
2. f	6. l	10. b	
3. j	7. i	11. m	
4. g	8. d	12. a	

ANATOMY AND PHYSIOLOGY REVIEW

1. Pineal gland—regulates sleep/wake cycles
2. Pituitary gland—controls the action of other endocrine glands
3. Thyroid gland—regulates metabolism
4. Parathyroid glands-increase calcium blood levels and regulate phosphorus balance
5. Thymus—production of T cells involved in immunity
6. Adrenal glands—medulla mimics sympathetic nervous system, cortex is involved in electrolyte regulation, synthesis of glucose, amino acids and fats during metabolism and supplement the sex hormones
7. Islets of Langerhans—primarily involved in controlling glucose levels
8. Ovaries—regulate female sex characteristics, functions, and menstruation
9. Testes—development of male sex characteristics

CORRECT THE FALSE STATEMENTS

1. True
2. False; fatty acids
3. True
4. True
5. False; kidney in adults
6. False; essential glands involved in calcium and phosphorus regulation
7. True
8. False; small, simple portion
9. False; Endocrine glands
10. True

MATCHING

1. d	4. b	7. b	10. a
2. c	5. d	8. c	
3. a	6. a	9. d	

MULTIPLE CHOICE

1. c	3. d	5. b	7. a
2. c	4. d	6. d	8. a

Chapter 21
The Sensory System

TERMINOLOGY REVIEW

1. d	5. p	9. b	13. j
2. e	6. c	10. a	14. h
3. n	7. i	11. k	15. f
4. g	8. o	12. m	16. l

ANATOMY REVIEW OF THE EYE

1. pupil
2. anterior chamber
3. iris

4. conjunctiva
5. posterior chamber
6. retina
7. choroid
8. sclera
9. optic disc
10. optic nerve
11. retinal blood vessel
12. vitreous body/vitreous chamber/vitreous humor
13. cornea

Light rays enter the eye and pass through the cornea, anterior chamber and aqueous humor, pupil (opening) lens, vitreous chamber and vitreous, retina, and optic disc.

ANATOMY REVIEW OF THE EAR

1. tympanic membrane
2. middle ear
3. incus
4. semicircular canals
5. inner ear
6. cranial nerve (CN) VIIII
7. cochlear portion of CN VIII
8. vestibular portion of CN VIII
9. cochlea
10. eustachian tube
11. stapes
12. malleus
13. external acoustic meatus or auditory canal
14. auricle or pinna

Sound waves enter the ear at the auricle, pass through the external auditory canal, tympanic membrane, malleus, incus, stapes, and enter the inner ear at the oval window. In the inner ear, the sound is transmitted through the cochlea in the fluids and hair cells of the organ of Corti. The nerve fibers carry the message to the acoustic nerve, the vestibular portion of CN VIII.

ANATOMY AND PHYSIOLOGY REVIEW

1. F	6. S	11. F	16. A
2. S	7. S	12. A	17. A
3. F	8. S	13. A	
4. A	9. F	14. S	
5. F	10. F	15. F	

MULTIPLE CHOICE

1. a	4. d	7. a	10. b
2. b	5. a	8. c	
3. d	6. c	9. c	

Chapter 22
The Cardiovascular System

TERMINOLOGY REVIEW

1. k	13. c	25. a	37. j
2. l	14. i	26. c	38. k
3. m	15. g	27. k	39. g
4. o	16. o	28. i	40. m
5. n	17. g	29. n	41. e
6. h	18. l	30. e	42. b
7. j	19. m	31. i	43. h
8. f	20. b	32. a	44. c
9. e	21. f	33. n	45. f
10. a	22. d	34. o	
11. b	23. j	35. l	
12. d	24. h	36. d	

CORRECT THE FALSE STATEMENTS

1. False; unidirectional
2. True
3. False; coronary arteries
4. True
5. False; mediastinum
6. False; apex of the heart
7. True
8. True
9. False; Arteries, veins
10. True

SHORT ANSWERS

1. They fit over the heart like a crown (corona).
2. Because of the crescent of half-moon shape of its cusps.
3. Any two of the following: number of pacemaker cells decrease in the SA node, decrease in fibers in bundle of His, and increase in ectopic heartbeats.
4. Tricuspid valve between right atria and right ventricle. Bicuspid or mitral between he left atria and left ventricle.
5. The greater the stretch the greater the force of contraction.
6. The autonomic nerves send input from cardiac center in the medulla to the heart.
7. You would explain what blood pressure is and the factors that influence it (see text).

ANATOMY REVIEW

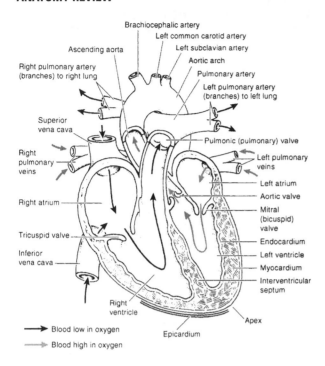

Right pulmonary artery (branches) to right lung

Ascending aorta

Brachiocephalic artery
Left common carotid artery
Left subclavian artery
Aortic arch
Pulmonary artery
Left pulmonary artery (branches) to left lung

Superior vena cava

Right pulmonary veins

Right atrium

Tricuspid valve

Inferior vena cava

Right ventricle

Pulmonic (pulmonary) valve
Left pulmonary veins
Left atrium
Aortic valve
Mitral (bicuspid) valve
Endocardium
Left ventricle
Myocardium
Interventricular septum
Apex
Epicardium

→ Blood low in oxygen
⇢ Blood high in oxygen

Chapter 23
The Hematologic and Lymphatic Systems

TERMINOLOGY REVIEW

1. h	11. d	21. b	31. f
2. k	12. o	22. n	32. g
3. b	13. g	23. l	33. e
4. l	14. i	24. d	34. d
5. n	15. j	25. o	35. a
6. m	16. j	26. a	36. b
7. f	17. c	27. f	37. c
8. a	18. h	28. e	
9. e	19. m	29. k	
10. c	20. i	30. g	

CORRECT THE FALSE STATEMENTS
1. True
2. True
3. False; watery
4. False; decrease
5. True
6. False; Incompatible
7. True
8. False; small intestine
9. True
10. False; inferior vena cava

11. True
12. True
13. True
14. False; capillaries
15. True

NUMBERS GAME

1. 55	4. 4	7. 45	10. 80
2. 120	5. 3	8. 10	
3. 25	6. 1	9. 6	

MULTIPLE CHOICE
1. b
2. a
3. d
4. d
5. c

Chapter 24
The Immune System

TERMINOLOGY REVIEW

1. l	7. d	13. b	19. j
2. i	8. f	14. e	20. d
3. j	9. m	15. c	21. b
4. k	10. g	16. g	22. i
5. e	11. h	17. h	23. f
6. c	12. a	18. a	

CORRECT THE FALSE STATEMENTS
1. False; B cells
2. True
3. True
4. False; Humoral immunity
5. False; tissue rejection
6. True
7. False; lung
8. True
9. False; Antigens
10. False, atrophy

COMPLETION
1. Interferon
2. Immunoglobulins
3. B
4. defense
5. over-reactive

CASE STUDY
After birth, the baby can receive protection through the mother's breast milk. This protection lasts up to 6 months, when the infant's own immune system begins to take over.

MULTIPLE CHOICE

1. a
2. a
3. d
4. b
5. b
6. c

Chapter 25
The Respiratory System

TERMINOLOGY REVIEW

1. o	12. i	23. e	34. l
2. f	13. a	24. o	35. b
3. j	14. l	25. h	36. n
4. k	15. h	26. a	37. f
5. e	16. f	27. n	38. d
6. n	17. j	28. g	39. h
7. g	18. l	29. m	40. c
8. b	19. i	30. d	41. i
9. m	20. b	31. j	42. g
10. d	21. k	32. k	43. m
11. c	22. c	33. e	44. a

CORRECT THE FALSE STATEMENTS

1. False; two layers
2. False; decrease
3. True
4. False; External respiration
5. True
6. False; The sinuses
7. True
8. False; a single layer of cells
9. True
10. True
11. False; is a passive process
12. False; The medulla's respiratory center
13. False; diffusion
14. True
15. True

MULTIPLE CHOICE

1. a
2. b
3. a
4. b
5. c

ANATOMY REVIEW

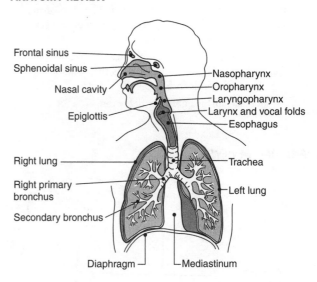

Frontal sinus
Sphenoidal sinus
Nasal cavity
Epiglottis
Nasopharynx
Oropharynx
Laryngopharynx
Larynx and vocal folds
Esophagus
Right lung
Right primary bronchus
Secondary bronchus
Trachea
Left lung
Diaphragm
Mediastinum

Chapter 26
The Digestive System

TERMINOLOGY REVIEW

1. f	12. i	23. c	34. j
2. n	13. k	24. j	35. a
3. b	14. o	25. g	36. e
4. c	15. d	26. l	37. i
5. m	16. b	27. d	38. k
6. a	17. n	28. i	39. d
7. h	18. a	29. m	40. h
8. g	19. e	30. k	41. b
9. e	20. o	31. c	
10. j	21. h	32. f	
11. l	22. f	33. g	

SHORT ANSWERS

1. Answers will vary. See Table 26-2
2. 24 to 36 hours
3. Moisten food particle to make food easier to swallow, begin to break down starch, prevent oral infections, assist in speech and tastes
4. Salty, sweet, sour, and bitter
5. Rugae allow the stomach to distend when food is eaten.
6. Water reabsorption
7. The liver stores fat-soluble vitamins, iron, and B complex. It also forms vitamin A.

8. The endocrine function of the pancreas is to secrete insulin and glucagons. The exocrine function of the pancreas is to produce pancreatic juices of amylase, trypsin, and lipase.

9. Mechanical digestion is the physical breakdown of food whereas chemical digestion is the breakdown of the chemical bonds in food.

10. To increase surface area for digestion.

MULTIPLE CHOICE

1. a
2. c
3. d
4. b
5. a

ANATOMY REVIEW

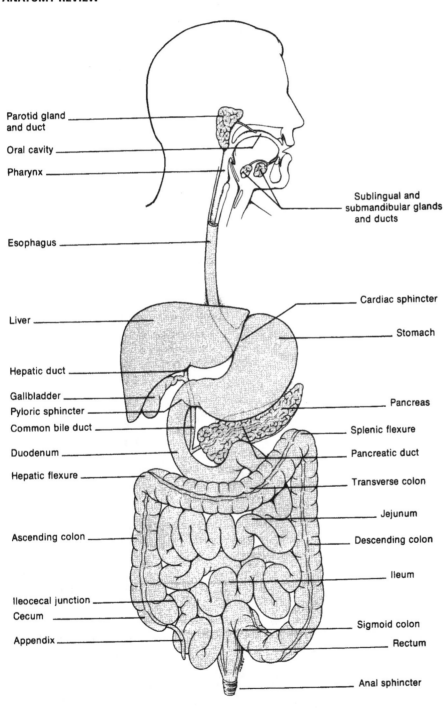

Parotid gland and duct

Oral cavity

Pharynx

Sublingual and submandibular glands and ducts

Esophagus

Cardiac sphincter

Liver

Stomach

Hepatic duct

Gallbladder

Pancreas

Pyloric sphincter

Common bile duct

Splenic flexure

Duodenum

Pancreatic duct

Hepatic flexure

Transverse colon

Jejunum

Ascending colon

Descending colon

Ileum

Ileocecal junction

Cecum

Sigmoid colon

Appendix

Rectum

Anal sphincter

Chapter 27
The Urinary System

TERMINOLOGY REVIEW

1. f	8. m	15. n	22. k
2. j	9. k	16. b	23. d
3. e	10. c	17. i	24. j
4. l	11. o	18. h	25. a
5. a	12. d	19. l	26. g
6. b	13. i	20. m	27. c
7. h	14. g	21. e	28. f

COMPLETION

1. 8
2. 1
3. 4
4. 5
5. 2
6. 95
7. 250, 400

CASE STUDY

Note color, clarity, and odor. Urine is initially a clear amber liquid with a characteristic odor. Abnormal products include blood, pus, or casts. You would compare the client's urine for normal characteristics versus abnormal characteristics.

SEQUENCING

6, 4, 2, 7, 1, 5, 3

CORRECT THE FALSE STATEMENTS

1. False; 1,000 times more acidic
2. True
3. False; glomerulus
4. False; efferent arteriole
5. True
6. True
7. False; increase blood volume
8. True
9. False; have a higher blood pressure
10. False; Tubular secretion

Chapter 28
The Male Reproductive System

TERMINOLOGY REVIEW

1. j	8. b	15. e	22. h
2. h	9. f	16. m	23. g
3. i	10. g	17. i	24. l
4. n	11. a	18. f	25. b
5. l	12. c	19. a	26. d
6. k	13. m	20. j	27. c
7. e	14. d	21. k	

CORRECT THE FALSE STATEMENTS

1. True
2. False; testes is lower
3. False; urine and semen
4. True
5. False; alkaline, acid
6. False; Testosterone
7. True
8. False; 2
9. True
10. True

CASE STUDY

The inguinal canal in men is an opening in the muscular abdominal wall. The inguinal canal is closed; however, it is a weak spot. The testicles descend down the inguinal canal into the scrotum before birth. Due to these reasons, the inguinal canal is a site of common herniation in men.

MULTIPLE CHOICE

1. a
2. d
3. d
4. b
5. c

Chapter 29
The Female Reproductive System

TERMINOLOGY REVIEW

1. d	9. j	17. b	25. h
2. k	10. g	18. j	26. a
3. o	11. a	19. o	27. l
4. i	12. f	20. i	28. e
5. n	13. b	21. k	29. g
6. e	14. l	22. c	30. n
7. m	15. c	23. d	
8. h	16. f	24. m	

COMPLETION
1. progesterone
2. oocyte
3. gonadotropin hormones
4. 16
5. ectopic pregnancy
6. 28
7. perimetrium, myometrium, endometrium
8. 14
9. clitoris
10. episiotomy

CORRECT THE FALSE STATEMENTS
1. True
2. True
3. False; Estrogens, and progesterone
4. True
5. False; estradial, estriol, and estrone
6. False; 300 to 400 oocytes
7. True
8. False; ovarian cycle
9. False; does not ovulate
10. False; follicular phase

Chapter 30
Basic Nutrition

TERMINOLOGY REVIEW

1. r	8. c	15. a	22. j
2. f	9. p	16. k	23. m
3. v	10. b	17. q	24. n
4. d	11. g	18. z	25. h
5. w	12. i	19. t	26. u
6. e	13. o	20. x	
7. y	14. s	21. l	

ACRONYM REVIEW

1. j	7. v	13. u	19. t
2. m	8. e	14. c	20. o
3. q	9. g	15. a	21. h
4. r	10. n	16. l	22. p
5. i	11. f	17. d	
6. s	12. k	18. b	

ANATOMY REVIEW

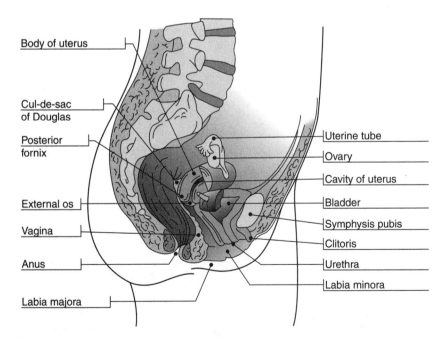

Body of uterus

Cul-de-sac of Douglas

Posterior fornix

External os

Vagina

Anus

Labia majora

Uterine tube

Ovary

Cavity of uterus

Bladder

Symphysis pubis

Clitoris

Urethra

Labia minora

LIFESPAN NUTRITION REVIEW

1. I	4. A	7. A	10. A
2. I	5. I	8. I	
3. A	6. A	9. A	

SHORT ANSWERS

1. BMI indicates that this client is obese, providing the client does not have a large percentage of muscle tissues as with an athlete. Teaching would include measures to decrease intake and increase physical activity, providing it is not medically contraindicated. Teaching should cover the Food Guide Pyramid and Dietary Guidelines for Americans and Guide to Daily Food Choices.

2. Complete proteins, as in all animal protein, provide all essential amino acid in sufficient quantities and proportions for growth and maintenance. Incomplete proteins, such as plant proteins, lack sufficient amount of one or more essential amino acids.

3. a. Carbohydrate—4 C, b. fat—9 C, c. protein—4 C, d. 60 C, e. 36 C, f. 40 C

4. Empty calories are foods that supply calories with few or no nutrients.

5. Adequate carbohydrates are needed in the diet so that the body does not burn its own protein for energy.

6. The four functions of water are: comprises a large percentage of cellular makeup, is one of blood's essential components needed in distributing nutrients, is a solvent, and is necessary for controlling body temperature.

7. Coronary artery disease, certain types of cancer, cerebral vascular accident, diabetes mellitus

FOOD PYRAMID

1. C, 2 to 4 servings
2. B, 3 to 5 servings
3. E, 2 to 3 servings
4. D, 2 to 3 servings
5. A, 6 to 11 servings
6. F, sparingly

MULTIPLE CHOICE

1. c	4. d	7. c	10. c
2. c	5. a	8. d	
3. b	6. c	9. a	

Chapter 31
Transcultural and Social Aspects of Nutrition

TERMINOLOGY REVIEW

1. d
2. g
3. c
4. a
5. e
6. f
7. b

NUTRITIONAL NEEDS REVIEW

1. I	4. I	7. A	10. A
2. I	5. A	8. A	11. I
3. A	6. I	9. A	12. A

MATCHING

1. c	4. e	7. c	10. d
2. a	5. b	8. b	
3. d	6. a	9. a	

MULTIPLE CHOICE

1. a
2. a
3. d
4. b
5. c

Chapter 32
Diet Therapy and Special Needs

TERMINOLOGY REVIEW

1. l	5. a	9. h	13. k
2. e	6. i	10. c	14. g
3. j	7. n	11. b	15. m
4. o	8. d	12. p	16. f

ACRONYM REVIEW

1. b	3. c	5. h	7. a
2. d	4. f	6. e	8. g

CORRECT THE FALSE STATEMENTS

1. True
2. False; both verbal and written instructions
3. True

4. True
5. False; Low-residue diets
6. True
7. False; are avoided
8. False; carbohydrate, meat and meat substitute, and fat groups
9. True
10. True
11. False; can only be used for a few days

MATCHING

1. c
2. d
3. a
4. e
5. b

SKILL DRILL

1. 4	4. 5	7. 1	10. 3
2. 2	5. 7	8. 10	11. 8
3. 12	6. 9	9. 6	12. 11

MULTIPLE CHOICE

1. d	4. b	7. b
2. b	5. a	8. a
3. c	6. b	9. d

Chapter 33
Introduction to the Nursing Process

TERMINOLOGY REVIEW

1. c	4. a	7. k	10. d
2. h	5. j	8. b	11. f
3. g	6. e	9. i	

SHORT ANSWERS

1. Trial and error has been used to distinguish between successful and unsuccessful treatments. It is also used in the laboratory to test solutions to problems. It is used with individuals only with safe guidelines.

2. Examination of facts with information already known, thereby being actively curious and critical of ideas for reasonableness. Form mental pictures of reality. Does not jump to conclusions. Forms own beliefs or ideas. Becomes open-minded and flexible to alternatives. Uses imagination and creativity to gather information and draw conclusions.

3. Critical thinking is a method of problem solving that is neither trial and error nor structured scientific problem-solving system; it uses a complicated mix of

inquiry, knowledge, intuition, logic, experience, and common sense.

4. The nursing process can help you to identify and treat client care problems. It allows for consistency among all nursing staff. It also allows for you to identify actual and potential problems. The nursing process helps avert costly and painful complications.

5. Nursing assessment, nursing diagnosis, planning, implementation, and evaluation

6. Based on scientific problem solving, systematic, client oriented, goal oriented, continuous, dynamic

MATCHING

1. c	4. d	7. c	10. e
2. e	5. b	8. d	
3. a	6. a	9. a	

FILL IN THE BLANKS

1. people
2. logical thought
3. actual, potential
4. measurable, observable

MATCHING

1. c
2. e
3. a
4. b
5. d

Chapter 34
Nursing Assessment

TERMINOLOGY REVIEW

1. d	4. b	7. e	10. j
2. a	5. i	8. h	
3. g	6. c	9. f	

SHORT ANSWERS

1. observation, interview, physical examination
2. visual, tactile, auditory, olfactory (examples will vary)
3. An admission interview is conducted on admission of a client to a healthcare facility. The nurse conducts an interview. A medical history is conducted by a physician.
4. systematic, continuous, analytical
5. client, family
6. Is there any other way in which I can be helpful to you? Is there anything else I should know?
7. Recognizing significant data—involves asking yourself which data items are pertinent to client care. Validating

observations—involves determining if your observations agree with what the client is experiencing; you also may consult colleagues or the nursing team leader. Recognizing patterns or clusters—involves noting what data are similar or have a pattern or connection. Identifying strengths and analyzing problems—includes looking for coping skills the client has for handling problems and noting which problems are actual and which are potential. Reaching conclusions—determining if the client has no problem, may have a problem but additional information is needed, is at risk for a problem, or has a clinical problem with a nursing diagnosis or medical diagnosis.

DATA COLLECTION MATCHING

1. O	5. S	9. O	13. S
2. O	6. S	10. S	14. O
3. S	7. S	11. O	15. S
4. O	8. O	12. O	

MULTIPLE CHOICE

1. b. This question could lead to more information about the severity of the client's problem.
2. b. Subjective data include information the client states. The other options in the question are objective data.
3. d. The client has the right to refuse to answer any question.
4. a. Biographic data include name, birth date, spouse, support person, children, address, occupation, financial status, insurance, and other such information.
5. a. Critical thinking is used by the nurse to draw conclusions and analyze information as well as to plan care.

Chapter 35
Diagnosis and Planning

TERMINOLOGY REVIEW

1. j	5. m	9. n	13. l
2. g	6. b	10. e	14. c
3. h	7. k	11. f	
4. a	8. d	12. i	

SHORT ANSWERS

1. Medical diagnoses are used to establish the disease process for a client. Nursing diagnoses focus on person and are used to determine how the client responds to the disease process.
2. Answers will vary
3. problem, etiology, and signs and symptoms
4. Answers will vary.
   Client will walk 20 feet in the hallway.

Client will have an absence of adventitious breath sounds.
Client will correctly state all current medications.
Client will express desire to quit smoking.
Client will correctly perform sterile dressing change.
5. Answers will vary.
6. Client-centered, specific, reasonable, measurable Examples will vary.

IDENTIFYING NURSING AND MEDICAL DIAGNOSES

1. a. N
   b. M
   c. N
   d. N
   e. M
   f. N
   g. N
   h. M
   i. M
   j. N
2. Answers will vary
   a. Impaired gas exchange
   b. Ineffective breathing pattern
   c. Impaired tissue perfusion
   d. Pain
   e. Impaired skin integrity
   f. Impaired physical mobility

MULTIPLE CHOICE

1. b. The Joint Commission on Accreditation of Healthcare Organizations, nursing home regulators, and Medicare require healthcare facilities to document the NCP within 12 to 24 hours or face severe penalties.
2. a. NCPs are constantly updated when the client's condition changes or as new data are obtained. NCPs are a permanent part of the client's record.
3. c. The RN usually writes the NCP but may be assisted by the LPN or other nurses.
4. c. The nurse establishes priorities first to focus planning on the client's most urgent needs.

Chapter 36
Implementing and Evaluating Care

TERMINOLOGY REVIEW

1. m	7. b	13. c	19. t
2. a	8. o	14. d	20. p
3. x	9. i	15. g	21. n
4. v	10. k	16. h	22. e
5. l	11. s	17. q	23. j
6. r	12. u	18. w	24. f

SHORT ANSWERS

1. a-D, b-I, c-I, d-D, e-ID, f-I, g-ID, h-D, i-I
2. do it, share it, and write it down

3. analyzing the client's response, identifying factors contributing to success or failure, and planning future nursing care

4. healthcare team, client, and family

5. Both involve planning the care for clients by setting priorities and organizing activities. They differ in that the CCP designates specific interventions for all members of the healthcare team. The CCP also designates alternative interventions if the ideal interventions do not work. The NCP does not list alternative interventions, but uses reassessment and critical thinking to modify the NCP if needed.

6. Third-party payers may refuse payment if adequate documentation is not completed.

7. See Box 36-1.

NURSING PROCESS REVIEW

1. c   4. e   7. b   10. e
2. a   5. d   8. a
3. b   6. c   9. d

MULTIPLE CHOICE

1. d. Discharge planning is a process and should be started immediately when the client is admitted to the facility. This ensures continuity of care.

2. c. Relating with clients is an interpersonal skill.

3. b. The nurse is accountable for all actions performed, whether they are dependent, interdependent, or independent.

4. d. Providing a back rub is providing nursing interventions and is the implementation phase of the nursing process.

5. a. Analyzing the client's response to nursing care is one step of evaluation.

6. b. A case manager is most helpful with high-risk clients and those whose care is more complex.

7. c. JCAHO and other federal and state regulatory agencies require QAC to evaluated safe and effective healthcare within the facility.

8. d. If the client's goals were not met, the nurse should revise the NCP after reassessing the client.

Chapter 37
Documenting and Reporting

TERMINOLOGY REVIEW

1. m   6. j   11. n   16. e
2. f   7. d   12. c   17. h
3. a   8. r   13. s   18. b
4. k   9. t   14. i   19. l
5. o   10. p   15. q   20. g

SHORT ANSWERS

1. assessment documents, plans for care and treatment, progress records, and plans for continuity of care

2. The nurse would cross out the incorrect information with a single line, enclose it in parentheses, and write ERROR and initials above it.

3. Mr. N. is a 70-year-old male with pneumonia and has a <u>history</u> of frequent respiratory infections. He is admitted to the unit. His orders include: <u>Diagnosis</u>— pneumonia, normal saline <u>intravenously</u> to run at 100 <u>milliliters/hour</u>, <u>bath room privileges</u>, regular diet, vital signs <u>four times a day</u>

   Alupent 0.3 mL in 3 mL NS <u>by</u> nebulizer, chest x-ray in <u>morning,</u>

   Levaquin 500 mg IV <u>every day</u>

4. D—1800 hours. Client stated, "I feel really hot." Client's skin is warm and diaphoretic. Her temperature is 101° Fahrenheit.

   A—1800 hours. Client was given Tylenol gr X po.

   R—1900 hours. Client's temperature decreased to 99.4° Fahrenheit.

5. Document what you see. Be specific. Use direct quotes. Be prompt. Be clear and consistent. Record all relevant

DOCUMENTATION SYSTEMS TABLE

	Manual Health Record	Electronic Health Record
Benefits	Documents client's relationship with facility Kept in central location and part at client's beside Documents assessment data, care plan treatment outcomes, and daily progress	Fast and convenient to use Uses a terminal at nurse's station, other offices, and/or cleint's room Documents assessment data, care plans, and nursing information as well as diet, laboratory and pharmacy order, billing information
Disadvantages	Care providers must enter information by hand in ink	Needs orientation to system Costly

information. Respect confidentiality. Record documentation errors.

Examples will vary.

6. See Nursing Skills Guidelines, Change-of-Shift Reporting

7. a—A, b—I, c—A, d—A, e—I, f—I, g—A

MATCHING

1. d	5. m	9. j	13. k
2. i	6. f	10. o	14. n
3. c	7. l	11. a	15. h
4. b	8. g	12. e	

Chapter 38
The Healthcare Facility Environment

TERMINOLOGY REVIEW

1. f	5. o	9. g	13. h
2. i	6. l	10. m	14. n
3. a	7. j	11. f	15. k
4. c	8. d	12. e	

FILL IN THE BLANKS

1. Coronary care unit
2. Pediatric
3. Rehabilitation unit
4. Emergency department
5. Obstetrics
6. Hospice
7. Central service supply
8. Quality improvement department
9. Housekeeping
10. chemical dependency unit

SHORT ANSWERS

1. furniture, linens, toilet equipment, other articles. Examples will vary.

2. Keep units clean and orderly. Arrange supplies efficiently. Minimize odors by removing bedpans, urinals, and soiled dressings promptly. Avoid using hygiene products with strong odors. Keep clothes clean and smoke free. Minimize noise to prevent frightening or overstimulating the client. Provide privacy for all clients. Ensure each client unit is thoroughly cleaned after a patient is discharged.

3. Answers will vary. Ensure that the procedure should be completed for the client. Provide for nurse and client safety at all times. Explain the procedures and be honest with the client about expected discomfort. Comfort the client. Document procedures. Ask for help when needed.

4.

Department Category	Examples and Abbreviations of Department	Function of Each Department
Diagnostic and Treatment Departments	1. Pathologists 2. Nuclear Medicine 3. Electroencephalography Department (EEG)	1. Determines the underlying nature of diseases through examination and study of tissues specimens 2. Performs diagnostic and radiation therapy 3. Records and determines electrical activity within a clients brain.
Direct Client Care Departments	1. Orthopedics (ORTHO) 2. Operating room (OR) and Post-anesthesia care unit (PACU)	1. Medical-surgical unit for musculoskeletal disorders 2. Care of surgical clients before, during, and after surgery
Specialized Client Care Departments	1. Intensive care unit (ICU) 2. Dialysis Unit	1. Provides care for critically ill clients 2. Provides care for clients who need dialysis
Support Services (nutritional therapy)	1. Dietary department diets 2. Parmacy Department 3. Admissopms Department and business office	1. Prepares meals and teaches about special 2. Dispenses medications

5. Orient the client to the client unit. Instruct the client on operation of the bed, lamp, call bell, television, and other equipment in the room. Perform any ordered procedures according to general guidelines for performing nursing procedures. Assist client with evening bath and other care before going to sleep.

Chapter 39
Emergency Preparedness

TERMINOLOGY REVIEW

1. e	4. l	7. j	10. g
2. k	5. i	8. a	11. f
3. h	6. d	9. b	12. c

FILL IN THE BLANKS

1. a. dry, b. Locked, c. transfer belt, d. obstacles, e. height, f. unopened, expired
2. emergency signal
3. a. read, b. protective, c. food, d. chemicals, e. indoors
4. substance's
5. prevention, safety
6. initiate, interpret
7. disaster, emergency

SHORT ANSWERS

1. Flammables, poisons, skin/eye irritants, carcinogens, and harmful physical agents
2. Cellular phones, amateur radio operators, television or radio broadcasts, runners, computers, contacts outside the affected area, pagers, portable or hand-held radios, police
3. Have flashlights, battery powered lamps and extra batteries on hand. Have a battery-powered radio on hand. Develop a plan where family members should meet during a power outage. Keep extra water, food, and medicines on hand. Ensure automobiles have a full tank of gas.
4. Include all of the items in the previous questions, plus strategies to keep warm. These would include blankets and shelter.

MATCHING

1. a
2. b, c
3. b, c
4. a, b, c

MULTIPLE CHOICE

1. b. A family escape plan from a house on fire should include a safe place to meet outside the home. This will ensure all family members are safe and accounted for.

2. b. The nurse should immediately assist the nursing assistant to ensure patient safety.
3. d. Side rails should be used with patients who are disoriented, confused, or sedated to prevent injury.
4. c. The nurse should try to get as much information as possible from the caller including where the bomb is.
5. b. The area should be cleared immediately to prevent injury to people in the area in case the package is the bomb. A suspicious package or item should never be touched or moved.
6. d. The client's safety is ensured first, before completing the other interventions. RACE is the acronym used to remember the correct order of procedures during a fire.

Chapter 40
Microbiology and
Defense Against Disease

TERMINOLOGY REVIEW

1. s	9. o	17. f	25. ff
2. x	10. n	18. dd	26. b
3. i	11. a	19. y	27. n
4. m	12. ee	20. q	28. bb
5. cc	13. z	21. l	29. p
6. e	14. g	22. d	30. j
7. u	15. v	23. h	31. r
8. w	16. aa	24. t	32. c

CORRECT THE FALSE STATEMENTS

1. False; organic nutrients
2. True
3. False; at normal
4. True
5. False; pathogenic
6. False; gram-positive and gram-negative
7. True
8. False; Spore-forming
9. True
10. False; should not be stopped, even if
11. False; reservoir, portal of exit, vehicle of transmission, portal of entry, susceptible host
12. False; Handwashing
13. True
14. True
15. True

MICROORGANISMS CLASSIFICATION TABLE

Microorganism	Characteristics	Virulence	Example of Microorganism of Disease
Algae	Resemble plants cells	Rarely cause human disease	Green scum found on sunlit water

Fungi
  a. Yeasts
 	
  b. Molds
	a. Single-celled, reproduce by budding
	
	b. Multicellular, fuzzy appearance, musty smell
		Can cause disease
		
		Multi-celled, common in environment
			Ringworm, tinea capitis, athlete's foot
			  a. thrush
			  b. molds on food

Protozoa	Single-celled, take in food and excrete wastes	Most are nonpathogenic	Pathogenic example: malaria, amoebic dysentery
Bacteria	Single-celled, do not have a true nucleus	Many bacteria can cause disease because of their capsule protection and makeup of cells	Answers will vary; see Table 40-1
Viruses	Smaller than bacteria, protein-covered sacs containing DNA or RNA must be in host cell to	Can cause a wide range of disease	Answers will vary; see Table 40-2

CHAIN OF INFECTION

Diagram includes the reservoir, portal of exit, vehicle of transmission, portal of entry, and susceptible host. Examples of stopping the spread of infection will vary.

Chapter 41
Nosocomial Infections and Medical Asepsis

TERMINOLOGY REVIEW

1. j	5. l	9. b	13. c
2. g	6. a	10. m	
3. h	7. f	11. i	
4. k	8. e	12. d	

SHORT ANSWERS

1. a. age, invasive therapy, frequent antibiotics, poor nutrition

   b. inactivity due to occupation, inadequate defenses due to cigarette smoking, invasive therapy of surgery

   c. age and trauma

   d. age, inactivity, invasive therapy including IV, catheter and surgery, fatigue

   e. poor nutrition, stress, broken skin, possibly poor health

2. Answers will vary. Handwashing, break the chain of infection, see Nursing Skill Guidelines: Preventing Infection

3. a. I
   b. A
   c. I
   d. A
   e. A
   f. I
   g. A
   h. I

4. bacteremias, GI infections, GU infections, respiratory infections, surgical site infections

5. Genitourinary infections

6. Clients should be taught handwashing techniques, hygiene practices, food handling, food preparation, food storage, aseptic techniques for self-care activities.

HANDWASHING SEQUENCING

6
9
2
11
4
8
10
1
7
3
5

MULTIPLE CHOICE

1. b. Genitourinary infections are the most common nosocomial infections.
2. a. Handwashing to remove soil and transient microorganisms is done with routine client care.
3. b. Handwashing should be completed for a minimum of 10 to 15 seconds.
4. c. Latex proteins attach to the powder in gloves and cause reactions through contact or breathing.
5. c. Soaps lower surface tension of the oil on the skin, which holds microorganisms and facilitates removal with rinsing.

Chapter 42
Infection Control

TERMINOLOGY REVIEW

1. l	5. e or i	9. b	13. f
2. g	6. c	10. d	14. h
3. j	7. e or i	11. m	
4. k	8. n	12. a	

SHORT ANSWERS

1. a. M, H; A mask must be worn when entering the room. Handwashing should be completed when exiting the room.

   b. H, Gl; Handwashing should be done before and after the examination. Gloves should be worn during the examination.

   c. H, Gl, M, G, E; all protective equipment would be needed to prevent exposure to splashed blood.

   d. N; No special protective equipment would be needed to talk with a client. Handwashing would be completed between clients.

   e. H, M, MC, Gl; Handwashing would be completed before and after transporting the client. The nurse would need a mask and gloves when entering the room. The client would need a mask when leaving the room.

   f. H, Gl, G; Handwashing will be done before entering the room and after care. Gloves should be worn before entering the room and removed before leaving the room. A gown would be needed to prevent exposure to feces in the bed or on linen.

   g. H, G, Gl, M, E; All equipment should be worn to prevent splashing contaminated body fluids on you during irrigation of the wound.

   h. H, M; A mask is needed when entering the client's room. Handwashing should be done before and after entering the room.

   i. H, Gl; Handwashing is done before and after the procedure. Gloves are needed during the procedure to prevent exposure to blood.

   j. H, Gl; Handwashing is done before and after giving medications. Gloves are applied before entering the room. Use disposable equipment and dispose of them in the room after administration.

2. The client would need airborne precautions. The client would need a private room with negative flow air pressure. The door would need to be kept closed and a mask would be needed by anyone entering the room.

3. Standard Precautions are used to reduce the risk of blood and moist body substances transmissions. They are used with all blood, body fluids, secretions and excretions (except sweat), nonintact skin and mucous membranes.

4. Place the client in a private room. Instruct healthcare workers and visitors they may not enter the room if they have a contagious disease. Anyone entering the room must thoroughly wash hands and wear a mask. Avoid invasive procedures. No fresh fruits, vegetables, or flowers are allowed in the room.

5. The infection control committee monitors and evaluates any infection occurring the facility. When the committee identifies the cause, it can take preventive measures.

MULTIPLE CHOICE

1. a. To prevent accidental needle sticks, do not recap, break, or remove the needle. Discard it immediately into a puncture-resistant container.
2. b. Standard precautions apply to all clients to prevent the transmission of disease.
3. c. The client should be placed in a private room on airborne precautions to prevent the transmission of the chickenpox to other clients or healthcare workers.
4. a. Pneumonia is spread by droplets during sneezing, coughing, talking, or procedures such as suctioning. Teach the client to use a tissue that helps to minimize the amount of disease-spreading droplets.
5. d. If no private room is available, a client on droplet or contact isolation may be placed in room with another client who is infected with the same organism.
6. c. Supplies are stored directly outside the client's room for easy access before entering the room.
7. b. Spending time with the client can help alleviate feelings of loneliness.
8. c. Using disposable equipment in the room will prevent transmission of disease to other clients.

Copyright © 2003 by Lippincott Williams & Wilkins. *Study Guide to Accompany Rosdahl & Kowalski's Textbook of Basic Nursing*, eighth edition, by Lazette Nowicki.

Chapter 43
First Aid

TERMINOLOGY REVIEW

1. v	12. b	23. s	34. ii
2. q	13. qq	24. k	35. m
3. mm	14. j	25. aa	36. e
4. a	15. cc	26. c	37. jj
5. ll	16. bb	27. o	38. u
6. pp	17. hh	28. kk	39. x
7. gg	18. nn	29. r	40. i
8. ee	19. d	30. l	41. y
9. dd	20. n	31. f	42. h
10. t	21. g	32. p	43. ff
11. w	22. oo	33. z	44. rr

CORRECT THE FALSE STATEMENTS

1. False; follow Standard Precautions whenever possible.
2. True
3. False; the tongue falling back and occluding the airway.
4. True
5. True
6. False; Do not, likely
7. True
8. False; homeless people, especially those who are mentally ill, inebriated, elderly, or physically debilitated.
9. False; a medical emergency
10. True
11. False; heat stroke
12. False; denial
13. True
14. True
15. False; Never induce vomiting, unless instructed to do so

SHORT ANSWER

1. Ensure the area is safe before administering assistance.
2. Medic Alert Tags are designed to provide medical information about victims' medical conditions to rescuers.
3. Use the following to help remember the order:
   A = airway and cervical spine
   B = Breathing
   C = Circulation and bleeding
   D = Disability
   E = Expose and examine
4. See Table 43-1.
5. The person's pulse will resume, pupils will constrict, color will improve, and breathing will start when resuscitation measures are successful.

6. Near-drowning victims may be submersed in cold water, which causes hypothermia and decreased metabolism.
7. RICE stands for rest, ice, compression, and elevation. The acronym is used in emergency procedures for sprains and strains.
8. A tourniquet should be used only as a last resort after direct and indirect methods have been used to stop the bleeding.
9. Always use the pressure point on the same side as the injured area.
   a. radial and ulnar
   b. temporal
   c. subclavian
   d. brachial
   e. femoral
   f. facial
10. Refer to Nursing Skill Guidelines: Giving First Aid in Poisoning and Overdose.
11. Factors would include: threat to harm self or others, suicidal thoughts with a plan, refusal to talk further, history of prior suicide attempts, severe depression, intoxication combined with suicidal or violent thoughts or actions, suicidal thoughts but no plan or injury. All of these factors should be reported to your supervisor.

MULTIPLE CHOICE

1. b. Good Samaritan laws provide protection when rescuers give reasonable assistance to the level of your training.
2. a. Early signs of shock include restlessness, panic, mental confusion, disorientation, weakness, and anxiety. The other signs indicate that shock is progressing.
3. a. When treating any emergency victim, always remember to assess airway first.
4. c. The rescuer should look, listen and feel for breathing for 3 to 5 seconds.
5. d. With initial unsuccessful ventilation, repositioning of the head is done; then try to ventilate again. After a second attempt at ventilating, if the airway is obstructed, the rescuer moves to back blows.
6. d. The neck and back should be immobilized to prevent further injury.
7. a. The object is helping to seal the chest wound and should not be removed.
8. c. The affected areas should be warmed slowly in tepid water.
9. a. These conditions prevent the body from cooling itself.
10. b. A person with a suspected fracture should not be moved to prevent further injury.
11. b. Back blows are used on infants to clear the airway; all other options are used with adults.
12. d. For severe anaphylaxis, epinephrine, adrenalin chloride, steroids, and theophylline may be used.

Chapter 44
Therapeutic Communication Skills

TERMINOLOGY REVIEW

1. j	6. g	11. l	16. k
2. h	7. r	12. o	17. i
3. q	8. m	13. p	18. f
4. e	9. n	14. c	
5. a	10. d	15. b	

CORRECT THE FALSE STATEMENTS

1. True
2. False; both the sender and the receiver of messages participate simultaneously
3. True
4. False; who is unconscious
5. True
6. True
7. False; point out the client's behavior or attitude that is underlying his or her words
8. False; "Mal"
9. True
10. False; do need to be

SHORT ANSWERS

1. The student should respond by informing the physician that he or she is a student and cannot take verbal orders. The student can direct the physician to the licensed nurse caring for the client.
2. Sender, message, medium, receiver, and interaction
3. Conveying attitudes of genuineness, caring, trust, empathy, and respect help build an atmosphere of harmony and rapport. Being nonjudgmental and respectful are essential for the client to trust the nurse and share information.
4. Culture, mental or physical disorders, and individual preferences can affect personal space. All information should be used, as well as asking the client, when interpreting personal space.
5. Open-ended questions could be used to determine pain level and client's perception of pain medications and his use of them.
6. a. O, b. C, c. O, d. O, e. C
7. a. "You've been having trouble sleeping, especially at bedtime."
   b. "You're not convinced about the dangers of smoking since the dangers haven't affected you."
8. a. "You seem anxious. You're concerned."
   b. "You don't feel like talking?"
9. Young child—consider development stage and possibly use role-playing.
   Visually impaired—ensure the client knows you are in the room and then explain the procedure.
   Client who is aggressive—see Box 44-1.

Client who speaks a different language—Special Considerations: Cultures.

10. Write down the message including date, time, and your name. Clarify the written message with the caller.

MULTIPLE CHOICE

1. b
2. d
3. c
4. d
5. a
6. b

Chapter 45
Admission, Transfer, and Discharge

TERMINOLOGY REVIEW

1. j	4. a	7. h	10. f
2. e	5. i	8. k	11. d
3. c	6. g	9. b	

SHORT ANSWERS

1. a. See Special Considerations: The Life Span for admission assessment for children. Treat the child and family members with respect. Remember that this is a frightening time and that the child may regress.
   b. Explain the transfer and reasons for the transfer. Remain calm and reassuring. Answer the client and families questions. Remember that this is a frightening time due the worsening of the client's condition. Follow In Practice: Nursing Care Guideline 45-2.
   c. Follow In Practice: Nursing Care Guideline 45-1 Discharge Preparation. Provide for adequate time for teaching. Present material in a nonrushed manner. Provide the information in written format as well as verbally.
2. a. T; b. D; c. D; d. T, D; e. A; f. A, T, D; g. A; h. A, D; i. A, T, D; j. T
3. Client complains of severe pain or seems uncomfortable, abnormal assessment findings, preliminary observations and assessment findings including vital signs, care and treatment that have already been completed
4. Answers will vary and can include assignment to a certain unit is temporary; change in condition; needs quieter environment; disturbing others; and new problem identified.
5. The staff should have the client sign a release form that absolves the physician and facility of responsibility should the client suffer complications. If the client refuses to sign the form, two witnesses should sign the form. The client should be discouraged from leaving.

CORRECT THE FALSE STATEMENTS
1. True
2. False; assumes no liability
3. False; in the hospital gown.
4. False; The healthcare facility can supply
5. True
6. True
7. True
8. False; Before transferring a client
9. True
10. False; seek assistance from other healthcare personnel

MULTIPLE CHOICE

1. c	3. c	5. d	7. a
2. d	4. b	6. c	8. a

Chapter 46
Vital Signs

TERMINOLOGY REVIEW

1. j	8. g	15. h	22. u
2. i	9. o	16. aa	23. q
3. m	10. l	17. p	24. t
4. a	11. n	18. r	25. s
5. e	12. f	19. z	26. w
6. d	13. k	20. x	27. v
7. c	14. b	21. y	

ACRONYM REVIEW

1. e	6. b	11. l	16. s
2. a	7. d	12. c	17. o
3. t	8. q	13. f	18. p
4. j	9. i	14. g	19. h
5. n	10. k	15. m	20. r

ASSESSMENT REVIEW

1. N	6. N	11. A	16. A
2. A	7. A	12. A	17. N
3. N	8. N	13. N	18. A
4. A	9. N	14. N	19. A
5. A	10. N	15. N	20. A

SEQUENCING

ORAL TEMPERATURE
3, 7, 1, 6, 2, 5, 4, 8, 9

RADIAL PULSE
3, 4, 6, 2, 5, 1

BLOOD PRESSURE
11, 1, 6, 4, 7, 14, 2, 8, 13, 3, 5, 10, 12, 15, 9

CASE STUDY
1. No. 190/100. Normal temperature is 98.6° F, normal pulse is 60 to 95 BPM, normal respirations are 12 to 18 per minute and normal BP reading is 120/80.
2. 130
3. Oral, easiest, least invasive, most comfortable
4. Terms such as regular, irregular, or weak could be used
5. Eupnea

MULTIPLE CHOICE

1. a	4. b	7. c	10. b
2. a	5. c	8. d	
3. b	6. a	9. c	

Chapter 47
Data Collection in Healthcare

TERMINOLOGY REVIEW

1. i	13. n	25. c	37. c
2. d	14. m	26. l	38. j
3. f	15. j	27. k	39. h
4. o	16. j	28. d	40. a
5. l	17. o	29. h	41. e
6. b	18. e	30. i	42. f
7. f	19. a	31. i	43. n
8. k	20. m	32. k	44. g
9. a	21. g	33. b	45. m
10. h	22. f	34. o	
11. c	23. n	35. d	
12. e	24. b	36. l	

CORRECT THE FALSE STATEMENTS
1. False; The nursing diagnosis
2. True
3. True
4. False; low intake of protein and vitamin C
5. True
6. False; UPT
7. True
8. False; shellfish or iodine
9. False; for analysis of urine and is part of screening
10. False; Spirometry and pulmonary function tests

ASSESSMENT REVIEW

1. A	9. N	17. N	25. A
2. N	10. A	18. A	26. N
3. A	11. N	19. N	27. N
4. A	12. N	20. A	28. N
5. N	13. A	21. N	29. N
6. A	14. A	22. N	30. A
7. A	15. A	23. A	
8. N	16. N	24. A	

MULTIPLE CHOICE

1. a
2. c
3. d
4. a
5. c

Chapter 48
Body Mechanics and Positioning

TERMINOLOGY REVIEW

1. i	11. f	21. i	31. h
2. e	12. k	22. e	32. a
3. b	13. l	23. c	33. m
4. j	14. d	24. o	34. q
5. m	15. f	25. l	35. b
6. c	16. b	26. i	36. d
7. g	17. d	27. n	37. e
8. n	18. h	28. g	38. j
9. h	19. g	29. p	39. c
10. a	20. a	30. k	40. f

SEQUENCING

DANGLING
6, 4, 2, 8, 9, 7, 3, 5, 1

MOVING CLIENT FROM BED TO STRETCHER
3, 6, 2, 5, 7, 1, 4,

MOVING CLIENT FROM BED TO WHEELCHAIr
5, 10, 3, 9, 2, 8, 4, 6, 1, 7

APPROPRIATE ACTIONS

1. A	4. I	7. A	10. A
2. I	5. I	8. I	11. I
3. A	6. A	9. A	

MULTIPLE CHOICE

1. c	4. b	7. a
2. d	5. a	8. b
3. c	6. d	9. c

Chapter 49
Beds and Bedmaking

TERMINOLOGY REVIEW

1. j	4. k	7. f	10. h
2. c	5. e	8. g	11. a
3. i	6. b	9. l	12. d

SEQUENCING

MAKING A CLOSED OR UNOCCUPIED BED
13, 5, 12, 15, 2, 4, 9, 6, 1, 10, 14, 7, 16, 8, 11

MAKING AN OCCUPIED BED
5, 2, 12, 9, 1, 11, 14, 3, 10, 13, 7, 4, 8, 6

CORRECT THE FALSE STATEMENTS

1. False; open or postoperative bed
2. True
3. False; immediately
4. True
5. True
6. True
7. False; fractures, extensive burns, and open or painful wounds
8. False; be down on the side the nurse is working on
9. True
10. False; side to side

COMPLETION

1. Prevent, assistive
2. Any two of the following: clients with fractures, extensive burns, or open or painful wounds
3. Support, correct alignment
4. Contractures, immobility, wounds
5. Pressure
6. Circle bed
7. Therapeutic beds

Chapter 50
Personal Hygiene and Skin Care

TERMINOLOGY REVIEW

1. g	3. c	5. f	7. a
2. b	4. h	6. d	8. e

NURSING ACTIONS

1. A	4. A	7. I	10. I
2. A	5. A	8. A	
3. I	6. I	9. A	

SEQUENCING

GIVING A BED BATH
6, 3, 4, 1, 8, 11, 2, 12, 7, 5, 9, 10

GIVING A BACK RUB
4, 12, 2, 6, 3, 5, 9, 7, 1, 11, 10, 8

CLEANING DENTURES
5, 8, 1, 7, 10, 2, 6, 9, 4, 3

MULTIPLE CHOICE

1. c	4. d	7. c
2. c	5. b	8. a
3. b	6. d	9. a

Chapter 51
Elimination

TERMINOLOGY REVIEW

1. b	8. e	15. c	22. e
2. n	9. m	16. c	23. a
3. a	10. g	17. m	24. j
4. h	11. l	18. i	25. f
5. o	12. k	19. k	26. b
6. f	13. i	20. d	27. g
7. d	14. j	21. h	28. l

ACRONYM REVIEW

1. f	4. h	7. i
2. e	5. a	8. b
3. d	6. c	9. g

ASSESSMENT REVIEW

1. A	6. A	11. A	16. A
2. A	7. A	12. A	17. A
3. N	8. A	13. N	18. A
4. N	9. N	14. A	19. N
5. N	10. A	15. N	20. N

SEQUENCING

ADMINISTERING AN ENEMA
11, 8, 3, 6, 9, 5, 10, 4, 1, 7, 2

REMOVING IMPACTED FECES
6, 2, 4, 7, 1, 5, 3

GIVING AND REMOVING THE BEDPAN
3, 5, 1, 7, 6, 8, 4, 2

CASE STUDY

1. The nurse should gather more information about the patient's voiding patterns, intake and output status, and physical examination of abdomen and external genitalia. The nurse should assess for any abnormal urinary symptoms such as frequency, urgency dysuria.

2. A plan of care would include helping Mrs. Ortez regain bladder control. Bladder training and Kegal exercise could be used to help the client. Teaching would include all items in In Practice: Nursing Procedure 51-3. The staff as well as the client and family would also need to be taught bladder retraining. It would be important to get all involved persons to understand the process and plan to successful help Mrs. Ortez.

MULTIPLE CHOICE

1. b	3. a	5. d	7. a
2. c	4. d	6. c	8. d

Chapter 52
Specimen Collection

TERMINOLOGY REVIEW

1. a	7. i	13. d	19. i
2. f	8. e	14. j	20. a
3. g	9. c	15. c	21. e
4. b	10. d	16. b	22. h
5. j	11. g	17. f	
6. h	12. k	18. l	

SEQUENCING

OBTAINING A URINE SPECIMEN FROM A RETENTION CATHETER:
5, 3, 1, 6, 2, 7, 4

COLLECTING A STOOL SPECIMEN:
2, 5, 3, 1, 4

MULTIPLE CHOICE

1. d	4. b	7. b
2. c	5. a	8. a
3. a	6. c	9. a

Chapter 53
Bandages and Binders

TERMINOLOGY REVIEW

1. i	4. c	7. h
2. a	5. g	8. b
3. f	6. d	9. e

SEQUENCING

APPLYING MONTGOMERY STRAPS:
7, 5, 1, 4, 2, 3, 6

APPLYING ANTIEMBOLISM STOCKINGS:
8, 4, 3, 1, 6, 5, 7, 9, 2

CORRECT THE FALSE STATEMENTS

1. True
2. True
3. False, stimulates blood return to the heart and prevents blood from pooling in the extremity
4. False, completed ever 2 hours
5. True
6. False, hold perineal or rectal dressings in place
7. True
8. False, may be used
9. False, Montgomery straps
10. False, return to normal color immediately when touched

MULTIPLE CHOICE

1. c
2. b
3. a
4. d
5. b

Chapter 54
Heat and Cold Application

TERMINOLOGY REVIEW

1. l	4. e	7. a	10. b
2. g	5. j	8. c	11. i
3. d	6. k	9. h	12. f

APPLICATION OF HEAT AND COLD THERAPY

1. C	4. H	7. H	10. H
2. C	5. C	8. C	
3. H	6. C	9. H	

FILL-IN-THE-BLANK

1. slowing, congestion
2. change
3. 3/4
4. clean gloves
5. petroleum jelly
6. heat loss, evaporation
7. breathing
8. axillae, groin
9. disinfected
10. physician's order

NURSING ACTIONS

1. I	4. A	7. I	10. A
2. I	5. I	8. I	11. A
3. A	6. A	9. A	

Chapter 55
Client Comfort and Pain Management

TERMINOLOGY REVIEW

1. i	6. g	11. b	16. e
2. k	7. a	12. e	17. b
3. f	8. d	13. d	
4. j	9. l	14. c	
5. h	10. c	15. a	

NURSING ACTIONS

1. I
2. A
3. A
4. A
5. I
6. I
7. A

CORRECT THE FALSE STATEMENTS

1. False, Perception
2. True
3. False, decreased blood supply to the muscle.
4. True
5. False, chronic or neuropathic pain
6. True
7. True
8. True
9. False, Gentle massage
10. True
11. False, breaking the cycle of pain as soon as possible.

MULTIPLE CHOICE

1. a
2. c
3. d
4. a
5. b

Chapter 56
Preoperative and Postoperative Care

TERMINOLOGY REVIEW

1. c	10. f	19. i	28. f
2. a	11. e	20. b	29. m
3. e	12. f	21. k	30. k
4. i	13. c	22. d	31. l
5. b	14. g	23. j	32. h
6. h	15. d	24. b	33. a
7. d	16. h	25. e	34. g
8. g	17. j	26. i	
9. j	18. a	27. c	

NURSING ACTIONS

1. A	5. A	9. A	13. I
2. A	6. I	10. I	
3. I	7. I	11. A	
4. A	8. A	12. A	

CORRECT THE FALSE STATEMENTS

1. True
2. False, emergency surgery
3. True
4. False, remain normal.
5. True
6. True
7. False, for all clients over age 40
8. True
9. False, hemorrhage, shock, hypoxia and hypothermia.
10. True

CASE STUDY

1. Assess Mr. J since he is displaying signs of shock. His pulse is at the high normal limits, respirations are low, and BP is low normal.
2. Assess the sequential machine for Mrs. P. Ensure that it is working or replace it. The machine is needed to prevent thrombophlebitis.
3. Instruct Mr. M to ambulate to help the flatus escape and relieve the pain.

4. Remove Mrs. H's catheter to assist her with normal elimination.

MULTIPLE CHOICE

1. b	4. b	7. a	10. d
2. a	5. c	8. d	
3. c	6. a	9. a	

Chapter 57
Surgical Asepsis

TERMINOLOGY REVIEW

1. k	5. j	9. m	13. e
2. i	6. b	10. l	14. g
3. h	7. f	11. a	
4. n	8. c	12. d	

CORRECT THE FALSE STATEMENTS

1. False, Sterile technique
2. True
3. False, cannot be used on plastic.
4. False, do
5. True
6. False, above the nipple line
7. False, 750 to 1,000 mL
8. True
9. False, open the flap toward the back of the table.
10. True

SEQUENCING

PUTTING ON STERILE GLOVES:
2, 4, 1, 5, 3

CATHETERIZING A FEMALE CLIENT:
4, 8, 15, 11, 2, 13, 16, 6, 10, 1, 3, 7, 14, 9, 5, 2

Chapter 58
Wound Care

TERMINOLOGY REVIEW

1. e	5. i	9. h	13. a
2. m	6. g	10. k	14. d
3. h	7. f	11. l	
4. c	8. b	12. j	

NURSING ACTIONS

1. I	4. I	7. I	10. A
2. A	5. A	8. A	
3. A	6. A	9. I	

SEQUENCING

CHANGING A STERILE DRESSING:
2, 8, 10, 1, 6, 7, 12, 9, 4, 3, 11, 5

IRRIGATING A STERILE WOUND:
1, 6, 4, 8, 2, 11, 3, 7, 9, 10, 5, 12

MULTIPLE CHOICE

1. b
2. c
3. c
4. b
5. a

Chapter 59
Care of the Dying Person

TERMINOLOGY REVIEW

1. g	6. h	11. g	16. h
2. f	7. c	12. i	17. a
3. d	8. e	13. j	18. b
4. b	9. i	14. e	19. f
5. a	10. d	15. c	

SHORT ANSWER

1. Answers may vary.
   a. Care of the mouth, nose, and eyes: swab the client's mouth with mouthwash to keep it clean, turn the client to promote drainage, free the nostrils of crust, moisten the tongue, wipe eyes with moist cotton balls.
   b. Breathing difficulties: turn the client onto the side or prop up client into a partially sitting position.
   c. Incontinent clients should be kept clean and dry.
   d. Nutrition may be provided through tube feelings or TPN.
   e. Odor control: keep dressings clean and dry, keep drainage bags emptied, and use subtle deodorizers.
2. Answers will vary. See Box 59-1. Failing circulation and failing senses are signs of approaching death.
3. A dead person's body should be cared for with respect and cleaned up. See In Practice: Nursing Process 59-1 for details.
4. Belongings should be sent home with the family. Ensure that you have the family members sign that they received the belongings. The funeral director may be given dentures and glasses.
5. The dying person should be treated with respect. The dying person is comforted knowing that his or her life was of value and that he or she made a difference in the world. Encourage family members to share their feelings of love with the dying person. Allow the dying person to care for himself or herself and to be as independent as possible.
6. Allow the son to verbalize his feelings and concerns. Assure the son that it is normal for a dying person to want to plan for his or her funeral. Discuss with the son that most dying people want permission from the family that is it okay for them to die.

CORRECT THE FALSE STATEMENTS

1. True
2. True
3. False, It is the nurse's responsibility
4. False, on their sides
5. False, 8 hours
6. False, keep a light on
7. True
8. True
9. True
10. False, acceptable.

Chapter 60
Review of Mathematics

TERMINOLOGY REVIEW

1. e	6. r	11. i	16. d
2. p	7. m	12. j	17. a
3. g	8. f	13. b	18. h
4. n	9. q	14. c	
5. o	10. l	15. k	

MATCHING

1. e
2. d
3. a
4. f
5. c

SHORT ANSWER

1. Because you are converting from a smaller to a larger unit, you would divide milligrams by 1,000 or move the decimal three places to the left.
2. First write the problem, second invert the divisor, and then multiply the numerators and denominators.
3. Smaller, half
4. Double-check the dosage conversions using a reference book or table; have another nurse double-check the calculations.

5. The nurse needs basic math skills to work with medications, calculate dosages correctly, and administer medications safely.
6. The product of the means equals the product of the extremes. The product of the means divided by one extreme yields the other mean. The product of the extremes divided by one mean yields the other mean.
7. The percent number becomes the numerator (drop the percentage symbol), and 100 is always the denominator.

MATCHING

1. b	5. c	9. c	13. c
2. a	6. a	10. a	
3. c	7. a	11. c	
4. b	8. b	12. a	

MULTIPLE CHOICE

1. d
2. a
3. d, Set up the problem: $(D)/(A) \times$ quantity $= 1/1$- divided by $1/200 \times 1$ tablet $= 1/100 \times 200/1 = 200/100 = 2$ tablets or gr $1/100 : 1$ tab $::$ gr $1/200 :$ Xtab $= 1/100 \times :: 1/200$, $X = 200/100 = 2$
4. d, $30\% = 30/100 \times 3,000/1 \rightarrow 30 \times 3,000/100 = 90,000/100 = 900$
5. b, $(D)/(A) \times$ quantity $= 60$ mg$/120$ mg $\times 5$ mL $= 0.5 \times 5 = 2.5$
6. c, Consult the table of equivalents and set up the problem; 1 tsp $: 5$ mL $:: 2$ tsp $: X \rightarrow X = 10$ mL
7. a, 50 mL $: 1$ hour $:: 250$ mL $: X \rightarrow 50X : 250$ mL $\rightarrow X = 250/50 = 5$ hours

Chapter 61
Introduction to Pharmacology

TERMINOLOGY REVIEW

1. n	7. q	13. l	19. b
2. k	8. t	14. h	20. c
3. o	9. s	15. a	21. j
4. w	10. p	16. g	22. i
5. r	11. u	17. e	23. d
6. v	12. m	18. f	

ACRONYM REVIEW

1. f	4. e	7. d	10. a
2. j	5. g	8. b	11. c
3. k	6. h	9. i	

ABBREVIATION REVIEW

1. BID = twice a day
2. IM = intramuscular
3. ou = both eyes
4. q = every
5. qd = every day
6. QID = four times a day
7. QOD = every other day
8. stat = immediately
9. subq = subcutaneous
10. susp = suspension

SHORT ANSWERS

1. Any three of the following would be correct: the drug classification, use, recommended dosage, desired effects, possible adverse or untoward effects, and route of administration.
2. Intramuscular, subcutaneous, intradermal, and intravenous
3. Any four of the following would be correct: age, gender, weight, condition, disposition and psychological state, method of administration, distribution, environment, time of administration, and elimination.
4. Physicians (MD), osteopaths (DO), dentists (DDS and DMD), physician assistants (PA), nurse practitioners (NP), midwives (CNM), and veterinarians (DVM)
5. At the end of the shift, the oncoming nurse counts the medications, and the outgoing nurse records. This ensures that all medications are there.
6. Therapeutic—amount of medication required to obtain a desired effect in the majority of people
   Minimal—smallest amount necessary to achieve a therapeutic effect
   Maximal—largest amount that can be given safely without causing an adverse reaction or toxic effect
   Toxic—amount of medication that causes symptoms of poisoning
   Lethal—amount of medication that will cause death

MULTIPLE CHOICE

1. a
2. b
3. a
4. c
5. b

Chapter 62
Classifications of Medications

TERMINOLOGY REVIEW

1. j	5. l	9. m	13. f
2. d	6. a	10. c	14. k
3. n	7. i	11. e	
4. g	8. b	12. h	

MEDICATION TABLE

Classification/Medication	Action/Use	Side Effects	Nursing Considerations
Penicillins (amoxicillin/[Amoxil])	Inhibit growth of bacteria; used to treat narrow spectrum of bacteria. Amoxil has extended spectrum of effectiveness.	Allergic reaction, sensitivity, generally few side effects	Take all of the medication; observe for reactions.
Hypnotics (phenobarbital/[Luminal])	Produce sedation and sleep (control seizures)	Drowsiness, lethargy, depression	Caution to avoid activities requiring alertness; watch for abuse; alcohol intensifies effect
Nonsteroidal anti-inflammatory drugs (NSAIDs)	Analgesic effect, anti-inflammatory action	Gastric upset	Administer with food
Adrenergic medications (epinephrine/[Adrenaline])	Mimic the actions of the sympathetic nervous system; used in treatment of anaphylactic reactions, asthma attacks	Nervousness, tachycardia, heart palpitations, nausea, tremors, headache	Reassure SE are short lived; used cautiously in clients with heart disease, hypertension, DM, or hyperthyroidism; contraindicated in pregnancy
Steroids (prednisone/[Delta-Cortef])	Anti-inflammatory agent	Cushingoid side effects	Instruct to take with food; do not discontinue abruptly
Narcotic analgesic (morphine)	Has a depressant effect on the brain; used to treat severe pain	Nausea, vomiting, constipation, respiratory depression	Administer antiemetic if needed; have Narcan available to counter effects of too much morphine; ensure client safety; monitor VS
Anticoagulants (heparin)	Increase the time it takes blood to coagulate; used to treat thrombophlebitis, prevent thrombus formation, and treat blood disorders	Excessive thinning of the blood	Monitor for bleeding (i.e., of the gums), bruising, occult blood

ACRONYM REVIEW
1. g   5. f   9. h   13. j
2. n   6. c   10. b   14. a
3. p   7. o   11. k   15. d
4. e   8. l   12. m   16. i

MATCHING
1. c   5. e   9. f   13. k
2. h   6. j   10. b   14. l
3. g   7. a   11. n
4. i   8. d   12. m

MULTIPLE CHOICE
1. a   4. a   7. c   10. c
2. d   5. b   8. d
3. b   6. b   9. d

Chapter 63
Administration of Medications

TERMINOLOGY REVIEW

1. m	6. s	11. o	16. k
2. p	7. j	12. i	17. f
3. t	8. d	13. r	18. n
4. c	9. e	14. l	19. g
5. h	10. a	15. b	20. q

ACRONYM REVIEW

1. i	7. s	13. j	19. d
2. u	8. h	14. v	20. a
3. b	9. f	15. q	21. e
4. o	10. p	16. k	22. l
5. g	11. w	17. r	23. c
6. n	12. t	18. m	

SEQUENCING

ADMINISTERING ORAL MEDICATION:
5, 7, 12, 2, 10, 4, 11, 6, 9, 1, 3, 8

DRAWING UP A MEDICATION FROM A VIAL:
4, 5, 3, 2, 1

GIVING A SUBCUTANEOUS INJECTION:
4, 6, 7, 10, 3, 9, 2, 5, 8, 1

ADMINISTERING MEDICATION THROUGH A G-TUBE:
3, 1, 7, 5, 2, 6, 4

MATCHING

1. b, h
2. d, i
3. e, i
4. a, h
5. c, i
6. f, i
7. g, i

CASE STUDY

The nurse should take measures to ensure that the most important medications are given first. The Capoten should be given first, followed by the other medications. The nurse could use the cough syrup as a liquid to swallow the other medications. The nurse should keep the medications separate to ensure that if the client does not take all the medications, the nurse can accurately document what was given as well as ensure that the most important medications are given first.

MULTIPLE CHOICE

1. c	4. b	7. b	10. b
2. a	5. c	8. a	11. c
3. b	6. d	9. a	

Chapter 64
Normal Pregnancy

TERMINOLOGY REVIEW

1. a	9. g	17. k	25. f
2. i	10. h	18. d	26. n
3. b	11. n	19. c	27. a
4. d	12. k	20. l	28. j
5. c	13. m	21. i	29. m
6. f	14. j	22. b	30. e
7. e	15. l	23. o	31. p
8. o	16. g	24. h	

ACRONYM REVIEW

1. h	4. f	7. e
2. i	5. g	8. b
3. d	6. a	9. c

ASSESSMENT REVIEW

1. probable
2. presumptive
3. probable
4. presumptive
5. positive
6. presumptive
7. probable
8. probable
9. positive
10. presumptive
11. presumptive
12. probable
13. presumptive
14. presumptive
15. probable

COMPLETION

1. 300
2. softener, fiber, laxatives
3. soap
4. not harmful
5. first
6. Morning sickness, frequent, small, dry
7. Antepartal classes
8. expectations, physical, emotional
9. seven, ten
10. Doppler, fetoscope

11. four weeks.
12. Rh negative
13. never recommended
14. Lamaze
15. wife, child

CASE STUDY

1. Assess the client for other presumptive signs of pregnancy. Complete a physical examination. LNMP date should be determined. Await results of pregnancy testing.
2. Instruct client on common discomforts of pregnancy using anticipatory guidance. See Table 64-1 for common discomforts of pregnancy and relief measures.
3. The client's developmental task is pregnancy validation, which means she will need to accept this pregnancy. She may display ambivalence, shock, and disbelief and may tend to focus on herself and the changes she is experiencing. Fear is common as well.

MULTIPLE CHOICE

1. b	5. a	9. c	13. c
2. b	6. a	10. d	14. b
3. c	7. a	11. d	
4. d	8. c	12. b	

Chapter 65
Normal Labor, Delivery, and Postpartum Care

TERMINOLOGY REVIEW

1. j	9. d	17. b	25. f
2. l	10. h	18. l	26. n
3. m	11. e	19. h	27. a
4. g	12. f	20. d	28. j
5. n	13. i	21. i	29. g
6. k	14. b	22. m	
7. c	15. o	23. k	
8. a	16. e	24. c	

STAGES OF LABOR REVIEW

1. c	4. a	7. c	10. c
2. a	5. d	8. d	
3. b	6. b	9. b	

ASSESSMENT REVIEW

1. N	7. A	13. N	19. N
2. A	8. N	14. A	20. N
3. N	9. N	15. A	21. N
4. N	10. A	16. N	
5. A	11. A	17. N	
6. A	12. N	18. A	

SHORT ANSWER

1. Longitudinal
2. Transverse
3. Any of the following: sharp, unremitting pain, prolonged contractions or failure of the uterus to relax, change in character of the fetal heartbeat, abnormal deceleration pattern, bleeding, extreme maternal exhaustion, cessation of labor after it has begun, hypotension or increased pulse rate of the mother, prolapse of the umbilical cord, irregular fatal heartbeat
4. See Table 65-1
5. The nurse should teach the client about breast care, nursing/feeding infant, perineal care, fundus observation, fluid intake, voiding, ambulation, engorgement, involution, infant care, follow-up care, and signs of complications. The nurse should include routine discharge instructions such as any medications, follow-up appointment, and referrals if needed.
6. Urinary catheterization may be needed to keep the bladder empty during labor to prevent trauma, urinary incontinence during delivery, and urinary retention in the immediate postpartum period.

CASE STUDY

1. The nurse will need to massage the fundus. See the nursing skill procedure for massaging the fundus. The procedure includes: cup hand around the uterine fundus, place other hand over the symphysis pubis to stabilize the uterus, rotate your hand gently over the fundus, observe for passage of clots, clean woman's vulva and perineum, apply clean perineal pad.
2. Instruct the client not to massage a firm fundus. Other instructions regarding routine postpartum care could be given.

MULTIPLE CHOICE

1. d	4. a	7. c	10. d
2. a	5. b	8. b	11. b
3. c	6. b	9. d	12. c

Chapter 66
Care of the Normal Newborn

TERMINOLOGY REVIEW

1. b	10. k	19. b	28. l
2. c	11. h	20. g	29. c
3. l	12. d	21. f	30. f
4. i	13. i	22. a	31. i
5. j	14. j	23. e	32. g
6. a	15. l	24. d	33. b
7. e	16. c	25. k	34. h
8. g	17. h	26. d	35. e
9. f	18. k	27. a	36. l

ASSESSMENT REVIEW

1. N	8. N	15. A	22. N
2. A	9. N	16. N	23. N
3. A	10. A	17. A	24. A
4. N	11. A	18. A	25. N
5. N	12. A	19. N	
6. N	13. N	20. A	
7. N	14. N	21. N	

SEQUENCING

WEIGHING A BABY:
3, 5, 1, 2, 4

BATHING A BABY:
3, 5, 9, 4, 6, 1, 7, 10, 2, 8

SHORT ANSWER

1. The first few breaths assist with the conversion from fetal to adult circulation, empty the lungs of liquid, and establish neonatal lung volume and function in the newborn.
2. Heart rate, respiratory rate, muscle tone, reflexes/irritability, color
3. Methods to identify newborns include immediate application of ID bands on mother, infant, and father; foot printing, electronic bracelets, documentation of newborn's information. It is essential to complete this information to ensure proper identification of the infant with the mother/parents as well as to prevent abduction of the infant.
4. Allow the mother/parents to spend as much time together as possible in the first hours of life. Encourage the family to interact and touch the infant.
5. See Box 66-1 on conserving heat.
6. The mother should be taught to swab the stump with alcohol with each diaper change, apply Triple Dye as ordered, do not place the diaper over the stump, and do not submerge the baby in water until the stump falls off.
7. Advantages of breastfeeding include better nutrition, less risk for allergies, reduced risk for infections. Breastfeeding also enhances bonding, promotes involution of uterus, delays ovulation, provides milk at correct temperature, is readily available, and is economical.
8. Bubbling the newborn is gently assisting the newborn to remove gas in the stomach to prevent regurgitation. The baby is held upright or prone over the knees and the back is gently patted. Bubbling should be done when switching breasts for the breast-fed infant and after 1/2 to 1 oz for bottle-fed infants. All infants should be bubbled at the end of each feeding.

MULTIPLE CHOICE

1. b	5. b	9. c	13. d
2. a	6. a	10. c	
3. c	7. a	11. c	
4. b	8. d	12. a	

Chapter 67
High-Risk Pregnancy and Childbirth

TERMINOLOGY REVIEW

1. j	10. e	19. f	28. h
2. g	11. h	20. c	29. d
3. f	12. c	21. a	30. k
4. d	13. a	22. b	31. f
5. l	14. j	23. g	32. j
6. i	15. i	24. d	33. e
7. b	16. j	25. g	34. c
8. n	17. e	26. i	35. a
9. m	18. h	27. b	

ACRONYM REVIEW

1. q	6. n	11. r	16. j
2. d	7. l	12. i	17. p
3. k	8. f	13. m	18. c
4. g	9. b	14. h	
5. o	10. a	15. e	

ASSESSMENT REVIEW

1. A	6. A	11. A	16. N
2. A	7. A	12. A	17. A
3. N	8. N	13. N	18. A
4. A	9. N	14. A	19. A
5. A	10. N	15. N	20. A

CORRECT THE FALSE STATEMENTS

1. True
2. False, ultrasound scan
3. False, Oxytocin
4. True
5. True
6. True
7. False, Mild preeclampsia
8. False, Diabetes mellitus
9. False, phototherapy.
10. True
11. True
12. False, PROM
13. False, the buttocks present with the knees bent and the feet next to the buttocks.
14. True
15. True
16. False, ambulate early.
17. False, postpartum hematoma.
18. True
19. True
20. True

MULTIPLE CHOICE

1. c
2. b
3. b
4. a
5. c

Chapter 68
The High-Risk Newborn

TERMINOLOGY REVIEW

1. c	8. h	15. i	22. k
2. j	9. a	16. j	23. f
3. g	10. m	17. g	24. a
4. i	11. l	18. b	25. c
5. e	12. d	19. h	
6. b	13. f	20. d	
7. k	14. l	21. e	

ACRONYM REVIEW

1. c	5. l	9. a	13. e
2. j	6. d	10. i	14. k
3. f	7. n	11. b	
4. h	8. o	12. g	

ASSESSMENT REVIEW

1. A	5. N	9. A	13. N
2. N	6. N	10. A	14. A
3. A	7. A	11. A	15. A
4. A	8. A	12. A	

NURSING ACTIONS

1. A	5. I	9. A	13. A
2. A	6. A	10. A	14. A
3. A	7. I	11. A	15. I
4. I	8. A	12. I	

MULTIPLE CHOICE

1. a
2. a
3. c
4. c
5. b
6. c

Chapter 69
Sexuality, Fertility, and Sexually Transmitted Diseases

TERMINOLOGY REVIEW

1. k	13. f	25. n	37. n
2. n	14. i	26. h	38. c
3. m	15. c	27. j	39. o
4. b	16. i	28. l	40. a
5. h	17. k	29. b	41. h
6. o	18. g	30. f	42. l
7. j	19. m	31. e	43. g
8. g	20. d	32. b	44. d
9. l	21. c	33. m	45. j
10. a	22. e	34. i	
11. e	23. a	35. f	
12. d	24. o	36. k	

SHORT ANSWER

1. Erectile dysfunction is the most common sexual dysfunction in males. Causes of the disorder can include medical causes such as STDs, chronic health disorder, open-heart surgery, prostate disorders, hormonal disorders, some medications, chemicals, and neurologic damage or disorders. Psychological factors can also be a cause.

2. Dyspareunia, vaginismus, chronic illnesses, and hormonal imbalances can cause female sexual dysfunction.

3. Rubin's test involves inflating the oviducts with carbon dioxide to determine tube patency. Hysterosalpingogram examines the fallopian tubes and uterus for problems. Curettage involves obtaining a uterine tissue sample to determine whether the uterine lining is normal.

4. EC must begin within 72 hours of unprotected sex. EC involves two doses 12 hours apart and is most effective if taken within 24 hours after intercourse.

5. Instruct the client that chemical barriers are more effective when combined with mechanical barriers. The client should follow the directions on the product closely and use before any genital–genital contact.

6. Risk factors for acquiring STDs include number of sexual partners, sexual freedom, being adolescent, and other factors for individual types of STDs.

7. Unprotected sex causes scratching or irritation of tissues and leads to fissures as a direct route for invasion of HIV.

8. a. HIV: treatment with medications to decrease viral loads
b. *Chlamydia*: tetracycline and doxycycline to treat client and partners simultaneously
c. Gonorrhea: treat with IM injections of ceftriaxone or cefixime; check for other STDs.
d. Syphilis: treat with benzathine penicillin G IM
e. HSV-2: treatment is palliative with antiviral medications; assess for cervical and prostate cancer

MULTIPLE CHOICE

1. a	3. c	5. d	7. d
2. b	4. a	6. d	8. c

Chapter 70
Fundamentals of Pediatric Nursing

TERMINOLOGY REVIEW

1. d	6. a	11. a	16. e
2. e	7. b	12. h	17. g
3. c	8. j	13. f	18. b
4. f	9. l	14. k	19. d
5. g	10. i	15. c	

FILL-IN-THE-BLANK
1. Play
2. milestone, delays
3. young
4. restraints, 1, 2, every
5. Never
6. protect

7. a. birth to 2 months; b. 2 months, 4 months, 6 months, 12 to 15 months; c. one recommended before school; d. two immunizations after the child's first birthday; e. 2 months, 4 months, 6 months, 15 to 18 months, 4 to 6 years

8. Any four of the following: restlessness, panic, tachycardia, tachypnea, nasal flaring, wheezing, stridor, change of color, expiratory grunt, retractions, gasping, shallow labored breathing, head bobbing.

9. infant seat
10. 104
11. speech, hearing, vision
12. privacy or protecting their modesty
13. protest, despair, denial
14. same time each day before feeding.
15. 30

SEQUENCING

USING AN OXY-HOOD:
3, 7, 9, 4, 5, 1, 6, 2, 8

MULTIPLE CHOICE

1. b	3. c	5. d	7. b
2. a	4. a	6. d	8. c

Chapter 71
Care of Infant, Toddler, Preschooler

TERMINOLOGY REVIEW

1. n	13. d	25. b	37. o
2. h	14. m	26. a	38. l
3. i	15. f	27. j	39. n
4. k	16. e	28. h	40. i
5. e	17. i	29. n	41. m
6. b	18. o	30. d	42. b
7. o	19. f	31. a	43. c
8. l	20. c	32. e	44. d
9. j	21. g	33. h	45. f
10. c	22. l	34. j	
11. a	23. k	35. k	
12. g	24. m	36. g	

ASSESSMENT REVIEW

1. A	5. A	9. A	13. A
2. A	6. A	10. A	14. A
3. N	7. A	11. A	15. A
4. N	8. N	12. N	

NURSING ACTIONS

1. I	5. A	9. A	13. I
2. A	6. I	10. I	14. A
3. A	7. I	11. A	15. A
4. I	8. A	12. A	

SEQUENCING

USING THE APNEA MONITOR:
5, 1, 4, 3, 7, 2, 6

LABELING

A. stenosis of pulmonary artery
B. aorta overriding both ventricles
C. ventricular septal defect
D. hypertrophy of right ventricle

MULTIPLE CHOICE

1. a
2. b
3. d
4. a
5. b

Chapter 72
Care of School-Age Child or Adolescent

TERMINOLOGY REVIEW

1. i	9. a	17. h	25. o
2. m	10. o	18. j	26. i
3. n	11. l	19. g	27. c
4. k	12. h	20. n	28. l
5. b	13. f	21. e	29. f
6. e	14. g	22. a	30. d
7. j	15. d	23. m	
8. c	16. b	24. k	

NURSING ACTIONS

1. A	4. A	7. I	10. A
2. A	5. I	8. A	
3. I	6. A	9. A	

LABELING

1. D, 2. C, 3. B

CORRECT THE FALSE STATEMENTS

1. True
2. False, hormonal changes during puberty
3. False, can lead to deformities, contractures, and impaired movement.
4. True
5. True
6. False, uncommon in children under 2 years of age.
7. True
8. False, Conflict, competition, and unacceptable aggression may be
9. True
10. True

MULTIPLE CHOICE

1. b
2. a
3. c
4. c
5. b

Chapter 73
Child or Adolescent With Special Needs

TERMINOLOGY REVIEW

1. e	11. h	21. d	31. h
2. i	12. d	22. h	32. c
3. f	13. l	23. l	33. a
4. b	14. k	24. i	34. i
5. j	15. c	25. m	35. e
6. g	16. b	26. e	36. f
7. o	17. o	27. n	37. g
8. n	18. j	28. k	38. b
9. a	19. a	29. g	39. d
10. m	20. f	30. c	

NURSING ACTIONS

1. A	4. A	7. I	10. I
2. I	5. A	8. A	
3. I	6. I	9. I	

CORRECT THE FALSE STATEMENTS

1. True
2. True
3. True
4. False, failure to gain in height and weight.
5. False, category X
6. True
7. False, fewer cases of pediatric HIV
8. False, *Pneumocystis carinii* pneumonia
9. True

SHORT ANSWERS

1. Children with Down syndrome have round, small, short heads, faces with flattened profile, and ears that are small and low set; children with fragile X syndrome have abnormally large heads, a face with a long, large, protruding jaw, and ears that are large and protruding.
2. Including the family, involving children in care, keeping up with school, and using community resources

Chapter 74
Skin Disorders

TERMINOLOGY REVIEW

1. r	10. q	19. v	28. j
2. t	11. k	20. i	29. d
3. ee	12. f	21. ff	30. n
4. bb	13. u	22. dd	31. cc
5. h	14. l	23. y	32. w
6. z	15. p	24. aa	33. x
7. gg	16. a	25. c	
8. g	17. s	26. o	
9. b	18. m	27. e	

MATCHING

1. d
2. c
3. a
4. b

SHORT ANSWER

1. The skins functions are: protection (keep out pathogens), thermoregulation (vasoconstriction or vasodilatation), sensation (respond to heat or cold), and communication (blushing). Examples will vary.
2. 47-12, papules; 47-13, vesicles; 47-14, fissures with dry scaly skin; 47-15, ulcer
   Documentation examples will vary.
3. Doing so could spread the infection to surrounding tissues, the blood stream, or the brain.
4. Both involve an allergic response by the body; however, angioedema is extensive and involves deep dermal and subcutaneous tissues.
5. Infections are the leading cause of death in burn victims. Protective isolation, handwashing, antibiotics, tetanus immunizations, and use of sterile gloves and supplies are some methods to prevent this complication.

6.

Disorder	Assessment Findings	How Disease Is Spread	Nursing Care
Venereal warts	Found in warm, moist body areas such as penis, foreskin, vagina, labial folds, and peri-anal areas	Sexual contact	Teach about prevention and spread of disease
Impetigo	Vesicles that ooze and develop golden-yellow crust	Contact with contagious individuals	Teach about spread of the disease
Scabies	Red spots with a row of blackish dots with tiny vesicles and depressions between the fingers, or on the wrist, front of the elbow, axillary folds, nipples, umbilicus, abdomen, genitalia, and gluteal cleft	Close personal contact; can also be transmitted through clothing, linens, or towels	Examine and treat all family members; have infected members bathe and towel dry to remove crusts and open infected spots; apply prescribed medication, leave on 12–24 hours before bathing
Lice	Presence of nits on hair of axillae, beard, eyebrows, eyelashes, head; pruritis	Contact with persons, clothes, bedding or over-stuffed furniture	Prevent spread of disease

7. Eschar is dead skin, which must be removed to expose living tissue. Eschar is removed by débridement using whirlpools, surgery, or enzymatic substances.

8. Types of dressings that can be used on burn victims include gauze, synthetic dressings such as Duoderm, Opsite, Vigilon, and Biobrane.

9. M basal cell carcinoma
   B pigmented nevi
   B angiomas
   M malignant melanoma
   B keloids
   M squamous cell carcinoma

10. Curettage, electrodessication, cryosurgery, and wide excision are all methods used to remove the cancerous tissues.

MATCHING

1. c

2. a

3. d

4. b

5. e

CASE STUDIES

1. a. Itching, dry powdery scales, inflammation
   b. Frequent shampoos using medicated shampoos such as Selsun Blue; instruct on a low-fat diet, exercise, sunlight, stress reduction, and adequate rest.
   c. Antihistamines may make client drowsy, and client should avoid activities that require alertness; may cause dry mouth; client should avoid alcohol; may cause nausea, diarrhea, constipation, and urinary retention.
   Selsun Blue should be left on scalp for 5 to 10 minutes and used according to manufacturer or physicians instructions.

2. a. airway—client could have inhalation burn breathing, may need resuscitation circulation, may be in shock and need fluids
   b. 13.5%
   c. 2,700 mL
   d. respiratory distress, fluid and electrolyte imbalances, impaired renal function, infection and pain
   e. This client is an older adult who may have respiratory and cardiovascular disease related to her smoking. She has impaired wound healing and diminished cardiovascular and respiratory function related to her age. All responses in item d will affect this client.

MULTIPLE CHOICE

1. b, Adhering to Standard Precautions will help protect the patient and nurse.

2. b, Antihistamines help relieve itching.

3. c, The patient may be developing angioedema.

4. c, Increased calories and protein help with wound healing.

5. b, Immobility prevents disturbing the graft and ensures that it will attach and grow.

6. c, Lice are easily transmitted.

7. d, Position promotes venous return and prevents edema.

8. c, 27%

9. b, Patient may be in shock

10. b

11. b, This can soothe the skin and relieve itching. Other interventions require an MD order.

12. c, Soaps containing lanolin can aggravate the condition.

13. d, Full-thickness burns damage all layers of skin and impair normal functioning.

14. b, 60 kg times 0.5 mg divided by 2 doses

15. a, Avoiding harmful effects of the sun's radiation can help prevent skin cancer.

16. b, May cause leukopenia.

17. c, Clothing and linens should be kept clean, Kwell shampoo is applied and then repeated in 1 week.

18. a, Fluid and electrolyte imbalances can result from shock.

Chapter 75
Fluid and Electrolytes

TERMINOLOGY REVIEW

1. i	6. k	11. a	16. a	21. b	26. e
2. l	7. d	12. e	17. j	22. m	
3. f	8. m	13. g	18. i	23. k	
4. b	9. h	14. g	19. l	24. d	
5. j	10. c	15. c	20. f	25. h	

ASSESSMENT REVIEW

1. E	4. E	7. D	10. E
2. E	5. D	8. D	11. E
3. D	6. D	9. E	12. D

SHORT ANSWER

1. CHF, thrombophlebitis, cirrhosis, low protein levels, sodium retention, inflammation, surgical stress

2. Potassium: 3.5 to 5.5mEq/L
   Sodium: 135 to 145 mEq/L
   Calcium: 9 to 10.5 mg/dL
   Magnesium: 1.5 to 2.5 mEq/L
   Phosphorus: 2.5 to 4.4 mg/dL

3. Imbalances in potassium can cause life-threatening cardiac dysrhythmias.

MATCHING

1. l	4. a	7. b	10. i	13. k
2. d	5. f	8. j	11. o	14. e
3. g	6. m	9. c	12. h	15. n

CORRECT THE FALSE STATEMENTS

1. True
2. False, cannot
3. True
4. False, sodium
5. True
6. True
7. False, hypochloremia
8. True
9. False, potassium deficit
10. True

MULTIPLE CHOICE

1. a
2. a
3. b
4. d
5. a

Chapter 76
Musculoskeletal Disorders

TERMINOLOGY REVIEW

1. l	8. d	15. b	22. e
2. g	9. a	16. c	23. g
3. c	10. m	17. k	24. h
4. h	11. j	18. m	25. f
5. e	12. i	19. j	26. d
6. k	13. f	20. a	
7. b	14. i	21. l	

CORRECT THE FALSE STATEMENTS

1. False; less expensive and invasive
2. True
3. True
4. False; should rest the joint for 1 day
5. True
6. False; elastic roller bandage
7. False; leg, ankle and arm.
8. True
9. False; 1-2 days
10. False; and stronger
11. False, primary
12. True
13. False; sprain

SHORT ANSWER

1. Plaster casts should be kept uncovered while drying. The client should be turned to dry the cast evenly. It takes 24 to 48 hours for the cast to dry. During that time, the nurse should handle the cast with palms only, not fingers. The nurse should not grasp a wet cast unless absolutely necessary. The client should be kept comfortable during this time and may complain of being hot or cold.
2. Petaling is covering the rough edges of a plaster cast with tape. It protects the client's skin from rough edges and plaster crumbs.
3. Explain procedure to the client. Wear protective gloves, eyewear and mask.
4. Signs and symptoms of infection.
5. MRI because the magnetic pull of the MRI could dislodge the implanted metal.
6. Arthroplasty is the repair or replacement of a joint. It can be used for the hip, ankle, knee, shoulder, elbow and wrist.
7. CMS checks involve checking the affected extremity for color, motion, and sensitivity (sensation). They are important because they are indicative of normal functioning versus signs of pressure in the affected extremity.
8. Teach the client the cause of the pain is damaged nerves in the stump. Encourage client to move the missing limb. Administer analgesics, TENS, visual imaging or ultrasound as indicated. Reassure client that the pain will disappear in time.
9. Nursing care should focus on monitoring neurovascular status. Other care would include administering anticoagulation therapy and antibiotics, ensuring a caffeine-free diet is followed, and wound care.
10. Maintain proper body alignment at all times. Use logroll method to assist with turning. Teach how to move from lying to sitting to standing and assist patient with this. Roll client to the side to place fracture bedpan under patient.
11. Many medications have serious side effects and the nurse must monitor for them. The nurse should assess the client to determine if the goals are being met. The goals are to relieve inflammation, relieve pain, maintain optimal functioning, and educate the client.
12. Drink at least 3 L of mixed fluids per day and do not take aspirin or other salicylate medications.
13. Intervertebral disk disease, tenosynovitis, carpel tunnel syndrome, lateral epicondylitis.

COMPARISON TABLE

Complications Related to Musculoskeletal Disorder	Description of Disorder	Nursing Care to Prevent Disorder
Neurovascular pressure	Pressure due to cast or splint. Check for edema, skin color, change in sensation, coolness, lack of distal pulse, slow capillary refill.	Complete CMS checks frequently. Handle casts and external fixation devices correctly. Monitor for correct functioning of equipment and traction. Teach client to report changes immediately. Teach client how to care for casts.

(continued)

COMPARISON TABLE *(continued)*

Complications Related to Musculoskeletal Disorder	Discription of Disorder	Nursing Care to Prevent Disorder
Wound infection	Overgrowth of organisms in a wound. Assess for elevated respirations. Assess for odor at site, increased WBCs, drainage, redness, swelling, and pain.	Observe for signs and symptoms of infection Use good hand washing and aseptic technique when changing dressings or emptying drains.
Osteomyelitis	Bone infection. Assessment findings include: acute—pus, pain, fever, flushed appearance, elevated WBCs and ESR, positive blood cultures, skin may be warm, red, and swollen; chronic—purulent drainage, pain, swelling, weakened bone on x-ray	Same as above.
Hypostatic pneumonia and alelectasis	Pneumonia is caused by status and atelectasis is collapse of a lung. Assessment findings include elevated temperature, tachycardia, cough, dyspnea, decreased oxygen saturation, pleural pain, and anxiety.	Turn, cough, deep breathe at least every 2 hours. Incentive spirometry every 2 hours. Exercise as ordered and tolerated. Suctioning, chest percussion and postural drainage as needed.
Embolism	Sudden blockage of one or more arteries. Signs of a fatty embolism include dyspnea, tachycardia, fever, petechial rash, hypoxemia, chest pain, and crackles. Assessment findings of pulmonary embolism include dyspnea, tachypnea, hypoxemia, chest pain, tachycardia, cough and hemoptysis.	Fatty embolism—keep fractures immobilized, minimize manipulation and support fractured bones when moving client. Pulmonary embolism—encourage active exercise and anticoagulant therapy as ordered, TED hose or pneumatic compression devices.
Deep vein thrombosis	Clots within the deep veins. Assessment findings include unequal leg circumference, pain, swelling, redness of the affected leg and positive Homans' sign	Apply TED house or pneumatic compression stockings, anticoagulant therapy as ordered, passive exercises or active exercises as soon as possible.
Hemorrhage	Loss of blood by damage to blood vessels. Signs include hypotension, tachycardia, change in mental status, anxiety, increased pain, decreased urine output.	Handle affected area as indicated. Monitor for early signs of hemorrhage.
Compartment syndrome	Inadequate or obstructed blood flow to muscles, nerves, and tissues. Can be caused by edema, hemorrhage, fracture or soft tissue injury. Assessment findings include pain unrelieved by medications, swelling, tightness and paresthesia.	Control swelling with elevation if not contraindicated. Apply ice. Complete neurovascular checks frequently. Teach client to monitor for syndrome.

MATCHING

1. c
2. e
3. d
4. f
5. a
6. b

FILL IN THE BLANK

1. Phantom limb pain
2. fasciotomy
3. prosthesis
4. Replantation
5. Intervertebral disk disease
6. decreases
7. women
8. Ankylosis
9. purines
10. primary, metastatic
11. butterfly rash

CASE STUDIES

1. a. Hemorrhage, infection, failure of the stump incisions to heal, and deformity of proximal structures
   b. Keep tourniquet near patient, observe for bleeding, use aseptic technique with dressing changes, monitor wound healing, use proper positioning, keep stump clean and dry
   c. Answers will vary. Some examples are pain, nausea, vomiting, constipation, urinary retention, pneumonia, atelectasis, and thrombophlebitis.
2. a. Complete musculoskeletal assessment, looking for inflammation, swelling, limited ROM and enlargement of joints. Assess laboratory values. Assess to see if she is having any side effects of the medication such as

elevated glucose, thinning skin, Cushing's syndrome, infection, or GI upset. Assess how the disorder has affected her ADLs. Assess knowledge of disorder, home environment for safety, diet and exercise patterns, and emotional status.
   b. Spend time with client and allow her to discuss her concerns. Determine if physical exercise or assistive aids would help her to become more mobile. Explore pain control measures and report findings to RN and MD.
   c. Answers will vary. Altered nutrition, Risk for infection, Self-care deficit, Altered sexuality patterns, Impaired physical mobility, Alteration in comfort, Body image disturbance, Impaired home maintenance management, Social isolation.
   d. Answers will vary.
   e. Answers will vary.

MULTIPLE CHOICE

1. a	4. b	7. b	10. a
2. c	5. c	8. a	
3. b	6. d	9. d	

Chapter 77
Nervous System Disorders

TERMINOLOGY REVIEW

1. m	8. f	15. g	22. e	29. d
2. n	9. o	16. l	23. c	
3. k	10. b	17. i	24. n	
4. c	11. a	18. a	25. k	
5. i	12. e	19. b	26. h	
6. d	13. l	20. m	27. g	
7. j	14. h	21. j	28. f	

COMPARISON CHART

Diagnostic Test	Description of Test	Nursing Care Before Test	Nursing Care After Test
Computed tomography scan	Noninvasive x-rays of a transverse body plane that feeds the information to a computer. May be used with or without contrast.	Check for allergies to iodine if contrast is used. Check for claustrophobia and ability to cooperate and lay still for 20–30 minutes. Children and older adults may need sedation.	If contrast dye is used, observe injection site for bleeding.
Magnetic resonance imaging	Uses magnetic fields instead of ionizing radiation to visualize the body areas.	Check if patient has any external or internal metal on the body. Check for claustrophobia, ability to cooperate, and ability to lay still 45–60 minutes. Explain procedure. Children and older adults may need sedation.	No special nursing care is required.

(continued)

COMPARISON CHART *(continued)*

Diagnostic Test	Description of Test	Nursing Care Before Test	Nursing Care After Test
Cerebral angiography	Radiopaque substance is injected into the carotid or femoral artery. X-rays are taken of the brain's blood vessels.	Obtain baseline neurological assessment. Check for allergies to dye. Ensure that consent is signed.	Apply sandbag or pressure to insertion site. Monitor for bleeding at site every 30 minutes. Monitor for allergies to dye or changes in neurologic status. Check legs for color, temperature, and pulse. Increase fluids.
Lumbar puncture	Hollow needle is inserted into the subarachnoid space in the lumbar region of spinal canal. This is done to check CSF pressure, obtain a sample, inject drugs, or perform special tests.	Ensure that permit is signed. Have client empty bladder. Obtain vital signs. Position on side with knees drawn to chest.	Keep supine for 6 hours. Monitor vital signs and neurologic status. Increase fluids. Check insertion site for leakage, hematoma, or edema.
Electro-encelphalogram	Electrodes are placed on the forehead and scalp, which records the electrical impulses of the brain.	Client may need sedation or be kept awake. Instruct client that he/she may need to follow commands during the test.	No specific care is required.

SHORT ANSWER

1. Teach that pain will be minimal, but surgery can be noisy. Instruct that the brain has no sensory nerves. Include routine perioperative teaching.
2. Neurologic history, speech patterns, LOC, neurologic status using Glasgow Coma Scale, muscle tone/strength, balance, coordination, reflexes, sensory function, signs of IICP, cranial nerve function and eye signs
3. Any change in LOC
4. All three involve pain in the head. Migraine and cluster headaches usually result from vascular disturbances, whereas symptomatic headaches can be from a large variety of causes. Migraine and cluster headaches may be unilateral.
5. Protect and observe the client. Make environment safe, loosen restrictive clothing, do not restrain, protect the head and airway, and monitor the seizure activity closely.
6. People who have repeated or continuous abnormal wrist positions such as physicians, secretaries, and computer operators. These movements cause edema and thus pressure on the nerve, resulting in pain, weakness, and abnormal sensations.
7. a. Fifth cranial nerve, excruciating spasmodic pain in jaw and parts of face lasting for 2 to 15 seconds.
b. Seventh cranial nerve, affects one side of the face, resulting in partial facial paralysis.
c. Follows the sensory nerve tracts, usually on the trunk of the body; appears as vesicular eruptions accompanied by itching, tenderness or pain, GI upset, and general malaise.
8. Congenital defects, tumors, or trauma
9. Paraplegia involves paralysis of the legs and lower body, whereas quadriplegia involves paralysis of all four extremities.
10. Encourage clients to be as independent and active as possible, avoid unnecessary stress and fatigue, protect from injuries, prevent constipation; teach clients how to take prescribed medications.
11. Menses usually resume in 3 months; discourage use of tampons, birth control pills, and intrauterine devices; and labor and childbirth may be dangerous.
12. Answers will vary. Skin breakdown—frequent turning; pneumonia—deep breathing, suctioning; urinary incontinence and retention—monitor Foley and bladder training; constipation—teach manual impaction removal; foot drop—change positions and perform active ROM.

CASE STUDIES

1. First priority: assess client with bacterial meningitis for changes in LOC, temperature, and notify RN/MD. Client's condition may be deteriorating
Second priority: assess client with craniotomy and check neurologic checks and pain level. Medicate if indicated and no change in neurologic status. This client would have some pain postoperatively, but changes in neurologic status could indicate IICP.
Third priority: assess client with ALS swallowing and assist with client's meal. This prevents aspiration.

Fourth priority: assess level of fatigue with client who has MS. This is an expected finding, but you need to determine if the weakness has increased.

2. a. Head bent forward, tremors of head and/or other body parts, rigidity, weight loss, akinesia, pill-rolling
b. Glaucoma and undiagnosed skin lesions because l-dopa is contraindicated with these disorders.
c. They promote activity and flexibility and allow the client to be independent and provide self-care activities.
d. Hemolytic anemia can develop in clients taking l-dopa.

3. The first priority is to complete a neurologic assessment to determine a baseline for the client and to assess the extent of the client's condition. The other interventions can be completed during the initial admitting nursing history.

MATCHING EXERCISE

1. e
2. c
3. a
4. d
5. b

MULTIPLE CHOICE

1. d	5. a	9. c
2. b	6. c	10. d
3. d	7. d	11. a
4. c	8. b	12. b

Chapter 78
Endocrine Disorders

TERMINOLOGY REVIEW

1. aa	11. s	21. v	31. w
2. dd	12. q	22. jj	32. g
3. p	13. bb	23. ee	33. z
4. x	14. u	24. d	34. b
5. k	15. cc	25. gg	35. j
6. y	16. f	26. h	36. e
7. kk	17. ii	27. mm	37. n
8. m	18. r	28. ll	38. l
9. c	19. a	29. hh	39. o
10. ff	20. i	30. nn	40. t

ASSESSMENT REVIEW

1. G	9. S	17. HE	25. HE
2. A	10. HE	18. HE	26. HO
3. A	11. HO	19. HO	27. HE
4. A	12. HE	20. HO	28. HO
5. DI	13. HE	21. C	29. HO, HE
6. S	14. HO	22. A	30. HE
7. DI	15. HE	23. A	
8. DI	16. HO	24. C	

MATCHING DIAGNOSTIC TESTS

1. d	4. c	7. i
2. h	5. e	8. f
3. g	6. b	9. a

CASE STUDIES

1. J.T. should be assessed first because of possible imbalance of calcium levels, which could be life-threateningly low. A.P. should also be assessed because this client's glucose levels could be very low. This client should be given a fast-acting carbohydrate such as 4 oz of orange juice. Both of these clients need constant attention until they have stabilized. You may have to illicit help from other staff. B.R. should be assessed to ensure that the client is not having any postoperative complications. Finally, G.S. should be assessed to see if the client is continuing with the 24-hour urine specimen.

2. Answers will vary but should include education about nutrition, exercise, glucose monitoring, medications, and general information. Teaching should focus on ensuring that the client is able to administer insulin and knows signs and symptoms of hyperglycemia and hypoglycemia and how to treat each, and should include review of a diabetic diet and resources such as cookbooks. A consult should be completed with the dietitian if it has not already been completed, including how to monitor blood glucose levels and education about his disease disorder. Supplemental handouts should be provided about the disease, foot care, and complications. Follow-up appointments should be made.

3. The ultra-lente insulin peaks at 4-6 hours. The client would be most at risk for hypoglycemic reactions at 12 to 2 PM and 10 to 12 PM.

MULTIPLE CHOICE

1. b, All interventions are appropriate; however, assessing the airway and ensuring the airway is patent are priority.
2. c, Desired dose divided by available dose multiplied by vehicle
3. d, An increase urine output will put the client at risk for fluid volume deficit.

4. b, The client with diabetes insipidus has difficulty concentrating urine and is at risk for fluid volume deficit and electrolyte imbalances.

5. b

6. d, Carbohydrates should be given to prevent the client's blood sugar from dropping any further. The client can quickly become unconscious as the blood sugar drops. The finger stick blood sugar could be obtained after giving carbohydrates.

7. a, Toenails should be cut only with a physician's permission and should be cut straight across to prevent ingrown toenails. Blunt-tip scissors should be used.

8. b

9. d, Weight gain, moon face, and increased facial hair are all symptoms of Cushing's syndrome.

10. b, The client with Cushing's syndrome may have an infection, and the high levels of glucocorticoids may mask the normal inflammatory process associated with infections.

11. a, A major complication of adrenal venogram is allergic reactions to the dye.

12. c, All options are mechanisms of oral hypoglycemic agents, but acarbose decreases glucose absorption from the intestine.

13. b, An excess of PTH causes an elevated calcium level, which can affect serum phosphorus levels.

14. c, The client with Addison's disease has imbalances resulting from decreased cortisol levels, which affect electrolytes (low sodium and high potassium) as well as hypoglycemia.

15. a, See Box 78-1 for other diagnostic criteria for diabetes mellitus.

16. b, The client with hypothyroidism needs to decrease total calories in the diet.

Chapter 79
Sensory System Disorders

MATCHING

1. d	4. b	7. c
2. g	5. e	8. f
3. a	6. h	9. i

SHORT ANSWER

1. Work over a soft or padded surface. To insert the eye: wear gloves, wet the prosthesis, lift upper eyelid, slip eye up under the top lid, hold the prosthesis while pulling down gently on the lower lid, slip the lower lid over the edge of the prosthesis, have client blink. To remove the prosthesis: pull down the lower lid, press inward on the bottom of the prosthesis, follow with care of the eye socket.

2. A cochlear implant is a surgically implanted device that emits an auditory signal to the auditory nerve tissue. The implant allows profoundly deaf individuals to perceive sound.

3. Most of the procedures are completed as an outpatient basis. Client and family teaching are essential to ensure client safety and uneventful recovery.

4.

	Preoperative Care	Postoperative Care
Eye Surgery	Sign consent Review postop procedures Review eye patching Remind awake during surgery Will need someone to drive Teach how to make meds	Leave dressings in place. Don't use meds until seen by surgeon. Client may wear shields while sleeping. Teach client how to remove mucus gently. Avoid sudden movements, bending, straining with stools, vomiting, coughing, sneezing, blowing nose, falls, jolts, and soap in the eye. Report excess drainage, sudden pain, or bleeding Stitches may be absorbable.
Ear Surgery	Review preoperative and postoperative procedures. Client may be awake. Teach client how to take meds. Sign consent.	Dressings and packs must remain in place. Watch for dizziness or prolonged nausea. Avoid vomiting, abrupt changes in position, sudden movement, straining, lifting, sneezing, coughing, and blowing nose. Observe for bleeding and complaints of pressure, pain, fever, headache, vertigo. Do not allow water into the ear. Follow surgeon's instructions for positioning.

5. The pinna is pulled superiorly and posteriorly in an adult and posteriorly and inferiorly in a child.

6. All contact lenses are designed to lie directly on the cornea to correct vision. They provide clearer vision than eye glasses. Hard contact lenses are made of rigid gas-permeable plastic and are very thin. Soft contact lenses are made of hydrophilic plastic. They are larger and more flexible than hard contact lenses. Both hard and soft contact lenses should be removed daily. Extended-wear soft contact lenses allow more gas to pass through and can be worn up to 2 weeks.

7. Prolonged wearing can cause infections (infectious keratitis) or injury (corneal abrasion).

8. Chronic open angle glaucoma–eye discomfort, temporary blurring of vision, halos around lights; narrow (closed) angle glaucoma—blurred vision, halos around lights, severe eye pain, nausea and vomiting; cataracts–impaired vision; retinal detachment—flashes of light, moving spots

9. Cochlear implants, lip reading, sign language, hearing aids

10. Similar assessment findings include some degree of hearing loss and pain. Different assessment findings include: serous otitis media may include crackling sensations; acute otitis media includes fever, inflamed and bulging eardrum; and chronic otitis media includes ringing in the ears and purulent drainage.

11. The nurse should assess the patient with Meniere's disease and determine whether she is currently having an attack and whether the medication can safely be given within prescribed time frame. The nurse should also make sure to administer the eye drops to the patient with glaucoma on time. The patient scheduled for surgery should be assessed regarding knowledge about surgery and postoperative care. His current assessment findings are expected in a patient with cataracts.

12. The Weber test results indicate sound in the left and right ear heard equally. Rinne results are air conduction greater than bone conduction, bilaterally.

CASE STUDY

1. Hearing problem
2. A thorough assessment of the client's hearing, including Rinne and Weber tests, will help confirm a hearing problem. Examination should include assessment of the external ear and checking for excess cerumen in the ear canal. Other important data should include current medical history and medication use, any recent trauma to the ears, and history of chronic respiratory or ear infections. The nurse should also determine how long he worked at the factory and the noise level to which he was exposed.
3. Document all pertinent assessment findings and share information with the RN and MD. If findings are positive indicating hearing loss, request hearing acuity evaluation.

4. Teach the wife to get her husband's attention before speaking. Teach her to face her husband when speaking and to speak slowly and clearly. If she needs to repeat information, repeat the entire phrase. Teach her to not chew, smoke, or put objects in her mouth or cover her mouth while talking. If possible, have her decrease background noises.

FILL-IN-THE-BLANK

1. in front
2. near, far
3. Braille
4. seeing eye dog or guide dog
5. Lions International
6. presbycusis
7. Otosclerosis
8. ototoxic
9. stapedectomy
10. polyethylene tube or PE tube

MULTIPLE CHOICE

1. a	4. c	7. c	10. b
2. b	5. b	8. c	
3. b	6. d	9. a	

Chapter 80
Cardiovascular Disorders

TERMINOLOGY REVIEW

1. s	13. ee	25. pp	37. mm
2. r	14. tt	26. h	38. bb
3. p	15. n	27. dd	39. hh
4. i	16. ss	28. d	40. j
5. w	17. g	29. cc	41. x
6. o	18. e	30. y	42. f
7. b	19. u	31. t	43. m
8. l	20. qq	32. ii	44. jj
9. gg	21. q	33. ll	45. z
10. oo	22. uu	34. aa	46. a
11. k	23. c	35. kk	
12. ff	24. nn	36. v	

ASSESSMENT REVIEW

1. N	6. A	11. A	16. A
2. A	7. N	12. N	17. A
3. N	8. A	13. N	18. N
4. N	9. A	14. A	19. A
5. A	10. A	15. A	20. N

DIAGNOSTIC TESTS REVIEW

1. i	6. c	11. k	16. p
2. l	7. m	12. j	17. b
3. o	8. e	13. n	
4. q	9. g	14. d	
5. f	10. a	15. h	

CASE STUDIES

1. a. The nurse has two clients who need immediate attention. Mrs. Garcia could be experiencing an embolism. She should be assessed, and the RN or MD notified immediately. Mr. Abe also needs attention because he could be experiencing another MI. He should be assessed, given nitroglycerin (if ordered), and the RN or MD notified. The nurse also needs to give Mr. Clooney his medication, but this is not a priority until the first two clients have been cared for. The nurse could ask a co-worker to medicate Mr. Clooney. The nurse should inform Ms. Crocker that her discharge instructions will need to be delayed until you address the other, more immediate concerns. Again, the help of a co-worker may be needed.

2. a. Intermittent claudication, b. The nurse may see tingling, numbness, coldness, difference in size, thin and shiny skin, and visible blood vessels. c, See Nursing Care Guideline 80-2: Caring for Clients with Peripheral Vascular Disease.

3. a. Decreased Cardiac Output and Fluid Volume Excess would be the two priority nursing diagnoses due to her medical condition of CHF and assessment findings (pulse—114, edema, bilateral crackles, JVD, weight gain). b. Administer medications as ordered to decrease the workload of the heart and to decrease excess fluid. Document assessment findings so that other health care team members will have the information. Place client on intake and output to evaluate the effectiveness of the medications. Provide mattress and chair padding to protect the client from skin breakdown. Locate a Doppler to assess pedal pulses, which can provide a basis for comparison of the client's progress. Prepare the client for an echocardiogram to evaluate the heart's size and function.

MULTIPLE CHOICE

1. b, Cardiac enzymes are elevated with damage such as with an MI.

2. d, The insertion site is usually the femoral artery, which is a large blood vessel. The nurse should monitor the site for bleeding because hemorrhage can be a complication.

3. c, It would be essential to determine the pregnancy status of the client before administering thrombolytics, which are contraindicated in a pregnant female.

4. c, A priority for cardiac surgery clients is to ensure adequate oxygenation of tissues. The tissues have been deprived of adequate oxygenation.

5. d, A diet high in saturated fats is associated with arteriosclerosis. The nurse should recommend a diet low in saturated fats.

6. a, Complications of HTN include MI, kidney damage, CHF, CVA, and other complications.

7. a, Nitrates and nitrites are vasodilators used to control angina.

8. c, Thiazides are diuretics, which cause increased urinary output to help control blood pressure.

9. d, Prolonged standing impedes venous return and should be avoided in a client with varicose veins.

10. d, Positioning the unresponsive person on the unaffected side prevents contractures and undue pressure on any part.

11. a, Aphasia is the inability to speak. Dysphasia is the inability to say what one wishes to say.

12. d, Loop diuretics cause potassium loss, so that potassium replacement is needed.

13. d

Chapter 81
Blood and Lymph Disorders

TERMINOLOGY REVIEW

1. h	8. f	15. p	22. o
2. e	9. c	16. i	23. m
3. l	10. a	17. e	24. g
4. d	11. j	18. l	25. c
5. k	12. b	19. b	26. h
6. g	13. f	20. n	27. k
7. i	14. a	21. d	28. j

ANEMIA COMPARISON

Type of Anemia	Description	Nursing Care
Iron deficiency	Most common type of anemia, caused by trauma, excessive menses, bleeding, pregnancy, or diet that lacks iron.	Assist with treatment of blood loss. Increase dietary iron. Instruct client how to administer iron at home.
Acute hemorrhagic	Develops after rapid and often sudden blood loss such as trauma, blood vessel rupture, aneurysm, or artery erosion by cancer lesion	Administer blood products as ordered. Administer IV fluids. Monitor status. Assess for signs of shock.
Pernicious	Person lacks intrinsic factor, which is produced in the stomach. Instrinsic factor is needed to absorb B_{12}, which is needed to absorb iron and protect nerve fibers. Develops slowly. Administer B_{12} intramuscularly, iron supplements, folic acid, and digestants Administer blood transfusions if needed.	Assess for early symptoms (infection, mood swings, GI disorders, and cardiac and renal problems) and for late symptoms (weakness, fatigue, tingling, and numbness, sore tongue, difficulty walking, abdominal pain, and loss of appetite and weight).
Aplastic	Bone marrow is underdeveloped or has failed. This results in decrease in RBCs, WBCs, and platelets. Caused by excessive radiation, toxicity to drugs, tumors, insecticides, chemicals, and environmental toxins. May also be autoimmune in origin.	Assist with bone marrow or stem cell transplantation. Protect from infection and bleeding. Follow sterile technique with invasive procedures. No rectal temperatures. Use reverse isolation as needed. Avoid injury. Teach client how to avoid infection and how to prevent bleeding.
Sickle cell	Genetic disease in which a person's RBCs become crescent shaped when exposed to decreased oxygen.	Prevent hypoxia and sickle cell crisis. Administer blood transfusions. Administer IV fluids. Assess pain level.

CORRECT THE FALSE STATEMENTS

1. True
2. False, anemia, neutropenia, and thrombocytopenia
3. True
4. False, prevent the progression of
5. True
6. True
7. False, bleeding.
8. False, may/usually
9. False, has extended to one or more extralymphatic organs or tissues.
10. True
11. True
12. True
13. False, hyperthermia/fever
14. False, blood culture
15. False, within the first 10 to 15 minutes of transfusion.

MULTIPLE CHOICE

1. d
2. a
3. b
4. a
5. c
6. b
7. d

Chapter 82
Cancer

TERMINOLOGY REVIEW

1. k	10. l	19. d	28. l
2. j	11. c	20. a	29. i
3. h	12. i	21. b	30. b
4. b	13. d	22. g	31. j
5. e	14. f	23. c	32. a
6. f	15. c	24. f	33. e
7. m	16. h	25. k	
8. a	17. g	26. h	
9. g	18. e	27. d	

SHORT ANSWER

1. Hormonal, chemical, viral, radiation related, immune, genetic
2. See Box 82-2
3. Radiation therapy may be used as the primary treatment, combined with chemotherapy, or as palliative treatment.
4. Time, distance, and shielding
5. The nurse should be alert for the seven warning signs of cancer. The nurse should be aware of signs and symptoms of cancer listed in the Nursing Assessment 82-1.

MEDICATION REVIEW

1. c	4. d	7. i
2. g	5. h	8. e
3. b	6. a	9. f

CORRECT THE FALSE STATEMENTS

1. False, primary site.
2. True
3. True
4. True
5. False, Hematopoietic growth factors
6. True
7. False, nearly all cancer clients.
8. False, Pain
9. True
10. True

CASE STUDY

The first priority is to notify the RN/MD that Mr. P is experiencing complications related to his cancer. The second priority is to discharge Ms. D because she is finished with her therapy. Mrs. L should be monitored and medicated on schedule to prevent reoccurrence of uncontrolled pain. Mr. J should be instructed about his surgery in the morning. The nurse should spend time with Mr. J and allow him to express his concerns about the surgery and cancer.

MULTIPLE CHOICE

1. c
2. b
3. a
4. a

Chapter 83
Allergic, Immune, and Autoimmune Disorders

TERMINOLOGY REVIEW

1. m	6. s	11. g	16. c
2. r	7. h	12. b	17. o
3. t	8. i	13. n	18. e
4. p	9. q	14. j	19. k
5. f	10. a	15. l	20. d

ASSESSMENT REVIEW

1. N	5. GI	9. GI	13. R
2. GI	6. N	10. R	14. R
3. S	7. GI	11. S	15. GI or N
4. R	8. S	12. N	

SHORT ANSWER

1. adverse reaction, drug allergy from the antigen–antibody response, and serum sickness
2. One method is avoidance of the substance. An example is avoiding a particular food that a person is allergic to. A second method is desensitization, which consists of giving minute doses of allergens subcutaneously to build up a tolerance. The third method is medications, such as antihistamines, which inhibit histamine's action within the body.
3. The exact reason is unknown, but thymic hormones, sex hormones, and corticosteroids are thought to play a significant role.
4. The differences are in body parts that are affected by the autoimmune disorder. Organ-specific affects one organ, systemic affects the entire body, and non–organ-specific affects one or more organs. See Table 83-1 for examples.
5. Symptomatic treatment is treating symptoms as they occur instead of treating the disease. Examples are using medications to treat pain and inflammation such as analgesics and corticosteroids.

CASE STUDIES

1. a. Physical examination will be done to identify any symptoms of allergic manifestations in any body systems.

   Laboratory tests such as complete blood count and differential count will be done to see if the client's body is producing an increased number of eosinophils, which are elevated during allergic responses. Skin testing will be done to identify the offending allergens.

b. Answers will vary: Sleep Pattern Disturbance related to coughing, chest tightness, and runny nose; Fatigue related to sleep deprivation; Knowledge Deficit related to treatment and self-management of allergy; Anxiety/Fear related to inability to breathe.

c. Client will report improved sleep/rest pattern. Client will report increased sense of well-being and feeling rested.
Client will report increased energy to complete ADLs.
Client will make modifications in lifestyle and environment to avoid allergens.

d. Ms. N should be taught that her medication may make her drowsy and to avoid activities where alertness is required. She should be taught how to minimize the dust mites in her home/work environment. See Box 83-2 teaching under implementation. She should be taught to avoid outdoor activities or to wear masks during her seasonal allergies.

2. a. Follow the ABCs of resuscitation, starting with the airway. Ensure that the airway is open to ensure that the client is able to breathe. Oxygen, endotracheal intubation, and suctioning may be needed to ensure an open airway. Without an open airway, adequate gas exchange is impossible. Support breathing and circulation if needed by initiating CPR if needed. Administer medications as ordered to support breathing and circulation.

b. The client should be taught to avoid iodine in any future diagnostic exams and in food such as shellfish and to wear a Medic Alert bracelet or necklace.

MULTIPLE CHOICE

1. b, Erythema and induration indicate which allergens the client is allergic to, by causing a local skin allergic reaction.
2. d, Antihistamines should be held before the appointment to ensure that the normal antigen–antibody response with release of histamine will occur.
3. a, Bronchial asthma is characterized by recurring paroxysms of dyspnea and wheezing. The other symptoms indicate allergic responses of other areas of the body.
4. a, Severe reactions can occur after desensitization, and clients should stay in the clinic for 20 minutes after injections.
5. b, Avoiding allergens will help reduce symptoms. Wearing a mask when outside during allergy season will help the client avoid allergy symptoms.
6. d, Ensuring that the client's airway is patent is the priority during anaphylaxis.
7. a, The client needs further teaching because results from desensitization take time to have an effect. Desensitization is usually started 3 months before allergy season.

8. c, A decrease in allergy symptoms indicates that the client has made necessary lifestyle, diet, and environmental changes to avoid allergic responses.
9. c, Serum sickness results 7 to 10 days after a client receives drug to which the client has no antibodies. Treatment includes antihistamines or corticosteroids.
10. d, The client is exhibiting signs and symptoms of rejection of the transplanted organ, and the RN or MD should be notified.

Chapter 84
HIV and AIDS

TERMINOLOGY REVIEW

1. p	7. a	13. b	19. g
2. n	8. x	14. i	20. w
3. k	9. e	15. d or j	21. h
4. q	10. r	16. f	22. o
5. u	11. v	17. j or d	23. c
6. t	12. s	18. l	24. m

ASSESSMENT REVIEW

1. B	6. A	11. B	16. H
2. H	7. B	12. A	17. B
3. A	8. N	13. A	18. B
4. B	9. B	14. B	19. B
5. N	10. N	15. B	20. A

CORRECT THE FALSE STATEMENTS

1. True
2. True
3. False, B cells, T cells
4. False, 10 years
5. True
6. False, can
7. False, within 3 weeks to 14 months
8. True
9. True
10. True
11. True
12. False, now treatable
13. False, after the client signs an informed consent.
14. True
15. False, Gastrointestinal problems

CASE STUDY

1. Categories are as follows, examples will vary, see Educating the Client 84-2.
Knowledge of the disease process, signs, and symptoms. The client probably knows the signs and symptoms, but review them and ensure that his partner knows them as well. Review progression of the disease and how important compliance with medication therapy is to slow the disease progression.

Knowledge of how HIV is and is not transmitted. Review sexual transmission of the disease with his partner. Review that HIV is transmitted through body fluids.

Infection control. Teach basic infection control and specific disposal of infected items. Instruct client to avoid exposure to ill individuals to prevent opportunistic infections, including people with colds.

Sharps disposal, care of contaminated objects. Prevent transmission of disease by correct disposal. Provide sharps containers.

Hygiene in the kitchen. Teach to clean kitchen/bath with bleach solution.

Medication side effects. Review all medications with client and partner.

Good nutrition, use of supplements. Teach to supplement diet with nutritious supplements. Encourage high-protein foods, avoid offensive odors and foods that the client does not like.

2. Use handouts that are available. Provide written information on what you cover with the client. Ensure that you allow adequate time to present the information as well as time to review with the client and partner. Provide aids that will help client keep medications organized such as weekly or daily pill containers.

MULTIPLE CHOICE

1. a, All HIV-positive individuals with fewer than 200 T cells now are considered to have a diagnosis of AIDS.
2. c, The Western blot test is specific for the detection of HIV and is completed if the ELISA is positive.
3. b, Women can have signs and symptoms of HIV that are often attributed to STDs, HPV, and PID. Women should be aware that HIV can be overlooked in them and attributed to these disorders.
4. d, Assessing for opportunistic infections will help determine the status of the client's immune system.
5. b, As a client's CD4 counts drop, opportunistic infections may develop.
6. c, The client must be aware of how the disease is transmitted to prevent spread of the disease.
7. d, The client with a CD4 count of less than 200 is at risk for obtaining an infection and should be placed on protective isolation.
8. a, Infectious material such as litter boxes, birdcages, and fish tanks should be avoided.
9. c, SOB, dyspnea, cough, chest pain, and fever are all associated with respiratory complications of AIDS.
10. b, Establish a baseline by assessing neurologic status. The client may have safety concerns related to impairment that need to be addressed.

Chapter 85
Respiratory Disorders

TERMINOLOGY REVIEW

1. tt	14. mm	27. k	40. p
2. ll	15. d	28. kk	41. i
3. cc	16. q	29. y	42. oo
4. dd	17. n	30. f	43. ee
5. pp	18. w	31. g	44. o
6. vv	19. j	32. c	45. h
7. jj	20. ff	33. r	46. x
8. z	21. bb	34. hh	47. a
9. rr	22. uu	35. ss	48. u
10. nn	23. l	36. t	49. s
11. b	24. v	37. gg	
12. qq	25. ww	38. aa	
13. e	26. m	39. ii	

PROCEDURE COMPARISON

Bronchoscopy	Thoracentesis	Thoracotomy
Before procedure Consent, throat is anesthetized, IV medications to promote relaxation, NPO for 6–8 hours, explain procedure to client, remove dentures, and check for loose teeth.	**Before procedure** Consent, sterile prep of skin, explain procedure to client, assist physician, emotional support for client	**Before procedure** Consent, explain procedure to client, routine preoperative instructions
After procedure NPO until gag reflex returns, vital signs until stable, position on side, note edema or bleeding, endotracheal tube at bedside, specimens to laboratory, soft foods for 24 hours, and rest for 24 hours.	**After procedure** Assess respiratory status and bleeding, monitor for bleeding and respiratory distress, monitor vital signs, ensure specimens are taken to laboratory.	**After procedure** Routine postoperative care and instructions. Assess respiratory status, monitor bleeding and respiratory distress.

1. Consent, explain procedure to client and answer questions, provide emotional support.

2. Assess respiratory status and for respiratory distress; assess for bleeding; monitor vital signs.

INFECTIOUS RESPIRATORY DISORDERS

Disorder	Location	Symptoms
Rhinitis	Nasal cavity, frontal and sphenoidal sinuses	Sneezing, nasal discharge, congestion, headache, sore throat, general malaise, cough, slight fever, blunted sense of taste and smell
Laryngitis	Larynx and vocal cords	Cough, hoarse voice and may lose voice
Streptococcal sore throat	Nasopharynx and laryngeal pharynx	General physical weakness, malaise, high fever, pus on the tonsils, headache
Bronchitis	Bronchi	Dry cough that becomes productive, fever, malaise
Pneumonia	Lung, alveoli	Sharp pain in chest, chill, fever, painful cough, tenacious sputum, pain on breathing, rapid pulse, rapid and difficult respirations, mental changes, elevated white blood cell count, person feels ill, may be cyanotic.
Pleurisy	Visceral and parietal pleura	Sharp pain with every breath, dry cough, SOB, exhaustion with slightest effort

ASSESSMENT REVIEW

    No complaints of pain when the chest is palpated
X Small mass palpated on the anterior chest
X Scoliosis
    Respiratory rate of 16 breaths/min, nonlabored
X Difficulty speaking in complete sentences because of SOB
X Barrel-shaped chest

    Chest rises and falls slightly with each breath
    Equal breath sounds on both sides of chest
X Cough
X Dyspnea
X Retractions
    Symmetric shape of chest
    High-pitched continuous musical sound on auscultation

ASSESSMENT REVIEW (continued)

<u>X</u> Low-pitched bubbling sound on auscultation
   Scapulae at the same level
   Relaxed breathing
   Low, soft-pitched blowing sound throughout
   lung fields on auscultation
<u>X</u> Expiration is longer than inspiration

MATCHING

1. f	4. d	7. i
2. c	5. b	8. h
3. a	6. e	9. g

SHORT ANSWERS

1. Skin testing is used to determine whether a person has been exposed to tuberculosis or other disorders such as histoplasmosis. It is also used to determine allergies to medications or allergens.
2. If there is suction applied to the system, there will be bubbling in the suction chamber, but not in the water-seal chamber. The system will be lower than the client's chest. The client will have breath sounds and not be in distress. The system will not have evidence of air leaks.
3. See Nursing Care Guideline 85-5.
4. The three types of tuberculosis are: pulmonary tuberculosis, which produces a tubercle in the lungs; Pott's disease or miliary tuberculosis, which affects the bones and joints; and, atypical tuberculosis, which is seen in clients who are immunosuppressed.
5. Methods to prevent the spread of tuberculosis include but are not limited to: educate the public, burn tissues used by infected people, follow guidelines for biohazardous waste disposal, trace active cases and start treatment, follow-up for infected clients, screening of at-risk groups, and isolation when infected.
6. Sleep apnea is characterized by more than five cessations of airflow for at least 10 seconds each per hour of sleep due to soft tissues at the back of the throat occluding the airway.
7. Sleep apnea treatment includes weight loss, smoking cessation, avoidance of alcohol before bedtime, elevation of HOB, CPAP, and possible surgery.
8. See text and Nursing Care Guideline 85-2.
9. Allergic rhinitis most commonly may be caused by pollen, dust, feathers, or animal dander.
10. Common causes of ARDS include aspiration, medication overdose, cardiac surgery, pancreatitis, end-stage renal disease, embolism, major surgery, and trauma.
11. Three categories of respiratory trauma include absence of air exchange, chest trauma, respiratory drug complications in drug poisoning, drowning, and pneumothorax. Examples will vary.
12. Bronchoscopy and biopsy are used to differentiate benign and malignant lung disorders.
13. Clients at risk for epistaxis include those with hypertension, certain blood disorders, cancer, rheumatic fever, and irritation or injury to the nose.

14. The priority would be to assess AJ and see what is causing the increased SOB. The RN and/or physician may need to be notified for complications that are developing. PD and TL should then both be medicated. Finally, DK's doctor should be notified.

MULTIPLE CHOICE

1. c, The anesthetic agent used to numb the throat prevents the client from coughing out secretions.
2. a, Low-pitched bubbling, moist sounds indicate air drawn through fluid in the large airways. This occurs with conditions such as pneumonia and pulmonary edema.
3. a, A sputum sample should be from the lungs and bronchi rather than mucus from the oral cavity.
4. a, D/A × Q = X 0.1 mg/1.0mg × 1 ml = 0.1 ml
5. b, Bronchial spasms that occur during an asthma attack produce wheezing. The client may also feel chest tightness and choking sensation, perspire, and become cyanotic. The client may have coughing with production of thick, white mucus as the attack subsides.
6. c, Cromolyn sodium is an antiasthmatic, antiallergic, and mast cell stabilizer. It is used for prevention of bronchial asthma and is not used during acute attacks.
7. c, Mrs. Smith is not responding to treatment and may be experiencing status asthmaticus, which is a medical emergency.
8. b, The bronchodilator should be used first to open the airways. The client should wait 5 minutes to ensure that the medication has a chance to work before the steroid inhaler is used.
9. d, Pursed-lip breathing will help prevent air trapping and allow the client to increase his oxygenation during the activity.
10. c, The older adult has weakened chest muscles and a diminished cough reflex that make coughing more difficult and less effective.
11. b, The client with any respiratory disorder should be discouraged from smoking because smoking can predispose the client to disorders or worsen existing conditions.
12. b, A client with active TB can transmit the disease to others. The priority intervention should be to place Mr. Ling on airborne isolation to prevent the transmission of the disease.
13. b, A client with sleep apnea has more than five cessations of airflow for at least 10 seconds each per hour of sleep. This causes the person to have a lack of oxygen. The results are that the client is extremely tired the next day. Other signs and symptoms include difficulty concentrating, memory loss, inability to perform one's job, and falling asleep.
14. c, Gloves prevent introducing pathogens into the client's respiratory tract.
15. a, Signs and symptoms of TB include cough, weight loss, and nocturnal diaphoresis. Other signs include lack of pain, thick sputum, and expectoration of blood, fatigue, and low-grade fever. As the disease progresses, the client may experience severe chest pains, persistent cough, and dyspnea.

16. c, The regimen for medication administration includes taking three medications for 2 months and two medications for 4 months (total of 6 months).
17. a, The client with chronic bronchitis develops the disease at age 30 to 40 years and has SOB, increased sputum, peripheral edema, and other manifestations. Other symptoms may be present. See Table 85-2.
18. b, The client's immediate need is to establish a more normal pattern of breathing to ensure adequate gas exchange.
19. d, Cigarette smoking causes or predisposes individuals to diseases of the respiratory system and other system. It is the single most common cause of disease.
20. b, Leukotriene antagonists block the inflammatory biochemical pathway, making airways less sensitive to asthma triggers.

CORRECT THE FALSE STATEMENTS

1. False, excess oxygen can be harmful.
2. True
3. True
4. False, may not be used
5. True
6. False, a metal cap screwed onto its top to protect the valve from damage.
7. True
8. False, Oxygen concentrators
9. False, Gloves
10. False, Assisted-breath ventilators

Chapter 86
Oxygen Therapy and Respiratory Care

TERMINOLOGY REVIEW

1. e	7. o	13. c	19. s
2. g	8. p	14. u	20. j
3. l	9. k	15. m	21. r
4. i	10. d	16. h	
5. t	11. q	17. n	
6. f	12. b	18. a	

OXYGEN TABLE

Type of Therapy	Description	Concentration and Flow Rate	Use	Nursing Considerations
Nasal Cannula	Two short tubes that fit into each nostril	24–44% 1–6 lpm/min	Small to moderate increases in oxygen concentration	Use with caution with irregular breathing patterns. Do not exceed 6 lpm/min. Monitor respiratory status. Encourage client to breathe through the nose. Use humidification. Monitor respiratory status.
Simple Mask	Transparent green mask with nipple adapter	40–60% 6–10 lpm/min	Low-flow oxygen	Use humidification. Put call signal in reach. Check for readness under straps. Use at least 6 lpm/min flow rate. Monitor respiratory status.
Partial rebreathing mask	Presence of a bag and absence of valves	60%–90% set as 12–15 lpm/min and adjust down to deflate bag with each breath.	Low-flow oxygen	Regulate flow rate to ensure bag deflates with each breath. Make sure that call signal is within reach. Check on client periodically. Monitor respiratory status.

(continued)

OXYGEN TABLE *(Continued)*

Type of Therapy	Description	Concentration and Flow Rate	Use	Nursing Considerations
Nonrebreather mask	Presence of valves on outside of mask and between mask and bag	90%–100% Adjust flow rate to keep bag inflated at least one-third full	Someone who needs very high concentrations of oxygen	Never leave client alone. Place on cardiac monitoring.Ensure bag deflates correctly.
Venturi mask	Mask that has hard plastic adapter with large "windows" on the adapters	24%–50% Flow rate varies with each manufacturer	Used when reliable and consistent oxygen enrichment is	Do not use a humidifier with this mask. Put call signal in reach. Assess for reddened areas. Monitor respiratory status.

MULTIPLE CHOICE

1. d, Blood in sputum or mucus should be reported immediately and could indicate bleeding in the respiratory tract or other serious complications.
2. c, The flow rate should be increased to keep the bag at least one third inflated to prevent the client from rebreathing carbon dioxide.
3. a, With anything that causes sedation, the nurse should assess for a depressed respiratory effort.
4. d, Respirations should be supported with an Ambu bag until the cause of the alarm can be identified to prevent hypoxia.
5. a, An abnormal ABG will demonstrate impaired exchange of gases and support the diagnosis.
6. a, Oxygen is necessary for anything to burn. In the presence of a fire (burning cigarette), oxygen allows flammable materials to burn faster and hotter and could cause an explosion.
7. b, As oxygen therapy increases oxygen levels, the client breathes more easily, pulse rate decreases, and an anxious attitude can become more relaxed.
8. b, Twill tapes should be removed after suctioning and after cleaning to ensure that the tracheostomy is not accidentally dislodged.

Chapter 87
Digestive Disorders

TERMINOLOGY REVIEW

1. d	12. i	23. n	34. e
2. g	13. b	24. k	35. k
3. o	14. m	25. o	36. h
4. c	15. k	26. d	37. a
5. f	16. e	27. a	38. f
6. a	17. j	28. g	39. j
7. j	18. i	29. b	40. c
8. e	19. m	30. c	41. i
9. h	20. h	31. b	
10. l	21. f	32. g	
11. n	22. l	33. d	

SEQUENCING

3,5,7,9,1,8,10,6,4,2

CORRECT THE FALSE STATEMENTS

1. True
2. True
3. False, chilled.
4. True
5. False, low-residue diet.
6. False, large bowel
7. True
8. False, swollen and may bleed occasionally.
9. True
10. False, bleeding/hemorrhage.
11. True
12. True
13. False, rarely, often
14. True
15. True

MULTIPLE CHOICE

1. c	4. c	7. a	10. a
2. a	5. a	8. d	11. b
3. b	6. c	9. d	

Chapter 88
Urinary

TERMINOLOGY REVIEW

1. f	11. d	21. b	31. e
2. h	12. n	22. m	32. h
3. o	13. b	23. e	33. d
4. i	14. k	24. c	34. c
5. l	15. e	25. h	35. i
6. c	16. i	26. g	36. a
7. g	17. d	27. k	37. g
8. a	18. f	28. a	38. f
9. m	19. j	29. h	
10. j	20. l	30. o	

ASSESSMENT REVIEW

1. A	4. N	7. N	10. A
2. A	5. A	8. A	11. A
3. N	6. A	9. N	12. A

SHORT ANSWERS

1. A culture and sensitivity are usually ordered together to determine whether an infection is present and, if so, what is the causative organism. Once the organism is identified, a sensitivity test will determine which antibiotics will destroy it.
2. a. Because of dehydration, edema and general tissue friability. Pruritus can cause the client to scratch skin.
   b. To assess for edema, urinary retention
   c. To help control edema and electrolyte imbalances
   d. To dilute urine and lessen dysuria
   e. To prevent disorders of immobility such as DVT, thrombosis, pneumonia, and UTIs
3. Oxybutinin, imipramine, and tolterodine
4. Care should focus on assessing for signs of bleeding, encouraging fluids, and straining urine.
5. The purposes of dialysis are to remove waste products, remove poisons and toxins, remove excess water, establish proper electrolyte levels, maintain acid–base balance, and instill medications.

DIAGNOSTIC COMPARISON CHART

Diagnostic Test	Description of Test	Nursing Care Before Test	Nursing Care After Test
Intravenous pyelogram	Series of x-rays are taken after client is injected with radiopaque dye.	Determine whether client is allergic to iodine or shellfish. NPO for 8–10 hours. Laxative night before test. Brush teeth in am, no swallowing water. Notify x-ray department, if client is diabetic or has decreased renal function.	Observe for reactions to dye. Force fluids for 24 hours. Monitor urine output.
Cytoscopy	Views the inside of the bladder using a tubular cytoscope. Can detect inflammation, bladder, openings of the ureter and urethra. Able to obtain urine specimens from each side to determine kidney disease.	Routine postoperative orders. Administer tranquilizer or sedative before exam. Instill Xylocaine jelly into the urethra. Check for allergies to lidocaine and so forth.	Sent specimens to laboratory. Administer analgesics. Sitzs baths. Encourage oral fluids. Instruct client that urine may be reddish colored for 24 hours. Report any signs of UTI or increasing bleeding.
Needle biopsy	Tissue sample of kidney is removed through large-bore needle.	Sedative. Place client in prone position with sandbag under abdomen.	Apply pressure to site. Flat in bed for 24 hours. Assess for signs of hemorrhage. Monitor VS.

6. Peritoneal dialysis involves instilling dialysate into the visceral cavity and using the peritoneum as a semipermeable membrane. Hemodialysis involves using an artificial semipermeable membrane outside the body. The client's blood is circulated outside the body.
7. See Box 88-2.
8. Feeling of a thrill and hearing the bruit.

CORRECT THE FALSE STATEMENTS

1. False, creatinine clearance test
2. False, BUN
3. True
4. False, cannot
5. True
6. False, Women, men
7. False, 2 to 3 weeks
8. True
9. True
10. False, always malignant.
11. True
12. False, ileal conduit
13. True
14. True
15. True

MULTIPLE CHOICE

1. a
2. a
3. d
4. a
5. b
6. c

Chapter 89
Male Reproductive Disorders

TERMINOLOGY REVIEW

1. t	8. q	15. z	22. n
2. j	9. g	16. d	23. aa
3. m	10. w	17. a	24. r
4. n	11. p	18. e	25. c
5. b	12. u	19. bb	26. i
6. k	13. f	20. y	27. x
7. l	14. v	21. o	28. s

ASSESSMENT REVIEW

1. A	6. A	11. A	16. N
2. N	7. A	12. N	17. N
3. A	8. N	13. A	18. N
4. A	9. A	14. A	19. A
5. N	10. N	15. N	20. A

SHORT ANSWER

1. Both exams are blood tests. The PSA detects glycoprotein that is found only in the tissue of the prostate gland. The free prostate-specific antigen determines the percentage of free PSA in the overall PSA.
2. The physician may order a prostatic biopsy after a suspicious rectal examination.
3. Explain to the client that the medication is a vasodilator used to help fill the penis with blood. It should be taken before intercourse. A baseline physical examination including blood pressure reading should be completed. Inform client of possible side effects such as priapism and hypotension.
4. Medications that can cause priapism include trazadone, chlorpromazine, prazosin, tolbutamide, antihypertensives, anticoagulants, and corticosteroids.
5. a. Accumulation of plaques or scar tissue along the corpora, which causes painful curvature of the penis when erect. b. Signs and symptoms include sudden severe scrotal pain, vomiting, abdominal pain, and nausea. c. Pain in the testicle or radiating to the other side, swelling and nagging dull pain in the scrotum, feels like a bag of worms when palpated. d. Enlarged scrotum, pain and swelling of the scrotum, often is asymptomatic.
6. The client should be instructed that antibiotic therapy will be for a long period of time and that he should take all antibiotics as ordered. This will help prevent the development of chronic bacterial prostatitis.
7. a. Suprapubic prostatectomy involves performing a cystostomy first and then removing the prostate. b. Perineal prostatectomy involves removing the prostate through the perineum. c. Nerve-sparing radical prostatectomy involves removing the prostate with an incision below the umbilicus and above the symphysis. d. Radical prostatectomy involves removing the prostate gland, seminal vesicles, and part of the urethra. e. Cyrosurgery involves freezing the prostate gland by an incision made in the perineum, and a tool is inserted into the area of the gland.
8. a. testicular; b. prostate; c. penile; d. testicular; e. prostate

CASE STUDIES

1. a. Additional assessment data would include assessing Joe for risk factors associated with testicular cancer, how he found the lump, when he discovered the lump, physical examination of Joe's testicles, and head-to-toe examination. b. Joe should be taught that no special

preparation is needed and that the test is relatively painless. c. Joe should have all the routine preoperative instructions for a client undergoing general anesthesia. He should be given the option to bank sperm, and the nurse should ensure that he understands that he will have the testicle removed. This could affect fertility but usually does not affect libido or ability to achieve organism. d. answers will vary, but can include Altered Urinary Elimination Pattern, Impaired Tissue Integrity, Altered Sexuality Patterns, Fear, Knowledge Deficit, Risk for Infection, Pain.

2. a. The physician would order PSA to rule out prostate cancer, urinalysis to rule out infection, digital examination to feel for the enlarged prostate, urodynamic testing, endoscopy and prostate ultrasound to assess nature and function of urinary system and prostate. b. Inform Mr. Smith that the physician is ordering diagnostic tests to determine the exact cause of his symptoms. Once the results are available and a diagnosis of BPH is made, discussing the differences between BPH and prostate cancer with Mr. Smith can be reassuring. Allow Mr. Smith to express his concerns.

MULTIPLE CHOICE

1. b, The American Urologic Association recommends all men older than 50 years of age to have an annual PSA and digital rectal examination.
2. d, The client will need to be prepared for surgery to prevent necrosis. Pain medications should not be given orally.
3. c, The scrotum is enlarged with a hydrocele and should be supported.
4. d, Flank pain could indicate a problem with the irrigation set-up or urinary retention due to clots. The system should be shut off and the RN or MD notified.
5. a, Endocrine disorders are one of the causes of ED. See Box 89-1 for other causes.
6. a, A nerve-sparing radical prostatectomy causes less

ED, incontinence, and bleeding than other methods.

7. b, Continuous bladder irrigation prevents blood clots form occluding the urinary catheter.
8. a, The client with prostate cancer receives GnRH medications to stop or decrease testosterone production and should have follow-up laboratory levels drawn.
9. b
10. a, The actual urinary output is calculated by subtracting the amount of irrigation solution from the total output.

Chapter 90
Female Reproductive Disorders

TERMINOLOGY REVIEW

1. s	12. n	23. cc	34. p
2. v	13. b	24. ff	35. t
3. bb	14. i	25. d	36. ii
4. hh	15. c	26. o	37. f
5. aa	16. g	27. jj	38. gg
6. q	17. ll	28. z	39. dd
7. m	18. l	29. w	40. k
8. u	19. j	30. e	41. nn
9. oo	20. h	31. kk	
10. x	21. y	32. v	
11. a	22. ee	33. mm	

ASSESSMENT REVIEW

1. N	6. A	11. A	16. A
2. A	7. N	12. A	17. A
3. N	8. A	13. A	18. N
4. N	9. A	14. N	19. N
5. A	10. N	15. A	20. A

DIAGNOSTIC TEST REVIEW

Diagnostic Test	Description of Test	Nursing Care Before Test	Nursing Care After Test
Laparoscopy	Surgical procedure done under general or spinal anesthesia. Small incision is made at umbilicus, adbomen is insufflated, and uterus and accessory organs are viewed.	Routine preoperative care, including explanation of test, consent, NPO	Postoperative instructions for signs of infection, caution until anesthesia is worn off

(continued)

DIAGNOSTIC TEST REVIEW *(Continued)*

Diagnostic Test	Description of Test	Nursing Care Before Test	Nursing Care After Test
Culdoscopy	Surgical procedure done with local, regional, or general anesthesia in which an instrument is passed through vaginal wall behind cervix to view pelvic contents.	Routine preoperative care	Routine postoperative carebased on type of anesthesia
Colposcopy	Magnifying speculum is inserted into vaginal vault.	Explain procedure to client.	Client may have mild cramping, and minimal bleeding or spotting. In-struct on signs of infection.
Cervical biopsy	A cervical tissue is ob-tained through punch procedure to examine tissue microsCopically.	Explain procedure to client.	Client may have minimal bleeding and cramping. Instruct on signs of infection.
Conization	Procedure done in the operating room with general or spinal anes-thesia. The surgeon removes a cone-shaped piece of the cervix for examination.	Routine preoperative instruction	Routine postoperative care. Client may have some bleeding. Watch for delayed bleeding and signs of infection.

Care common before all tests includes obtaining informed consent, explaining the procedure, and ensuring that the client prepared for the exam. All tests needing anesthesia have routine preoperative care in common.

Care common after all tests includes watching for signs of infection. Clients who have had anesthesia need routine postoperative care.

CASE STUDIES

1. a. The order of assessment would be: the postoperative client, the new admission, the client to be discharged, and the new admission.

   b. The postoperative client should be assessed for ABCs, bleeding, VS, neurologic status, pain level, dressing, and a head-to-toe assessment. The new admission should be assessed for pain, fever, nausea, vomiting, and admission history. The client to be discharged should be assessed for knowledge about discharge instructions including follow-up care, signs of infection, and pain medication. The preoperative client should be assessed for baseline knowledge, preoperative and postoperative instructions, emotional status, and concerns.

2. a. This client is at risk for postoperative complications including respiratory complications such as pneumonia, atelectasis; bleeding and hemorrhage; urinary tract infection; paralytic ileus; and infection.

   b. The client's pain should be thoroughly assessed for location, quality, rating on a pain scale, and duration. The client's VS should be assessed, the client should be checked for bleeding, and a head-to-toe assessment should be performed to observe for postoperative complications. If all assessment data are stable, the client may need an increase in pain medication, or it could be the vaginal packing causing her to have back pain. The LVN should share the information with the RN/MD.

3. See Educating the Client 90-1: Prevention of Vaginal Infections for teaching guidelines.

MULTIPLE CHOICE

1. c, This type of surgery removes both ovaries, and the client will have surgically induced menopause.

2. d, Shoulder pain is not uncommon after a laparoscopy owing to the gas instilled into the abdomen during surgery.

3. c, The client should avoid coffee, tea, chocolate, and cola drinks, which can aggravate cyst formation.

4. a, The client should continue to examine the chest wall and scar because these are common sites of recurrence.

5. c, The nurse should make a referral to Reach to Recovery to help the client with postoperative exercise and answer common questions about the breast cancer experience.

6. c, The client is expressing concern about her body and how her husband will perceive her changes.
7. b
8. b, See Educating the Client 90-2: Breast Self-Examination.

Chapter 91
Gerontology

TERMINOLOGY REVIEW

1. j	7. d	13. e	19. i
2. e	8. g	14. g	20. h
3. f	9. i	15. j	21. d
4. b	10. c	16. f	
5. a	11. c	17. b	
6. h	12. k	18. a	

ASSESSMENT REVIEW

1. N	5. N	9. A	13. A
2. A	6. A	10. A	14. N
3. N	7. A	11. N	15. N
4. A	8. N	12. A	16. A

CORRECT THE FALSE STATEMENTS

1. False, Chronic illnesses
2. True
3. False, 24 hours a day, 7 days a week.
4. False, 1 gram of protein for each kilogram of body weight.
5. True
6. True
7. False, straight across.
8. False, enlarged prostate gland obstructing urine flow.
9. True
10. True

MULTIPLE CHOICE

1. d
2. a
3. c
4. d
5. b

Chapter 92
Dementias

TERMINOLOGY REVIEW

1. j	7. i	13. e	19. i
2. m	8. g	14. h	20. a
3. l	9. a	15. c	21. j
4. f	10. h	16. g	22. b
5. c	11. b	17. e	23. f
6. d	12. k	18. d	

ASSESSMENT REVIEW

1. E	5. L	9. F	13. F
2. A	6. E	10. A	14. A
3. L	7. F	11. A	15. L
4. F	8. E	12. L	

NURSING ACTIONS

1. A	3. I	5. A	7. I
2. A	4. I	6. A	8. I

FILL-IN-THE-BLANK

1. Any three of the following: genetic, viral, toxic, immunologic, trauma, biochemical, or nutritional.
2. Short-term, long-term
3. cerebral cortex atrophy, loss of neurons, changes in brain cells
4. faster, stepwise, conditions
5. Toxic, metabolic
6. express

Chapter 93
Psychiatric Nursing

TERMINOLOGY REVIEW

1. c	13. m	25. f	37. a
2. l	14. j	26. m	38. d
3. o	15. h	27. c	39. n
4. f	16. g	28. o	40. f
5. n	17. b	29. k	41. g
6. e	18. i	30. h	42. l
7. a	19. a	31. k	43. c
8. k	20. d	32. m	44. h
9. i	21. n	33. j	45. i
10. g	22. e	34. o	
11. d	23. l	35. b	
12. b	24. j	36. e	

CORRECT THE FALSE STATEMENTS

1. False, About half of all adults
2. True
3. True
4. False, Perseverate
5. True
6. False, Psychotropic
7. True
8. False, Positive reinforcement
9. True
10. False, bone marrow suppression.

COMPLETION

1. depressive
2. anhedonia
3. bipolar disorder
4. Any one of the following examples is accurate
   Personality disorder: paranoid, schizoid, schizotypal, antisocial, borderline, histrionic, avoidant, dependent
   Anxiety disorder: panic attacks, phobias, obsessive-compulsive, posttraumatic
   Psychosis: schizophrenia, brief psychotic, other substance induced psychosis
5. remotivation
6. Pet
7. extrapyramidal
8. civil, vulnerable, advocacy.
9. physical care, teaching life, occupational
10. no information status

MATCHING

1. d
2. a
3. b
4. c
5. c

Chapter 94
Substance Abuse

TERMINOLOGY REVIEW

1. i	11. h	21. j	31. c
2. a	12. l	22. f	32. d
3. f	13. k	23. g	33. j
4. m	14. c	24. e	34. e
5. d	15. i	25. a	35. b
6. e	16. d	26. i	36. f
7. b	17. h	27. k	37. a
8. g	18. l	28. h	
9. c	19. b	29. g	
10. j	20. k	30. l	

ASSESSMENT FINDINGS

1. A, S, H	5. C, H	9. A,C,H, S	13. A, C, H
2. H	6. A, C, H	10. C, H	14. H
3. A, S	7. C, S	11. H	15. A
4. A, C, H	8. A	12. C	

SHORT ANSWER

1. The APA define substance abuse as a maladaptive pattern of substance use leading to clinically significant impairment or distress with one or more of the following in a 12-month period: failure to fulfill role obligations, use that presents a danger, recurrent use-related legal problems, continued use despite related interpersonal problems.
2. Physical factors, genetic factors, emotional and psychological factors, and coexisting mental illness can be contributing factors to development of chemical dependency.
3. The four concepts of management of all dependencies are recognition, intervention, treatment, and recovery.
4. Comfort and safety are the most important goals in detoxification management.
5. An appropriate diet would include small, carefully planned fluids and feedings to prevent refeeding syndrome.
6. Alcohol is absorbed in the proximal small intestine, which can impair the absorption of other nutrients.
7. The stages of alcohol withdrawal are: autonomic hyperactivity, neuronal excitation, sensory-perceptual disturbances, and delirium tremens.

MULTIPLE CHOICE

1. b
2. c
3. d
4. b
5. d

Chapter 95
Extended Care

TERMINOLOGY REVIEW

1. e	6. d	11. f	16. j
2. f	7. b	12. i	17. a
3. g	8. e	13. c	18. k
4. c	9. b	14. g	
5. a	10. h	15. d	

CORRECT THE FALSE STATEMENTS

1. False, are usually levels of care.
2. False, subacute care facilities.

3. True
4. True
5. True
6. False, Therapeutic swimming
7. False, is covered by private insurance, third-party payers, Medicare, Medicaid, and individual resources.
8. True
9. False, respite care
10. True

SHORT ANSWER

1. Subacute care facilities, medically complex care facilities, short-term rehabilitation units, and long-term facilities make up ECFs.
2. 2 to 4 weeks
3. Nursing functions include IV therapy, cardiac monitoring, ventilator care, peritoneal dialysis, and management of severe wounds.
4. Clients who require more specialized or high-tech care than is provided in an SNF are cared for in a medically complex nursing unit.
5. LTC facilities must provide room, board, and nursing care, with emergency medical care available. Additional services include activities and services.
6. Common recreational activities in LTC include crafts, playing cards, games, outings in the community, sports activities, musical programs, dance, and other social activities.
7. The CM oversees the client's care, is a client advocate, and may be responsible for overseeing the client's money.
8. Clients are kept safe by utilizing locked or alarmed units. Mattresses can have a warning system that detects when the client gets out of bed.
9. ICFs provide few services but are less expensive than the SNF.
10. People who need room, board, and minimal supervision would be well suited to live in a board-and-care home. Clients who need help or supervision taking their medications would be suited to live in a supervised group home.

Chapter 96
Rehabilitation Nursing

TERMINOLOGY REVIEW

1. g	7. d	13. i	19. j
2. e	8. k	14. m	20. h
3. h	9. j	15. d	21. l
4. c	10. a	16. g	22. k
5. f	11. b	17. b	23. c
6. i	12. e	18. f	24. a

NURSING ACTIONS

1. A	6. I	11. I	16. I
2. A	7. I	12. A	17. A
3. I	8. A	13. A	18. A
4. A	9. A	14. I	19. I
5. I	10. I	15. I	20. A

MULTIPLE CHOICE

1. a
2. c
3. b
4. d

Chapter 97
Ambulatory Nursing

TERMINOLOGY REVIEW

1. g	5. l	9. e	13. j
2. f	6. h	10. p	14. o
3. d	7. i	11. b	15. m
4. a	8. n	12. c	16. k

NURSING ACTIONS

1. A	4. I	7. A	10. A
2. I	5. I	8. I	
3. A	6. A	9. I	

SHORT ANSWER

1. Answers will vary. See Box 97-1 for details.
2. Answers will vary. Any of the following are acceptable: laparoscope, arthroscope, laser, fiberoptics, ultrasound, MRI, CT scans, stent placements, operating microscope.
3. Benefits include decreased risk for postoperative complications related to smaller incisions, less time under anesthesia or use of local anesthesia. Client is able to recover in familiar, relaxing home setting.
4. The nurse is responsible for teaching the following: preoperative preparation, referral to appropriate sources for equipment, giving instructions by telephone and in writing, instruct clients to call if any change in their condition, type of anesthesia, useful relaxation equipment such as radio with headphones, what to expect after surgery, provide tour of operating suite, instruct to have arrangements for a ride home and a caregiver, and provide postoperative instructions.
5. The nurse can provide a relaxed, friendly environment. The nurse can ensure that preoperative and postoperative teaching is completed. The nurse can instruct the client that radios or tapes can be used

during the surgery. Keeping the client informed and educated about the procedure will help the client relax.

Chapter 98
Home Care Nursing

TERMINOLOGY REVIEW

1. d	3. b	5. c	7. e
2. h	4. a	6. f	8. g

NURSING ACTION

1. A	4. I	7. I	10. I
2. I	5. I	8. A	11. I
3. A	6. A	9. I	12. A

CORRECT THE FALSE STATEMENTS
1. True
2. False, given on a short-term, long-term or intermittent basis
3. False, are one type of agency
4. True
5. False, Cardiac disorders
6. False, intermittent
7. True
8. False, may
9. True
10. False, Case manager

MULTIPLE CHOICE
1. b
2. d
3. c
4. a

Chapter 99
Hospice Nursing

TERMINOLOGY REVIEW

1. e	8. b	15. d	22. g
2. i	9. m	16. f	23. l
3. f	10. l	17. c	24. e
4. a	11. h	18. k	25. h
5. o	12. j	19. i	26. m
6. k	13. c	20. j	27. a
7. g	14. n	21. b	28. d

CORRECT THE FALSE STATEMENTS
1. True
2. False, willingness, ability, and motivation of primary caregivers to provide care.
3. False, no more than 6 months
4. True
5. True
6. False, Volunteers
7. False, need
8. True
9. True
10. False, Less medication
11. True
12. False, every 2 to 3 days.
13. True
14. True

MULTIPLE CHOICE
1. c
2. b
3. c
4. a
5. d
6. c
7. d

Chapter 100
From Student to Graduate

TERMINOLOGY REVIEW

1. g	3. c	5. e	7. a
2. h	4. b	6. f	8. d

LICENSE REVOCATION REVIEW

1. X	4. -	7. X	10. X
2. -	5. -	8. X	
3. X	6. X	9. -	

NURSING ACTION

1. I	3. A	5. A	7. I
2. A	4. I	6. A	8. A

CORRECT THE FALSE STATEMENTS
1. True
2. True
3. False, physiologic integrity
4. False, all four phases of the nursing process
5. True
6. False, study throughout the time spent in the basic nursing program.
7. True
8. True
9. True

10. True
11. False, keep the area well lighted
12. False, "stat" orders first.

MULTIPLE CHOICE

1. a
2. b
3. c
4. d
5. c

Chapter 101
Career Opportunities and Job Seeking Skills

TERMINOLOGY REVIEW

1. e	3. b	5. f	7. d
2. h	4. g	6. a	8. c

CORRECT THE FALSE STATEMENTS

1. True
2. False, advantage of private duty nursing
3. False, triage
4. True
5. True
6. True
7. False, networks
8. False, advantage
9. True
10. False, 5 minutes
11. False, 2 to 4 weeks
12. True

SHORT ANSWER

1. Answers will vary and may include any six of the following: hospitals, ECFs, public health, community health centers, private duty, travel nurse, hospice care, substance abuse programs, MHC, physician's office, correctional facilities, ambulatory surgery centers, HMO, telehealth, occupational health, armed forces, schools, parish nursing, and working overseas.
2. Answers will vary and may include any five of the following: practical nursing programs, operating room, dialysis, hyperbaric medicine, pharmaceutical sales, veterinary clinics, chiropractic clinics, specialty clinics, emergency rescue, self-employment.
3. The nurse in correctional facilities monitor inmates with special needs, give medications, assist with diabetic management, perform routine health screening, provide health-related counseling, and consult physicians for referrals.

4. The Internet can be used to obtain a job by searching for posted jobs through employment services, on-line magazines, facility websites, or classified ads. Applying for positions can often be done at facilities' websites on-line. Nurses can post their resume on websites in which employers review and contact qualified applicants. The Internet can be used to speed up the job search process.
5. Answers will vary. See Box 101-1, Factors to Consider When Looking for a Place of Employment.
6. A cover letter should convince the employer that you are the best candidate for the job. The letter should include the position for which you are applying, qualifications for the position, and availability for and how to contact you for an interview.
7. Items to include in a resume are education, previous employment, work experience, special skills or training, honors, volunteer positions, references, and career objective.
8. Items will vary. See Box 101-3, Guidelines for the Job Interview.

Chapter 102
Advancement and Leadership in Nursing

TERMINOLOGY REVIEW

1. n	5. l	9. g	13. f
2. h	6. e	10. d	14. b
3. c	7. a	11. k	
4. i	8. m	12. j	

NURSING ACTION

1. A	5. I	9. I	13. A
2. A	6. A	10. A	
3. I	7. A	11. I	
4. A	8. A	12. I	

MULTIPLE CHOICE

1. b
2. d
3. b
4. a
5. c

PROGRAM LICENSE AGREEMENT

Read carefully the following terms and conditions before using the Software. Use of the Software indicates you and, if applicable, your Institution's acceptance of the terms and conditions of this License Agreement.
If you do not agree with the terms and conditions, you should promptly return this package to the place you purchased it and your payment will be refunded.

Definitions

As used herein, the following terms shall have the following meanings:
"Software" means the software program contained on the diskette(s) or CD-ROM or preloaded on a workstation and the user documentation, which includes all accompanying printed material.
"Institution" means a nursing or professional school, a single academic organization that does not provide patient care and is located in a single city and has one geographic location/address.
"Geographic location" means a facility at a specific location; geographic locations do not provide for satellite or remote locations that are considered a separate facility.
"Facility" means a health care facility at a specific location that provides patient care and is located in a single city and has one geographic location/address.
"Publisher" means Lippincott Williams & Wilkins, Inc., with its principal office in Philadelphia, Pennsylvania.
"Developer" means the company responsible for developing the software as noted on the product.

License

You are hereby granted a nonexclusive license to use the Software in the United States. This license is not transferable and does not authorize resale or sublicensing without the written approval or an authorized officer of Publisher.
The Publisher retains all rights and title to all copyrights, patents, trademarks, trade secrets, and other proprietary rights in the Software. You may not remove or obscure the copyright notices in or on the Software. You agree to use reasonable efforts to protect the Software from unauthorized use, reproduction, distribution or publication.

Single-User license

If you purchased this Software program at the Single-User License price or a discount of that price, you may use this program on one single-user computer. You may not use the Software in a time-sharing environment or otherwise to provide multiple, simultaneous access. You may not provide or permit access to this program to anyone other than yourself.

Institutional/Facility license

If you purchased the Software at the Institutional or Facility License Price or at a discount of that price, you have purchased the Software for use within your Institution/Facility on a single workstation/computer. You may not provide copies of or remote access to the Software. You may not modify or translate the program or related documentation. You agree to instruct the individuals in your Institution/Facility who will have access to the Software to abide by the terms of this License Agreement. If you or any member of your Institution fail to comply with any of the terms of this License Agreement, this license shall terminate automatically.

Network license

If you purchased the Software at the Network License Price, you may copy the Software for use within your Institution/Facility on an unlimited number of computers within one geographic location/address. You may not provide remote access to the Software over a value-added network or otherwise. You may not provide copies of or remote access to the Software to individuals or entities who are not members of your Institution/Facility. You may not modify or translate the program or related documentation. You agree to instruct the individuals in your Institution/Facility who will have access to the Software to abide by the terms of this License Agreement. If you or any member of your Institution/Facility fail to comply with any of the terms of this License Agreement, this license shall terminate automatically.

Limited warranty

The Publisher warrants that the media on which the Software is furnished shall be free from defects in materials and workmanship under normal use for a period of 90 days from the date of delivery to you, as evidenced by your receipt of purchase.

The Software is sold on a 30-day trial basis. If, for whatever reason, you decide not to keep the software, you may return it for a full refund within 30 days of the invoice date or purchase, as evidenced by your receipt of purchase by returning all parts of the Software and packaging in saleable condition with the original invoice, to the place you purchased it. If the Software is not returned in such condition, you will not be entitled to a refund. When returning the Software, we suggest that you insure all packages for their retail value and mail them by a traceable method.

The Software is a computer assisted instruction (CAI) program that is not intended to provide medical consultation regarding the diagnosis or treatment of any specific patient.

The Software is provided without warranty of any kind, either expressed or implied, including but not limited to any implied warranty of fitness for a particular purpose of merchantability. Neither Publisher nor Developer warrants that the Software will satisfy your requirements or that the Software is free of program or content errors. Neither Publisher nor Developer warrants, guarantees, or makes any representation regarding the use of the Software in terms of accuracy, reliability or completeness, and you rely on the content of the programs solely at your own risk.

The Publisher is not responsible (as a matter of products liability, negligence or otherwise) for any injury resulting from any material contained herein. This Software contains information relating to general principles of patient care that should not be construed as specific instructions for individual patients.

Manufacturers' product information and package inserts should be reviewed for current information, including contraindications, dosages and precautions.

Some states do not allow the exclusion of implied warranties, so the above exclusion may not apply to you. This warranty gives you specific legal rights and you may also have other rights that vary from state to state.

Limitation of remedies

The entire liability of Publisher and Developer and your exclusive remedy shall be: (1) the replacement of any CD which does not meet the limited warranty stated above which is returned to the place you purchased it with your purchase receipt; or (2) if the Publisher or the wholesaler or retailer from whom you purchased the Software is unable to deliver a replacement CD free from defects in material and workmanship, you may terminate this License Agreement by returning the CD, and your money will be refunded.

In no event will Publisher or Developer be liable for any damages, including any damages for personal injury, lost profits, lost savings or other incidental or consequential damages arising out of the use or inability to use the Software or any error or defect in the Software, whether in the database or in the programming, even if the Publisher, Developer, or an authorized wholesaler or retailer has been advised of the possibility of such damage.

Some states do not allow the limitation or exclusion of liability for incidental or consequential damages. The above limitations and exclusions may not apply to you.

General

This License Agreement shall be governed by the laws of the State of Pennsylvania without reference to the conflict of laws provisions thereof, and may only be modified in a written statement signed by an authorized officer of the Publisher. By opening and using the Software, you acknowledge that you have read this License Agreement, understand it, and agree to be bound by its terms and conditions. You further agree that it is a complete and exclusive statement of the agreement between the Institution/Facility and the Publisher, which supersedes any proposal or prior agreement, oral or written, and any other communication between you and Publisher or Developer relative to the subject matter of the License Agreement.

Note

Attach a paid invoice to the License Agreement as proof of purchase.

Installing the Student Self Study CD-ROM

System Requirements

This program will run on any IBM-PC or compatible computer that *minimally* includes:

Pentium 100 MHz CPU;
32 MB RAM (64 recommended);
Microsoft Windows;
SVGA display supporting 256 colors (16 bit recommended);
12X CD-ROM drive;
800 x 600 monitor resolution;
Microsoft compatible mouse;
5 MB of hard-disk space

Note: In order to run this program, you must have Macromedia Flash Player installed on your PC. If you do not currently have this program installed, it is a free download available at: .

Running the program:

Insert the CD-ROM into your disk drive. Double click on the **RosdahlQB.exe** file to launch the program.